Herbal Drugs: Synthesis, Interactions and Applications

Herbal Drugs: Synthesis, Interactions and Applications

Edited by Melissa Gould

SYRAWOOD
PUBLISHING HOUSE
New York

Published by Syrawood Publishing House,
750 Third Avenue, 9th Floor,
New York, NY 10017, USA
www.syrawoodpublishinghouse.com

Herbal Drugs: Synthesis, Interactions and Applications
Edited by Melissa Gould

International Standard Book Number: 978-1-68286-732-7 (Hardback)

Cataloging-in-Publication Data

Herbal drugs : synthesis, interactions and applications / edited by Melissa Gould.
p. cm.
Includes bibliographical references and index.
ISBN 978-1-68286-732-7
1. Materia medica, Vegetable. 2. Herbs--Therapeutic use. 3. Medicinal plants.
4. Alternative medicine. I. Gould, Melissa.
RS164 .H47 2019
615.321--dc23

Printed in China.

TABLE OF CONTENTS

PREFACE

Herbalism develops on the science of botany, to develop drugs or diet supplements for the maintenance of health, disease prevention and treatment. Herbal medicine is widely practiced in different parts of Asia and Africa. The use of herbal remedies is more common for patients with cancer, diabetes, asthma, end-stage renal disease, etc. Sometimes, synthetic and herbal drugs can interact causing toxicity to the patient. Essential oil extracts, salves, creams, lotions, etc. can be applied topically. Aromatherapy is also a herbal treatment and works through the direct inhalation of vapors. Herbal medicine is also administered in the form of herbal teas, decoctions, infusions, tinctures, etc. The aim of this book is to present researches that have transformed this discipline and aided its advancement. It is a vital tool for all researching and studying this field. It aims to shed light on some of the unexplored aspects of herbal drugs, their synthesis and applications.

Various studies have approached the subject by analyzing it with a single perspective, but the present book provides diverse methodologies and techniques to address this field. This book contains theories and applications needed for understanding the subject from different perspectives. The aim is to keep the readers informed about the progresses in the field; therefore, the contributions were carefully examined to compile novel researches by specialists from across the globe.

Indeed, the job of the editor is the most crucial and challenging in compiling all chapters into a single book. In the end, I would extend my sincere thanks to the chapter authors for their profound work. I am also thankful for the support provided by my family and colleagues during the compilation of this book.

Editor

Antioxidant effects of strawberry fruits at two phenological stages

Gita Amini*, Saeed Irian, Ahmad Majd, Sedigheh Mehrabian

Deparment of Plant Biology, Faculty of Biological Sciences, Kharazmi University, Tehran, Iran;

Email:** ***gita.amini85@gmail.com

ARTICLE INFO

Topic: *Physiology & Food Health*

Key words:

Fragaria vesca *L.*

Antioxidant activity

Phenolic compounds

ABSTRACT

Background & Aim: Strawberry (*Fragaria vesca* L.) is a plant belonging to the Rosaceae family with medicinal properties, including antioxidant activity. The present study aimed at investigating the antioxidant properties of strawberry.

Experimental method: To examine the antioxidant effect, fruit extracts at two phonological stages of growth (ripe and unripe strawberry) were prepared. In addition, four different solvents, including 80% ethanol, 80% methanol, acetone and distilled water were used for the preparation of plant extracts. In total, eight different plant extracts were prepared and their properties comparatively studied. To study the antioxidant effect, potassium ferricyanide and reducing power determination method were used.

Results & Discussion: Results indicated that strawberry fruit had antioxidant effects in both of two stages. That is due to the presence of the higher pigments and phenolic compounds in ripe fruit than unripe fruit.

Recommended applications/industries: The results of present indicated the red fruit had the highest antioxidant activity.

1. Introduction

Nowadays, the advantage of using medicinal drugs is obvious for everyone, while chemical drugs have many side effects. In current world, the human environment is full of mutative materials that are the agent of many diseases such as cancer. Plants are very effective in preventing such diseases with trapping free radicals and having antioxidant effects (Zeng *et al.*, 2010).

Strawberry (*Fragaria vesca* L.), belongs to the family Rosaceae, is widely consumed, both as fresh fruit and as an ingredient in processed products. It is a very rich source of bioactive compounds including vitamin C, E, β-carotene, and phenolic compounds (phenol acids, flavan-3-ols, flavonols, and anthocyanins) (Oszmianski & Wojdylo, 2009). The major phenol compounds are procyanidins, ellagitanins, catechin, and *p*-coumaroyl esters (Aaby *et al.*, 2005).

Strawberries are unique with highly desirable taste, flavour, excellent dietary sources of ascorbic acid, potassium, fiber and other secondary metabolites and also simple sugar sources of energy (Wang & Galletta, 2002). Various beneficial biological effects of strawberry fruits consumption have been documented, such as an increase of the serum antioxidant capacity in humans (Cao *et al.,* 1998), anti-carcinogenic activity (Carlton *et al.,* 2001; Wedge *et al.,* 2001), anti-thrombotic effects (Naemura *et al.,* 2005), etc.

The strawberry is one of the most commonly consumed berries. Its high nutritional value has long been correlated to the relevant content of antioxidant micronutrients, such as vitamin C and folate, and more recently to the high variety and content of antioxidant polyphenolic constituents, such as flavonoids, hydrolysable and condensed tannins, and phenolic acids (da Silva Pinto *et al.*, 2010; Seeram *et al.*, 2006). Glucose is the most common sugar substituent in strawberry, but rutinose, arabinose and rhamnose have also been tentatively identified. Other minor anthocyanins, include acylated derivatives with the following organic acids: malic, malonic, succinic, or acetic acids (Lopes-da-Silva *et al.,* 2007).

Significant increases in the plasma total antioxidant capacity (TAC) have already been reported after acute intake of strawberries. In addition, anti-haemolitic effects of strawberry extracts have been recently demonstrated *in vitro*, revealing that part of the antioxidant properties of strawberry bioactive compounds could lie in their localisation within cell membranes. A significant increase in fasting plasma TAC and in serum vitamin C concentrations were progressively observed during the period of strawberry supplementation. An enhanced resistance to haemolysis was also observed in both AAPH-treated and untreated erythrocytes, collected during and after the period of strawberry consumption. The results obtained in this work suggest that regular consumption of antioxidant-rich strawberries may exert an improvement on the plasma antioxidant status (Tulipani *et al.*, 2011). In addition, epidemiological studies have shown that high fruit and vegetable consumption has health benefits in the prevention of chronic diseases (Ness & Powles, 1997; Steinmetz & Potter, 1991). Several studies have suggested that the phytochemical content and antioxidant / free radical scavenging effect of fruits and vegetables contribute to their protective effect against chronic and degenerative diseases (Heinonen *et al.,* 1998; Record *et al.,* 2001). Strawberry extracts were found to have higher antioxidant activity, as indicated by the oxygen radical absorbance capacity assay, than extracts from plum, orange, red grape, kiwifruit, pink grapefruit, white grape, banana, apple, tomato, pear, and honeydew melon (Meyers *et al.*, 2003).

Increase in the consumption of foods rich in antioxidants, micronutrients and phytochemical has long been proposed as a preventive measure to decrease the risk of several chronic diseases caused by oxidative stress. In particular, the improvement in plasma antioxidant status (and the increase in serum antioxidants) has been recognized as a potential tool to prevent the development of cardiovascular, proliferative, degenerative and other diseases (Kay & Holub, 2002).

Anthocyanin increasing concentrations in ripe strawberries is a well-known phenomenon (Ferreyra *et al.*, 2007; Given *et al.*, 1988; Wang and Lin, 2000). The main anthocyanin found in strawberries is pelargonidin 3-glucoside, with cyanidin 3-glucoside and pelargonidin 3-rutinoside present as minor components (Gil *et al.,* 1997). Therefore, there is a lack of research evidence from *in vivo* protracted strawberry consumption studies. We carried out a 16-day pilot study where 12 healthy subjects ingested 500 g of antioxidants-rich strawberries daily, and we evaluated the potential effects of fruit consumption on biomarkers of plasma and cellular antioxidant status.

2. Material and Methods

2.1. Plant Samples

Unripe and ripe fruits of strawberry were collected from the strawberry farm in Rasht, northern Iran on April 2012. The fruits were dried in shadow and then were powdered and stored at 25 °C until use.

2.2. Ethanol and methanol extracts of strawberry

For preparation of ethanol and methanol extraction, 1 g autoclaved power of strawberry was added to 10 ml of 80% ethanol and methanol, separately. Then, the extracts were filtered from filter paper. By this way ethanol and methanol extracts of strawberry was produced. The extracts were stored at fridge for 48 h until use.

2.3. Acetone and distilled water extracts of strawberry

For preparation of ethanol extraction, 1 g autoclaved power of strawberry was added to 10 ml of acetone and distilled water, separately. Then, the extracts were filtered from filter paper. By this way acetone and distilled water extracts of strawberry was produced. The extracts were stored at fridge for 48 h until use.

2.4. Control samples

Control samples used in this assay were acetone, distilled water, methanol and ethanol solvents.

2.5. Measurement of fruit antioxidant activity

Reducing power of both extracts of strawberry were measured by method of ferric reducing power. According to this method, the reduction of Fe^{3+} to Fe^{2+} was determined by measuring absorbance of the Prussian blue complex. This method is based on the reduction of (Fe^{3+}) ferricyanide in stoichiometric excess relative to the antioxidants. For this purpose,

10% concentrations of distilled water extract, ethanol, methanol, and acetone extracts of strawberry were mixed with 2.5 ml of 0.2 M sodium phosphate buffer (pH 6.6) and 2.5 ml (1%) of potassium ferricyanide $[K_3Fe(CN)_6]$. The mixture was incubated at 50 °C for 20 min. After 20 min of incubation, the reaction mixture was acidified with 1 ml of trichloroacetic acid (10%). Finally, 2.5 ml of $FeCl_3$ (0.1%) was added to this solution. Distilled water was used as blank and for control. Absorbance of this mixture was measured at 700 nm using a spectrophotometer. Increased absorbance indicates ferric reducing power capability of sample.

2.6. Statistical analysis

Antioxidant assays were repeated three times, and the data were analyzed by statistical software, SPSS (ver. 17) and Excel software. And related graphs were drawn.

3. Results & Discussion

In figures 2a, 2b, and 2c, control, unripe and ripe solvents of strawberry have been shown, respectively. Results indicate that control sample had not antioxidant effect, whereas the fruit had antioxidant activity at both of phenological stages. But in ripe fruit was higher than unripe. Because phenol compounds such as anthocyanins are the higher in ripe fruit. After adding $Fecl_3$, the color of Prussian blue was observed in ripe and unripe extracts (Fig 3b and Fig 3c). And Prussian blue did not observe in control sample (Fig 3c).

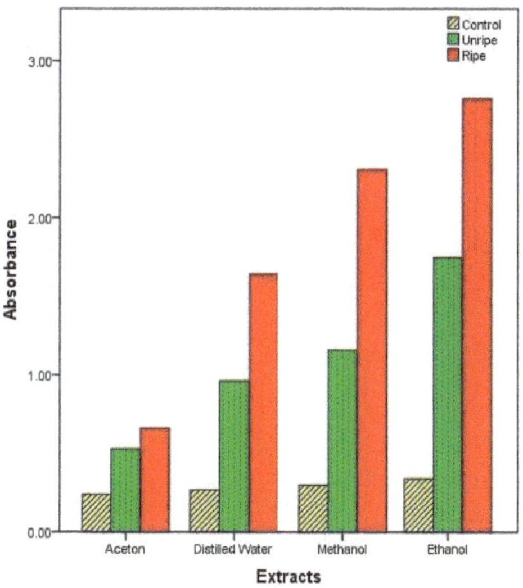

Fig 1. Comparison of the rate of absorbance within four different solvents at 700 nm

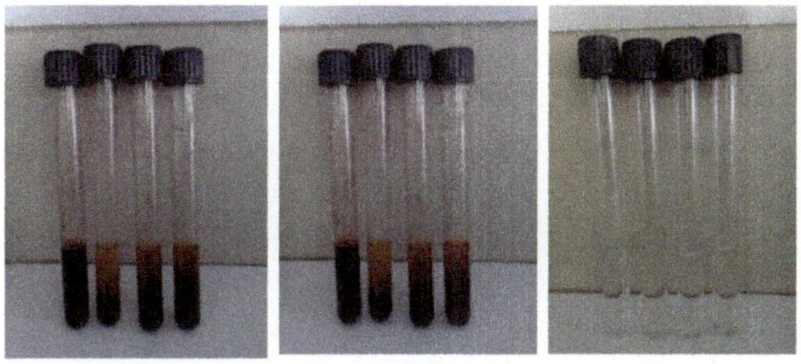

c b a

Fig 2a: From right to left respectively ethanol, methanol, acetone and distilled water of control solvent; **ʏb:** From right to left respectively ethanol, methanol, acetone and distilled water of unripe fruit; **2c:** From right to left respectively ethanol, methanol, acetone and distilled water of ripe fruit

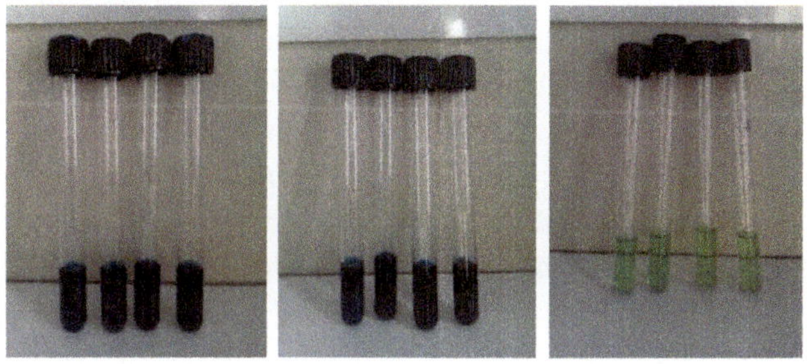

c b a

Fig 3a: From right to left respectively ethanol, methanol, acetone and distilled water of control solvent after adding $Fecl_3$; **3b:** From right to left respectively ethanol, methanol, acetone and distilled water of unripe after adding $Fecl_3$; **3c:** From right to left respectively ethanol, methanol, acetone and distilled water of ripe fruit after adding $Fecl_3$

Table 1. Comparison evaluation of antioxidant effects between different extracts at 700 nm

Samples / Extracts	Control	Unripe extract	Ripe extract
Ethanol	0.34	1.75	2.76
Methanol	0.30	1.16	2.31
Distilled water	0.27	0.96	1.63
Acetone	0.24	0.53	0.66

The rate of absorbance was measured at 700nm (Table 1) and comparison graph of control and ripe and unripe extracts was drawn (Fig 1). Among extracts, respectively ethanol, methanol, distilled water and acetone extracts of ripe and unripe fruit had the most effect. The rate of absorbance also was in low level in ripe acetone extracts because effective materials of fruit dissolve very little in acetone solvent.

In aerobic cells, ROS produces during the normal aerobic metabolic process (Chance *et al.*, 1979; Halliwell *et al.*, 1989). It has estimated that 1-5% of consumed oxygen by cells can produce ROS (Chance *et al.*, 1979). In addition, to endogenic production ROS could be produced by exogenous factors such as ionizing radiation, diet and foreign materials. Oxidative stress could be arise by extra production of ROS or deficiency in antioxidant action or repairing mechanism which causes reversible or irreversible damage to the vital micro molecules of cells such as lipids, proteins and DNA (Davies *et al.*, 1987). It has shown that unrepaireble oxidative stress plays the role in several chronic diseases like cancer (Ames *et al.*, 1993). Cells have several mechanisms for inactivation of ROS and repair and replacing the damaged molecules to maintain the cell homeostasis (Yu, 1994).

Some studies (Heinonen *et al.*, 1998; Vinson *et al.*, 2001) have pointed out that strawberry generally possesses a high level of antioxidant activity, which could be linked to the levels of phenolic compounds in the fruit. Wang and Jiao (2000) showed that strawberry juice exhibited a high level of antioxidant capacity against free radical species including superoxide radicals, hydrogen peroxide, hydroxyl radicals, and singlet oxygen.

Various beneficial biological effects of strawberry fruits consumption have been documented, such as an increase of the serum antioxidant capacity in humans (Cao *et al.*, 1998), anti-carcinogenic activity (Carlton *et al.*, 2001; Wedge *et al.*, 2001), anti-thrombotic effects (Naemura *et al.*, 2005), etc. These beneficial effects have been mostly attributed to the phenolic compounds that are found in large quantities in strawberry fruits (Hannum, 2004). This is especially true for the wild strawberry (*Fragaria vesca* L.) which has a several times higher antioxidant capacity than the average of the most common, cultivated strawberry varieties (Scalzo *et al.*, 2005).

Reduction capacity of a compound may serve as a significant indicator of its potential antioxidant activity. Antioxidant compounds are able to donate electrons to reactive radicals, reducing them into more stable and unreactive species (Gülçin *et al.*, 2003). Reducing power of methanol, ethanol, distilled water and acetone extracts of strawberry was investigated by ferric reducing power assay. Antioxidant compounds cause the reduction of ferric (Fe^{3+}) form to the ferrous (Fe^{2+}) form because of their reductive capabilities. Prussian blue-colored complex is formed by adding $FeCl_3$ to the ferrous (Fe^{2+}) form. Therefore, reduction can be determined by measuring the formation of Prussian blue at 700 nm (Chung *et al.*, 2002). In this assay, yellow color of the test solution changes to green or blue color depending on the reducing power of antioxidant samples. A higher absorbance indicates a higher ferric reducing power.

As shown in Fig 1, the ethanol and methanol extracts of strawberry showed increased ferric reducing power and following this, distilled water and acetone showed little antioxidant activity. According to results of the present study, ferric reducing power of ripe fruit extract was higher than unripe. In addition, among the extracts, the rate of absorbance in ethanol extract was higher than others. Fe (III) reduction is often used as an indicator of electron-donating activity, which is an important mechanism of phenolic antioxidant action (Dorman *et al.*, 2003).

(Yellow complex) $Fe_4\,[Fe\,(CN_6)]_3 \longrightarrow K_3[Fe(CN_6)]$
(Prussian blue)

In the most of plants, antioxidant activity and trapping the free radicals is due to the phenolic compounds which cause the reduction of Fe^{3+} in potassium ferricyanide. Because there are a lot of hydroxyl group in the structure of phenolic compounds.

4. Conclusion

Our results indicate the extracts from red fruit of strawberry have the highest antioxidant activity that is due to the presence of the higher pigments and phenolic compounds in ripe fruit than unripe fruit.

5. References

Aaby, K., Skrede, G. and Wrolstad, R. E. 2005. Phenolic composition and antioxidant activities in flesh and achenes of strawberries (*Fragaria ananassa*). *Journal of Agricultural and Food Chemistry*., 53: 4032–4040.

Ames, B. M., Shigena, M. K. and Hagen. T. M. 1993. Oxidants, antioxidants and the degenerative diseases of aging. *Proceedings of the National Academy of Sciences of the United States of America*., 90: 7915-7922.

Bursal, E. and Koksal, E. 2010. Evaluation of reducing power and radical scavenging of water and ethanol extract from sumac (*Rhus coriaria* L.). *Food research International*., 1356-1361.

Cao, G., Russell, R.M., Lischner, N. and Prior, R. L. 1998. Serum antioxidant capacity is increased by consumption of strawberries, spinach, red wine or vitamin C in elderly women. *Journal of Nutrition.*, 128: 2383–2390.

Carlton, P. S., Kresty, L.A., Siglin, J. C., Morse, M. A., Lu, J., Morgan, C., Stoner, G. D. 2001. Inhibition of N- nitrosomethylbenzylamine- induced tumorigenesis in the rat esophagus by dietary freeze-dried strawberries. *Carcinogenesis.,* 22: 441–446.

Chung, Y. C., Chang, C. T., Chao, W. W., Lin, C. F. and Chou, S. T. 2002. Antioxidative activity and safety of the 50% ethanolic extract from red bean fermented by *Bacillus subtilis* IMR-NK1. *Journal of Agriculture and Food Chemistry.*, 50: 2454–2458.

Da Silva Pinto, M., de Carvalho, J. E., Lajolo, F. M., Genovese, M. I. and Shetty, K. 2010. Evaluation of antiproliferative, anti-type 2 diabetes, and antihypertension potentials of ellagitannins from strawberries (*Fragaria ananassa* Duch.) using in vitro models. *Journal of Medicinal Food..* doi:10.1089/jmf.2009.0257.

Davies, K. J. 1987. Protein damage and degradation by oxygen radicals. I. General aspects. *Journal of Biological Chemistry.,* 262: 9895-9901.

Dorman, H. J. D., Peltoketo, A., Hiltunen, R. and Tikkanen, M. J. 2003. Characterisation of the antioxidant properties of de-odourised aqueous extracts from selected Lamiaceae herbs. *Food Chemistry.*, 83: 255–262.

Eberhardt, M. V., Lee, C. Y. and Liu, R. H. 2000. Nutrition – Antioxidant activity of fresh apples. *Nature.*, 405(6789): 903–904.

Ferreyra, R. M., Vina, S. Z., Mugridge, A., Chaves, A. R. 2007. Growth and ripening season effects on antioxidant capacity of strawberry cultivar Selva. *Scientia Horticulturae.*, 112: 27–32.

Gil, M. I., Holcroft, D. M., Kader, A. A. 1997. Changes in strawberry anthocyanins and other polyphenols in response to carbon dioxide treatments. *Journal of Agricultural and Food Chemistry.*, 45: 1662–1667.

Given, N. K., Venis, M. A. and Grierson, D. 1988. Phenylalanine ammonia-lyase activity and anthocyanin synthesis in ripening strawberry fruit. *Journal of Plant Physiology.*, 133: 25–30.

Gülçin, İ., Oktay, M., Kireççi, E. and Küfrevioğlu, Ö. İ. 2003. Screening of antioxidant and antimicrobial activities of anise (*Pimpinella anisum* L.) seed extracts. *Food Chemistry.*, 83: 371–382.

Halliwell, B. and Gutteridge, J. M. C. 1989. *Free Radicals in Biology and Medicine,* 2nd ed.; Clarendon Press: Oxford, U.K.

Harding, A. H., Wareham, N. J., Bingham, S. A., Khaw, K., Luben, R., Welch, A., *et al.* 2008. Plasma vitamin C level, fruit and vegetable consumption, and the risk of new-onset type 2 diabetes mellitus: The European prospective investigation of cancer – Norfolk prospective study. *Archives of Internal Medicine*, 168(14): 1493–1499.

Heinonen, M. I., Meyer, A. S. and Frankel, E. N. 1998. Antioxidant activity of berry phenolics on human low-density lipoprotein and liposome oxidation. *Journal of Agricultural and Food Chemistry.*, 46: 4107–4112.

Hannum, S. M. 2004. Potential impact of strawberries on human health: a review of the science. *Critical Reviews in Food Science & Nutrition.*, 44: 1–17.

Kay, C. D. and Holub, B. J. 2002. The effect of wild blueberry (Vacciniun angustifolium) consumption on postprandial serum antioxidant status in human subjects. *British Journal of Nutrition.*, 88: 389–397.

Lopes-da-Silva, F., Escribano-Bailon, M. T., Pérez Alonso, J. J., Rivas-Gonzalo, J. C. and Santos-Buelga, C. 2007. Anthocyanin pigments in strawberry. *Learning with Technologies.*, 40:374–382.

Meyers, K. J., Watkins, C. B., Pritts, M. P. and Liu, R. H. 2003. Antioxidant and antiproliferative activities of strawberries. *Journal of Agricultural and Food Chemistry.*, 51: 6887–6892.

Naemura, A., Mitani, T., Ijiri, Y., Tamura, Y., Yamashita, T., Okimura, M. and Yamamoto, J. 2005. Anti-thrombotic effect of strawberries. *Blood Coagulation Fibrinolysis.*, 16: 501–509.

Ness, A. R. and Powles, J. W. 1997. Fruit and vegetables, and cardiovascular disease: a review. *International Journal of Epidemiology.*, 26: 1–13.

Oszmianski, J. and Wojdylo, A. 2009. Comparative study of phenolic content and antioxidant activity of strawberry puree, clear, and cloudy juices. *European Food Research*

Pe´rez, A. G., Olı´as, R., Espada, J., Olı´as, J. M. and Sanz, C. 1997. Rapid determination of sugars, nonvolatile acids, and ascorbic acid in strawberry and other fruits. *Journal of Agricultural and Food Chemistry.*, 45: 3545–3549.

Rastall, R. A., & Maitin, V. 2002. Prebiotics and synbiotics: Towards the next generation. *Current Opinion in Biotechnology.*, 13: 490–496.

Record, I. R., Dreosti, I. E. and McInerney, J. K. 2001. Changes in plasma antioxidant status following consumption of diets high or low in fruits and vegetables or following dietary supplementation with an antioxidant mixture. *British Journal of Nutrition.*, 85: 4459–4464.

Rouanet, J. M., Decorde, K., Del Rio, D., Auger, C., Borges, G., Cristol, J. P., *et al.* 2010. Berry juices, teas, antioxidants and the prevention of atherosclerosis in hamsters. *Food Chemistry.*, 118(2): 266–271.

Scalzo, J., Politi, A., Pellegrini, N., Mezzetti, B. and Battino, M. 2005. Plant genotype affects total antioxidant capacity and phenolic contents in fruit. *Nutrition.*, 21: 207–213.

Seeram, N. P., Lee, R., Scheuller, H. S. and Heber, D. 2006. Identification of phenolic compounds in strawberries by liquid chromatography electrospray ionization mass spectrometry. *Food Chemistry.*, 97: 1–11.

Steinmetz, K. A. andPotter, J. D. 1991. Vegetables, fruit, and cancer. I. Epidemiology. *Cancer Causes and Control.*, 2: 325–357.

Tulipani, S., Josè, M., Alvarez-Suarez, A., Franco Busco, B., Stefano Bompadre, C., Josè, L., Quiles, D., Bruno Mezzetti, E. and Maurizio, B. 2011. Strawberry consumption improves plasma antioxidant status and erythrocyte resistance to oxidative haemolysis in humans. *Food Chemistry.*, 128: 180–186

Valko. M, Leibfritz. D., Moncola. J., Cronin, M., Mazura. M. and Telser, M. 2007. Free radicals and antioxidants in normal physiological functions and human disease. *The International Journal of Biochemistry & Cell Biology.*, 39: 44-84

Vinson, J. A., Su, X., Zubik, L. and Bose, P. 2001. Phenol antioxidant quantity and quality in foods: Fruits. *Journal of Agricultural and Food Chemistry.*, 49: 5315–5321.

Wang, S. Y. and Galletta, G. J. 2002. Compositional change in Colletotrichum (Anthracnose) infected strawberry fruit. *Acta Horticulturae.*, 567: 815–819.

Wang, S. Y. and Lin, H. S. 2000. Antioxidant activity in fruits and leaves of blackberry, raspberry, and strawberry varies with cultivar and developmental stage *Journal of Agricultural and Food Chemistry.*, 48: 140–146.

Wedge, D. E., Meepagala, K. M., Magee, J. B., Smith, S. H., Huang, G. and Larcom, L. L. 2001. Anticarcinogenic activity of strawberry, blueberry, and raspberry extracts to breast and cervical cancer cells. *Journal* of *Medicinal Food.*, 4(1): 49-51.

Yu, B. P. 1994. Cellular defenses against damage from reactive oxygen species. *Physiological Reviews.*, 74: 139-162.

Zeng, L. B., Zhang, Z. R., Luo, Z. H. and Zhu, J. X. 2010. Antioxidant activity and chemical constituent of essential oil and extracts of *Rhizoma Homalomenae. Food Chemistry.*, 125: 456- 463.

2

Antibacterial activity of essential oils from *Thymus vulgaris*, *Trachyspermum ammi* and *Mentha aquatica* against *Erwinia carotovora in vitro*

Mehrdad Jafarpour*, **Ahmad Reza Golparvar, Amin Lotfi**

Agriculture Faculty, Isfahan (Khorasgan) Branch, Islamic Azad University, Isfahan, Iran;
***Email:** *jafarpour@khuisf.ac.ir*

ARTICLE INFO

Topic: *Plant Pathology*

Key words:
- ✓ Erwinia carotovora
- ✓ *Essential oil*
- ✓ *Growth inhibitor*
- ✓ *Antibacterial*

ABSTRACT

Background & Aim: The aim of this study was to assess the bactericidal effect of three medicinal plant species, including *Thymus vulgaris*, *Trachyspermum ammi*, and *Mentha aquatica* on *Erwinia carotovora* growth.
Experimental: This research was done in a factorial to completely randomized design with three concentrations, and three replicates on nutrient agar culture medium.
Results &Discussion: Results of this study indicated that the essential oils from the studied plants were effective against *Erwinia carotovora.* At 300 ppm concentration, diameter of growth inhabitation was 43 mm. Results indicated the essential oil from *T. ammi*, especially at 300 and 400 ppm concentrations had the highest antibacterial activity against *Erwinia carotovora* with 43.00 and 46.67 mm diameter of growth inhabitation. In addition, there was no significant difference between 300 and 400 ppm concentrations of *M. aquatica* and at concentrations of 200, 300, and 400 ppm for *T. vulgaris.*
Recommended applications/industries: The overall results indicated the essential oils, especially *Trachyspermum ammi* have antibacterial activity against *Erwinia carotovora*; it seems that the essential oils can be employed in manufacturing desirable bactericidal agents.

1. Introduction

In recently years, due to increased interest of the public in consuming natural substances also prevalence of digestive and respiratory diseases and types of cancer, extensive investigations have been performed to use essential oils. Essential oils, also called ethereal or volatile oils, are in fact aromatic oily liquids obtained of plants. Phenolic compounds are mainly responsible for exhibiting bactericidal properties of essential oils. Essential oils, in addition to exhibiting bactericidal properties also show anti-parasite characteristics, a property related to the type of active ingredient of the essential oil (Burt, 2004).

Trachyspermum ammi is an herbaceous annual from the Apiaceae (Umbelliferae) family also known as *Carum copticum*. Medicinal part of this plant is the fruit that containing 2% essential oil. Its fruit essential oil called Ajowan is yellow-colored with a thymol scent (Amin, 1993). Analysis of the Persian anise reveals such ingredients as thymol, *p*-cymene, β-pinene, γ-terpinene, and sabinene (Mirzavand, 1991).

Thyme is one of the oldest medicinal and condiment plants officially introduced from 16th century as a medicinal plant. This woody perennial belongs to the family Lamiaceae. The genus *Thymus* includes numerous species being very different from the viewpoint of their chemical type, quality and quantity of active substances. Thyme essential oil is a yellow liquid, lighter than water, aromatic, with a strong, acrid taste exhibiting bactericidal and fungicidal properties. Chemical analysis of essential oil from thyme reveals existence of various phenolic compounds, monoterpene hydrocarbons and alcohols however, its bactericidal properties is mostly attributed to thymol and carvacrol both being phenolic compounds with bactericidal properties which at the same time are irritant and caustic (Ghasemi Pirbalouti, 2009).

Mentha aquatica is a medicinal plant belonging to the family Lamiaceae. Plants of this family include about 160 genera and over 3000 species grown almost all over the world especially in the Mediterranean region. Menthol in essential oil has antibacterial activity (Omid-Beiguy, 2009).

Erwinia carotovora (Sym. *Pectobacterium carotovorum*) is a plant pathogen belonging to the Family Enterobacteriaceae. It is a Gram- negative, rod-shaped bacterium (Barras *et al.*, 1994). The species is a plant pathogen with a diverse host range, including many agriculturally and scientifically important plant species. It produces pectolytic enzymes that hydrolyze pectin between individual plant cells. This bacterium is a ubiquitous plant pathogen with a wide host range (carrot, potato, tomato, leafy greens, squash and other cucurbits, onion, etc.), able to cause disease in almost any plant tissue it invades. It is a very economically important pathogen in terms of postharvest losses, and a common cause of decay in stored fruits and vegetables (Toth *et al.*, 2003).

In Iran, in spite of frequency of natural resources, not much attention has been paid to medicinal plants. Therefore, paying scientific attention to this subject is crucial. In this study, antibacterial activity of the essential oils from *Trachyspermum ammi*, *Thymus vulgaris,* and *Mentha aquatica* against growth of the bacterium *Erwinia carotovora* was investigated.

2. Materials and Methods

2.1. Plant materials

In this study, essential oils of three medicinal plants, including *Trachyspermum ammi*, *Thymus vulgaris,* and *Mentha aquatica* (growing at Zagros mountains, Iran) prepared from Atran Daru Agro-Industry Co., Isfahan, Iran.

2.2. Antibacterial test

Gram-negative *Erwinia carotovora* bacterium (PTCC: 1675) was obtained from the Iranian organization of Scientific and Industrial Research, Biotechnology Research Institute. To study the antibacterial properties of essential oils, the pitted-plate method was used. To do so, the nutrient agar (NA) culture medium was prepared and via carbibauer procedure, the intended bacterium was cultured on it in solid form. Before culture, to assess the level of microorganisms via carbibauer procedure, standard microbial suspension with 0.5 Mc-Farland was prepared in which suspension there are about 1.5×10^8 CFU/ml bacteria. Then the above said suspension was diluted to reach the 1.5×10^6 CFU/ml density. Then 5 μl of the above said solution equal to 10^4 microorganisms was with-drown and transferred to the plates and employing sterile swab was solid or broom cultured. Then using the sterile Pasteur pipette bottom, pits were made in the culture medium and then the bottom of each pit was closed using a drop of molten NA culture medium. Then, 100, 200, 300, and 400 ppm of each essential oil were added to each of the pits. Plates were refrigerated for 1-2 h and then incubated for 16-20 h at 27 ºC. As a result around some of the pits no-growth halos were formed resulting from diffusion of essential oils from the pits to the culture medium preventing growth of bacteria sensitive to such substances. The diameter of growth inhabitation was measured employing calipers and the best concentration of each concentration was determined.

2.3. Statistical analyses

The data was statistically analyzed by SPSS (19.0) software, using a completely randomized design. Means of the traits were separated by Duncan's multiple range test at $p \leq 0.05$ level.

3. Results and discussion

Results indicated that species, concentrations, and interaction of essential oils × species were significant ($p \leq 0.05$) against *Erwinia carotovora* bacterium. The essential oil from the studied plants against *Erwinia* was effective at 300 and 400 ppm concentrations with diameter of growth inhibition 43.00 and 43.67 mm, respectively.

Results this study indicated the essential oil from *T. ammi*, especially at 300 and 400 ppm concentrations had the highest antibacterial activity against *Erwinia carotovora* with 43.00 and 46.67 mm diameter of growth inhabitation (Table 2). In addition, there was no significant difference was seen between the concentrations of the essential oil from *T. ammi* at 300 and 400 ppm concentrations. Compared with other plants at different concentrations and the controls however, there was a significant difference (Table 2). Iacobellis et al. (2005) reported the antibacterial activity of the essential oil from anise by agar diffusion method against different bacteria (*Rhodotorula*, *Erwinia*, *Xanthomonas*, and *Agrobacterium*).

Table 1. Variance analysis of essential oils at different concentrations against *E. carotovora*

Source variation	d.f	DI (mm)
Species	2	1457.22**
Concentration	4	1306.81**
Concentration × Species	8	143.02**
Error	30	5.28
CV	-	11.86

Table 2. Comparison means of antibacterial activity of essential oils (EOs) at various concentrations against *E. carotovora*

DI (mm)			Concentrations of EO (ppm)
T. vulgaris	*M. aquatica*	*T. ammi*	
0^f	0^f	0^f	0
22.67^c	6.33^e	27.33^b	100
13.33^d	13.67^d	31.00^b	200
26.33^{bc}	14.33^d	43.00^a	300
30.67^b	15.33^d	46.67^a	400

The essential oil from *M. aquatica* at 300 and 400 ppm concentrations had 14.33 and 15.33 mm diameters of growth inhabitation against *Erwinia carotovora*, respectively. No significant difference ($p \leq 0.05$) was seen between these concentrations, however, the best treatment was found at 300 ppm concentration (Table 2). Results a study by Preuss et al. (2005) indicated the inhibitory and lethal effect of mountain mint and some other essential oils against *Escherichia coli*, *Helicobacter pylori*, *Anthracis* and *Mycobacterium* of leek. The essential oil from mountain mint revealed, except on *Anthracis bacillus*, a lathed effect on other tested microorganisms.

The essential oil from *T. vulgaris* at 300 and 400 ppm concentrations had antibacterial activity with 26.33 and 30.67 mm diameter of growth inhabitation against studied bacteria, respectively. Results a study by Karami et al. (2010) indicted the essential oils from thyme and savory having carvacrol and thymol, as the main constituents, at 0.05 M concentration in the culture medium had 5.6 to 7 mm diameter of growth inhabitation against *Erwinia*.

Phenolic compounds present in essential oils exhibited the most bactericidal properties. These compounds both diffuse in the cell membrane and also can play a role in clotting of cellular contents (Dorman & Dianne, 2000). For instance, thymol and cravacrol as the main constituents in the essential oils from *Trachyspermum ammi* and *Thymus vulgaris* have antimicrobial activity (Nostro *et al*., 2000).

4. Conclusion

According to the findings of this study, the essential oil *T. ammi* and *T. vulgaris* had antibacterial activity against *Erwinia carotovora*. The present study suggests that the essential oil of *T. ammi* is a potential source of natural antibacterial agents. After this screening experiment, further work should be performed to describe the antibacterial activities in more detail as *in vivo*.

5. References

Omidbeygi, R. 2009. *Product and processing of medicinal* plants. five edition, volume 1. Tehran. Astane Ghodse Razavi Press. 248 p. (In Persian)

Amin G. H. 1993. *Iranian traditional medicine plant. Ministry of Health and Educational Medical*

Science, Research Express, Tehran, Iran, (1): 115. (In Persian)

Barras. F., Van Gijsegem, F. and Chatterjee, A. K. 1994. Extracellular enzymes and pathogenesis of soft-rot Erwinia. *Annual Review of Phytopathology*., 32: 201-34.

Burt, S. 2004. Essential oils: their antibacterial properties and potential application in foods-a review. *International Journal of Food Microbiology*., 94: 223-253.

Dorman, H. J. D. and Dena, S. G. 2000. Antimicrobial agents from plants: Antibacterial activity of plant volatile oils. *Journal of Applied Microbiology*., 88: 308-316.

Ghasemi Pirbalouti, A. 2009. *Iranian medicinal and aromatic plants*. Islamic Azad University Publishers, Shahrekord, Iran, 550.

Iacobellis, N. S., Lo Cantore, P., Capasso, F., & Senatore, F. 2005. Antibacterial activity of *Cuminum cyminum* L. and *Carum carvi* L. essential oils. *Journal of Agricultural and Food Chemistry*., 53(1), 57-61.

Karami-Osboo, R., Khodavandi, M. and Aliakbari, F. 2010. Antibacterial effect of effective compounds of Satureja hortensis and Thymus vulgaris essential oils against Erwinia amylovora. *Journal of Agricultural and* Food Chemistry., 12: 35-45. (In Persian with English Summary).

Mirzavand-Brojeni, S. 1991. *Evaluation and comparative study on Macroscopic and Phytochemical Characteristics of Standard Sedde of Anison and Carum copticum*. Presented for the Ph.D., Isfahan, Medical Sciences University. (In Persian)

Nostro, A., Germano, M. P., Angelo, V. D., Marino, A. and Cannatelli, M. A. 2000. Extraction methods and bioautography for evaluation of medicinal plant antimicrobial activity. *Letters in Applied Microbiology*., 30: 379-384.

Preuss, H. G., Echard, B., Enig, M., Brook, I., Elliott, T. B. 2005. Minimum inhibitory concentrations of herbal essential oils and monolaurin for gram-positive and gram-negative bacteria. *Molecular and Cellular Biochemistry*., 272: 29-34.

Toth, I. K., Bell, K. S., Holeva, M. C. and Birch, P. R. 2003. Soft rot erwiniae: from genes to genomes. *Molecular Plant Pathology*., 4(1): 17-30.

Antibacterial activity of different extracts from the aerial parts and roots of *Stachys lavandulifolia* Vahl harvested at two stages of growth

Saman Mahdavi[*1], **Yousef Mehmannavaz**[2], **Masoud Taheri**[3]

[1]*Department of Microbiology, Maragheh Branch, Islamic Azad University, Maragheh, Iran;*
Email:** ***S.Mahdavi@iau-Maragheh.ac.ir

[2]*Department of Animal Science, Maragheh Branch, Islamic Azad University, Maragheh, Iran;*

[3]*Department of Botany, Marand Branch, Islamic Azad University, Marand, Iran;*

ARTICLE INFO

Topic: *Food Health*

Key words:

- ✓ *Alcoholic extract*
- ✓ *Antimicrobial activity*
- ✓ Stachys lavandulifolia *Vahl*

ABSTRACT

Background & Aim: Nowadays, the application of traditional medicine and herbal medicinal plants instead of chemical and synthetic drugs has captured the attention of the researchers. The purpose of this study was to investigate the antimicrobial effects of the aquatic, ethanolic and methanolic (80%) extracts of the aerial and root parts of *Stachys lavandulifolia* Vahl which were taken from the countryside of Marand (Eastern Azerbaijan, Iran) in two generative and vegetative phases against standard strains of microorganisms.
Experimental: Antimicrobial activity of the alcoholic and aquatic extracts from different parts of *S. lavandulifolia* was investigated against standard strains of *Staphylococcus aureus* (ATCC 6538), *Escherichia coli* (ATCC 8739), *Pseudomonas aeruginosa* (ATCC 9027) through well-plate and micro-dilution methods. Ampicillin as antibacterial agent was used as positive control.
Results & Discussion: Results of antimicrobial properties of *S. lavandulifolia* extracts revealed that the aquatic extract of the plant had no antibacterial effects. While the ethanolic and methanolic (80%) extracts showed the growth inhibition effect against standard strains of examined microorganisms. Their effect against Gram-positive bacteria was higher than Gram-negative bacteria. The antimicrobial activity of the ethanolic extract from the inflorescence of *S. lavandulifolia* was higher than the alcoholic extract of the roots.
Recommended applications/industries: The overall results indicated the ethanolic extract of the inflorescence of *Stachys lavandulifolia* has the best antimicrobial effects and it can be employed in manufacturing desirable bactericidal agents.

1. Introduction

Among *Iranica flora*, nearly all plant species have important role in traditional medicine. Almost 9000 plant species exist in *Iranica flora* out of which more than 500 species are extensively used in traditional medicine due to antimicrobial and anticancerous properties (Parsa, 2001; Sengul *et al.*, 2005). In fact, it is common for Iranian people to use some plant species for treatment of infectious diseases and other health problems (Adiguzel *et al.*, 2005). For centuries, herbal medicinal plants have been known due to curative properties or disease treatments (Skaltsa *et al.*, 1999). In addition, there is a vital need for discovering the new antimicrobial compounds (with different chemical structures) in order to deal with re-emerging infectious diseases. Thus, researchers have increasingly paid attention to traditional medicine and have looked for better herbal drugs against the microbial infectious diseases (Parekh and Chanda, 2007). Today, great interest towards traditional medicines has been arisen and even there have been increasingly immense demand for some drugs with herbal origin. This rehabilitation of interest towards herbal drugs could be mainly because of the common belief that herbal medicine is healthy and is more reliable than expensive synthetic drugs that have usually side effects (Nair and Chanda, 2007). This view was a source of motivation for research on new antimicrobial substances out of various herbal medicinal plants.

From this perspective, the effect of different plant extracts on pathogen microorganisms has captured the attention of researchers (Cordell, 2000). The species of *Stachys* L. genus in traditional and local medicine have been explored for the treatment of genital tumors, spleen sclerosis, inflammatory tumors, and cancerous ulcers (Skaltsa *et al.*, 1999). *Stachys lavandulifolia* Vahl. is a medicinal plant belonging to the Lamiaceae family and is used as an herbal tea. It is worth noting that the flowering shoots of the herb is extremely important in treatment of diseases such as digestive problems, headache, and stomachache, gastritis, and nerve disorders. Moreover, *S. lavandulifolia* can relieve the primary disminorey problems and reduce the intensity and the time of pain. It also decreases tiredness and nausea caused by primary disminorey, but it has no effect on vomiting (Seyyed-Javadi *et al.*,1998). The quick review of studies showed that there has been no research on antimicrobial activity of *S. lavandulifolia*. Therefore, the purpose of this study was to investigate the antimicrobial effects of the aquatic, ethanolic, and methanolic (80%) extracts of the aerial parts and roots of *S. lavandulifolia* collected from Marand (Eastern Azerbaijan, Iran) at two generative and vegetative phases against standard bacterial strains.

2. Materials and methods

2.1. Plant material

Samples of *S. lavandulifolia* at two generative and vegetative phases were collected during April to June 2013 from Mishudagh region in East Azerbaijan. The plant was identified according to the sample at Herbarium, Department of Plant Biology of Islamic Azad University of Marand Branch (No.19405).

2.2. Preparation of extracts

The collected the plants were separated into two parts, including the aerial organs (stem, leaf, petiole, and flower) and root organs. The samples were kept in shade and were dried far from the direct light of sun. Then, the electronic powdering apparatus was used to powder this plant and the extraction was performed (Kursat and Erecevit, 2009; Dugler and Aki, 2009). Various extracts included aquatic, ethanolic and methanolic (80%) extracts.

2.3. Examined microorganisms

In this research, the antimicrobial studies were done against three standard bacterial strains as follows: *Staphylococcus aureus* (ATCC 6538), *Escherichia coli* (ATCC 8739), and *Pseudomonas aeruginosa* ATCC 9027.

2.4. Antimicrobial activity by Well-plate assay

In this method, the inoculation of 100 μl microbial suspension was fulfilled into surface of the plate with a sterile pipette. All culture plates were allowed for dry for about 5 min. The same diameter wells produced on Mueller-Hinton agar. Then, 100 μl the extracts were poured in well separately [one well was allocated to distilled water, ethanol and methanol (80%)]. Later, plates were put in incubator for 18-24 h at 37 °C and then the diameter of zone of growth inhibition were measured that results from diffusion of the extracts into the medium surrounding the wells with millimeter ruler. Additionally, ampicillin disc was used as standard control antibiotic (Shafiee, 1992; Kursat and Erecevit, 2009).

2.5. Antimicrobial activity by micro-dilution assay

The identification of the minimal inhibitory concentration (MIC) was performed with some modifications (Zyoda and Porter, 2001). Then the minimal bactericidal concentration (MBC) was determined. Then, ampicillin as a standard antimicrobial agent was considered in this method. In addition, their dilutions (0.25 to 128 μg/ml) were similar to plates of microliter (Dugler and Aki, 2009).

2.6. Statistical analysis

This study was performed within the framework of factorial experiment 2 ×3 ×2, including two organs of the plant, three extracts (aquatic, ethanolic, and methanolic), and two stages of growth with a completely randomized design with three replications. After analysis of variance in procedure of GLM of SAS software, means comparison was performed by Tukey method ($p \leq 0.05$). Means of the antibacterial activity of the extracts with standard antibiotic were compared using Dunet test at $p \leq 0.05$.

3. Results and Discussion

In this study, the antimicrobial activity of the aquatic, ethanolic, and methanolic (80%) extracts of *S. lavandulifolia* were investigated against the standard strains of bacteria and the antimicrobial capacity of these extracts was evaluated through the existence or non-existence of diameter zone of inhibition. In well-plate assay, the aerial and root organs of *S. lavandulifolia* were determined in two generative and vegetative phases against standard strains of microorganisms through aquatic, ethanolic, and methanolic extracts. Results of this study indicated that the different extracts had a significant growth inhibition effect against examined microorganisms in comparison with standard control antibiotic. The extracts from the aerial parts of *S. lavandulifolia* collected at generative stage had the largest zone of growth inhibition against studied bacteria (Table 1).

In comparison, the extracts of the herb with standard antibiotic showed that the ethanol extract from the aerial parts of *S. lavandulifolia* at vegetative stage acts like antibiotic, while the ethanol extract from the aerial parts at generative stage acts higher than ampicillin (Table 2).

Comparison of minimal inhibitory concentration (MIC) in two groups showed that there was no significant difference between standard antibiotic and ethanol extract of *S. lavandulifolia* (Table 3). The aquatic extract from the aerial parts of *S. lavandulifolia* at the vegetative phase had no antimicrobial effect. Regarding to the antimicrobial effects of different extracts of the plant, the findings revealed that the ethanolic, methanolic, and aquatic extracts from the aerial parts had the higher antimicrobial effect than the extracts from the roots, especially at the generative phase. Results of plate-well assay indicated that *Staphylococcus aureus* was the most sensitive in comparison with other studied bacteria. Probably, some components in the extracts, including phenols, flavonoids, monoterpenes (β-phellandrene, α-pinene, β-pinen, myrcene, and β-ocimene) and sesquiterpenes (germacrene-D and Spathulenol) are caused to antimicrobial activity in *S. lavandulifolia* (Javidnia *et al.*, 2004). The phytochemical analysis of *S lavandulifolia* has proved the presence of some secondary metabolites such as diterpenes, phenyl ethanoidglycosides, flavonoids, and saponis (Khanavi *et al.*, 2005) in a way that flavonoids might be responsible for antimicrobial activity (Saeedi *et al.*, 2008).

In present study, both ethanolic and methanolic extracts could be regarded as organic solvent with favorite polarity because they were able to solve antimicrobial compounds in the plant. In fact, those extracts that were provided during the generative phase of this plant showed more antimicrobial properties. In addition, the generative phase is important for survival of the species so that the above-mentioned substances may increase in this phase. From physicochemical perspective, the cell wall structure of Gram-negative bacteria was more complex than that of Gram-positive bacteria. For this reason, Gram-negative bacteria indicated more resistance against antimicrobial substances. Gram-negative bacteria have external hydrophilic membrane due to presence of lipopolysaccharide (LPS) molecules. The small solution substances of molecules are able to pass this external membrane of bacteria through numerous porin proteins. Thus, this membrane might be regarded as a barrier against macromolecules and hydrophobic compounds, and toxic drugs and it is important for evaluation of the antimicrobial compounds in plants. In total, Gram-positive bacterium (*S. aureus* ATCC 6538) showed more sensitivity towards the extracts as compared to Gram-negative bacteria. These findings are in agreement with results of a study on *Stachys inflata* by Maleki et al. (2001).

The ethanolic and methanolic extracts have a great amount of bactericide properties even in high dilutions, in exception of *E.coli*, which showed a static reaction and was resistant to the extracts. These findings are in agreement with results of a research by Rasooli and Mirmostafa (2002). It has been shown that extracts depend on species, type of chemical substance of the plant and the climate condition. As a result, the antimicrobial activities of extracts in various plant species were different from each other (Lawrence *et al.*, 2005; Chi-kuen and Chi-Chiu, 2006).

Table 1. Simple and interaction effects of organs, extracts and stages of growth of *Stachys lavandulifolia* on the zone diameter of growth inhibition of studied bacteria

Factor		*S. aureus* ATCC 6538	*E. coli* ATCC 8739	*P. aeruginosa* ATCC 9027
Organ	Aerial	11.67a¶	6.33a	9.17a
	Root	4.83b	2.67b	4.05b
	SEM	0.204	0.192	0.219
Extract	Ethanol	13.00a	7.00a	10.25a
	Methanol	10.75b	6.00b	8.83b
	Water	1.00c	0.50c	0.75c
	SEM	0.250	0.236	0.268
Stage	Vegetative	6.50b	3.67b	5.55b
	Generative	10.00a	5.33a	7.67a
	SEM	0.204	0.192	0.219
Organ×Extract	Aerial × Ethanol	18.50a	9.50a	14.00a
	Aerial × Methanol	14.50b	8.50a	12.00b
	Aerial × Water	2.00d	1.00c	1.50d
	Root × Ethanol	7.50c	4.50b	6.50c
	Root × Methanol	7.00c	3.50b	5.67c
	Root × Water	0.00e	0.00c	0.00d
	SEM	0.353	0.333	0.379
Organ × Stage	Aerial × Vegetative	9.00b	5.00b	7.33b
	Aerial × Generative	14.33a	7.67a	11.00a
	Root × Vegetative	4.00d	2.33c	3.78c
	Root × Generative	5.67c	3.00c	4.33c
	SEM	0.289	0.272	0.309
Extract × Stage	Ethanol × Vegetative	11.00c	6.00bc	9.00b
	Ethanol × Generative	15.00a	8.00a	11.50a
	Methanol × Vegetative	8.50d	5.00c	7.67c
	Methanol × Generative	13.00b	7.00b	10.00ab
	Water × Vegetative	0.00f	0.00d	0.00d
	Water × Generative	2.00e	1.00d	1.50d
	SEM	0.353	0.333	0.379
Organ × Extract × Stage	Aerial × Ethanol × Vegetative	16.00c	8.00b	12.00c
	Aerial × Ethanol × Generative	21.00a	11.00a	16.00a
	Aerial × Methanol × Vegetative	11.00d	7.00b	10.00d
	Aerial × Methanol × Vegetative	18.00b	10.00d	14.00b
	Aerial × Water × Vegetative	0.00i	0.00h	0.00h
	Aerial × Water × Generative	4.00g	3.00f	3.00f
	Root × Ethanol × Vegetative	6.00h	6.00e	6.00e
	Root × Ethanol × Generative	9.00e	7.00e	7.00e
	Root × Methanol × Vegetative	6.00h	5.33e	5.33e
	Root × Methanol × Generative	8.00f	6.00e	6.00e
	Root × Water × Vegetative	0.00i	0.00h	0.00h
	Root × Water × Generative	0.00i	0.00h	0.00h
	SEM	0.500	0.536	0.536

¶ Different letters in above of means in any column represent significant statistical difference ($p \leq 0.05$)

Table 2. Comparison of antibacterial activity the extracts of *Stachys lavandulifolia* with standard antibiotic against the studied bacteria

Treatments	*S. aureus* ATCC 6538	*E. coli* ATCC 8739	*P. aeruginosa* ATCC 9027
Aerial × Ethanol × Vegetative	2.00ns	0.00ns	0.00ns
Aerial × Ethanol × Generative	7.00*	3.00ns	4.00*
Aerial × Methanol × Vegetative	-3.00*	-1.00ns	-2.00ns
Aerial × Methanol × Vegetative	4.00*	2.00ns	2.00ns
Aerial × Water × Vegetative	-14.00*	-8.00*	-12.00*
Aerial × Water × Generative	-10.00*	-6.00*	-9.00*
Root × Ethanol × Vegetative	-8.00*	-4.00*	-6.00*
Root × Ethanol × Generative	-5.00*	-3.00*	-5.00*
Root × Methanol × Vegetative	-8.00*	-5.00*	-6.67*
Root × Methanol × Generative	-6.00*	-4.00*	-6.00*
Root × Water × Vegetative	-14.00*	-8.00*	-12.00*
Root × Water × Generative	-14.00*	-8.00*	-12.00*

Table 3. Comparison of the ethanolic extract of *Stachys lavandulifolia* Vahl and standard antibiotic against standard strains of bacteria by *t*-student test.

Treatment	*S.aureus* ATCC 6538	*E.coli* ATCC 8739	*P. aeruginosa* ATCC 9027
Ampicilin	9.33	115.33	4.67
Ethanolic extract	18.67	271.33	37.33
t-value	1.18	1.09	2.30
p-value	0.302	0.338	0.145

Results of this study indicated that the ethanol was the best solvent to extract of the plant. Indeed, our findings were in consistent with findings of other studies concerning the antimicrobial effects of ethanolic extracts (Jonathan and Fasidi, 2003; Saeedi *et al*., 2008). It is worth noting that the slight variations between our findings and other researchers might be due to several reasons such as intraspecific variation for producing secondary metabolites and differences in extracted protocols that were used for discovering the active metabolites and even differences in evaluation methods (Dugler and Aki, 2009).

4. Conclusion

The findings of this research indicated that the extracts of *Stachys lavandulifolia* Vahl contain some compounds with antibacterial properties that can be used as an herbal drug for treatment of infectious diseases. Obviously, most species of *Stachys* genus were particularly native and were traditionally used by local people in different regions of Iran. However, little evidence is available about the application of such plants. As a result, ethno-botanical studies in various parts of Iran are essential for recording all traditional medicinal knowledge that was experienced among local people.

5. References

Adiguzel, A., Gulluce, M., Sengul, M., Ogutcu, H., Sahin, F. and Karaman, I. 2005. Antimicrobial effects of *Ocimum basillicum* (Labiatae) extract. *Turkish Journal of Biology*., 29: 155-160.

Chi-Kuen, Ch. and Chi-Chiu, L. 2006. Risk of active tuberculosis among school children in Hong Kong. *Archives of Pediatrics and Adolescent Medicine*., 160: 247-251.

Cordell, G.A. 2000. Biodiversity and drug discovery- a symbiotic relationship. *Phytochemistry*., 55: 463-480.

Dugler, G. and Aki, C. 2009. Antimicrobial activity of the leaves of endemic *Stachys pseudopinardii* in Turkey. *Tropical Journal of Pharmaceutical Research*., 8(4): 371-375.

Javidnia, K., Mojab, F. and Mojahedi, S.A. 2004. Chemical constituents of the essential oil of *Stachys lavandulifolia* Vahl from Iran. *Iranian Journal of Pharmaceutical Research*., 3: 61-63.

Jonathan, S.G. and Fasidi, I.O. 2003. Antimicrobial activities of two Nigerian edible marofungi, *Lycoperdon pusilum* and *Lycoperdon giganteum*. *African Journal of Biomedical Research*., 6: 85-90.

Khanavi, M., Sharifzade, M., Hadjakhoondi, A. and Shafiee, A. 2005. Phytochemical investigation and anti-inflammatory activity of aerial parts of *Stachys byzantina* C. koch. *Journal of Ethnopharmacology*., 97: 463-468.

Kursat, M. and Erecevit, P. 2009. The antimicrobial activities of methanolic extracts of some Lamiaceae members collected from Turkey. *Turkish Journal of Science and Technology*., 4(1): 81-85.

Lawrence, S.J., Korzenik, J.R. and Mundy, L.M. 2005. Probiotics for recurrent *Clostridium difficile* disease. *Journal of Medical Microbiology*., 54: 905-906.

Maleki, N., Garjani, A., Nazemiyeh, H., Nilfouroushan, N., Eftekhar Sadat, A.T., Allameh, Z. and Hasannia, N. 2001. Potent anti-inflammatory activity of hydroalcoholic extract from aerial parts of *Stachys inflata* on rats. *Journal of Ethnopharmacology*., 75: 213-218.

Nair, R. and Chanda, S.V. 2007. Antibacterial activities of some medicinal plants of western region of India. *Turkish Journal of Biology*., 31: 231-236.

Parekh, J. and Chanda, S.V. 2007. In vitro antimicrobial activity and phytochemical analysis of some Indian medicinal plants. *Turkish Journal of Biology*., 31:53-58.

Parsa, A. 2001. *Iranica Flora*. Tehran university press, Iran. (In Persian)

Rasooli, I. and Mirmostafa, S.A. 2002. Antimicrobial reports of *Thymus pubescens* and *Thymus serpyllum* essential oil. *Fitoterapia*., 73: 244-250.

Saeedi, M., Morteza-Semnani, K., Mahdavi, M.R., Rahimi, F. 2008. Antimicrobial studies on extracts of four species of *Stachys*. *Indian Journal of Pharmaceutical Sciences*., 70(3): 403-406.

Sengul, M., Ogutcu, H., Adiguzel, A., Sahin, F., Kara, A.A., Karaman, I., Gulluce, M. 2005. Antimicrobial effects of *Verbascum georgicum* Bentham extract. *Turkish Journal of Biology*., 29:105-110.

Seyyed-Javadi, H.E., Olphati, F., Hadizadeh, M., Azerbaijani, S. 1998. The study on effects of *Stachys lavandulifolia* Vahl on primary dismenorey and its signs. *Edrak Scientific Journal*. Qazvin Medical Science University., 12: 3 (in Persian)

Shafiee, A. 1992. *Chromatography and spectrometry*. Tehran university press, Iran (in Persian).

Skaltsa, H.D., Lazari, D.M., Chinou, I.B. and Loukis, A.E. 1999. Composition and antimicrobial activity of the essential oils of *Stachys candida* and *Stachys chrysantha* from southern Greece. *Planta Medica*., 65: 255-256.

Zyoda, J.R. and Porter, J.R. 2001. A convenient microdilution method for screening natural products against bacteria and fungi. *Pharmaceutical Biology*., 39: 221-225.

4

In vitro anti-fungal activity of watercress (*Nasturtium officinale*) extract against Fusarium solani, the causal agent of potato dry rot

Jafar Nikan[1*], Hadi Khavari[2]

[1] *Plant Protection Research Department, Agricultural and Natural Resources Research Centre of Hamadan, Hamadan, Iran;*
[*]**E-mail:** *JNikan@gmail.com*

[2] *University of Applied Science and Technology of Hamadan, Hamadan, Iran;*

ARTICLE INFO

Topic: *Plant Pathology*

Key words:

- *Potato Dry Rot*
- *Growth Inhibition*
- *Natural Fungicide*

ABSTRACT

Background & Aim: The aim of this study was to assess the antifungal effect of the watercress extract on the growth of *Fusarium solani*, the causal agent of potato dry rot.
Experimental: This research was done in a completely randomized design with three concentrations and four replicates on potato dextrose agar (PDA) culture medium.
Results: Results of this study indicated that all concentrations of alcoholic extract of watercress can significantly inhibit mycelia growth of *Fusarium solani* on PDA medium. Among different concentrations of watercress extract, the highest inhibition zone of the fungus (26.1 mm in diameter) was obtained at dose of 600 mg/ml. The rate of growth inhibition was concentration dependent. However, no significant difference in the rate of growth inhibition of the fungus by watercress extract was seen between the 500 mg/ml and 400 mg/ml or between 400 mg/ml and 300 mg/ml of the plant extract.
Recommended applications/industries: The overall results of this experiment indicated that the alcoholic extract of watercress can inhibit mycelia growth of *Fusarium solani* in a dose dependent manner. It seems therefore, that the watercress extract has the potential to be employed for manufacturing natural fungicidal compounds. It is recommended that the experiment to be tested on potato tubers (*in vivo* conditions).

1. Introduction

Potato (*Solanum tuberosum* L.) is as the fourth most important crop in the world (Anonymous, 2012). Dry rot caused by various species of *Fusarium* spp., is a post-harvest disease of significant importance in potato (Stevenson *et al.*, 2001; Al-Mughrabi, 2010). Crop losses attributed to this disease has been estimated up to US$ 100 m per year (Rowe, 1993). Moreover, most species of *Fusarium* produce toxins that are dangerous to man and livestock (Marasas *et al.*, 1984). *Fusarium solani* has been reported as the most pathogenic

Fusarium species causing potato dry rot in Hamadan province of Iran (Sharifi *et al.*, 2009; Soheili-Moghadam and Hosseinzadeh, 2013).

Potato dry rot is commonly controlled by the proper handling of potato tubers to minimize the amount of wounds on tubers, proper storage to heal the wounds and chemical control of the pathogen. The fungicides thiabendazole and fludioxinil (Maxim-based products) have been recommended for seed treatment and for post-harvest use on tubers, respectively (Murdoch and Wood, 1972; Kirk and Wharton, 2008). Biological control of the disease has also been investigated and some bio-control agents been introduced (El-Kot, 2008; Gould *et al.*, 2008). However, effective and efficient management of crop pests is generally achieved by the use of synthetic pesticides (Kiran *et al.*, 2006). On the other hand, due to increased awareness about the risks associated with the use of pesticides including: the advent of pesticide resistant pests, ecological impact of pesticide application on the environment and particularly consumer concerns about pesticide residue in crops (Viana *et al.*, 1996; Nikan and Morowati, 2013), much attention is being focused on the alternative methods of pest control. Natural plant extracts have been recommended as suitable alternative choices to synthetic chemicals (Suhr and Nielsen, 2003; Ownagh *et al.*, 2010; Bahraminejad *et al.*, 2010; Mangang and Chhetry, 2012; Jafarpour *et al.*, 2013).

Babu et al. (2008) studied the effect of some plant extracts on the control of *Fusarium solani* f.sp. Melongenae *in vitro*. All the plant extracts showed significant reduction in the growth of the pathogen. Among the different extracts, 20% of *Azadirachta indica* was found most effective.

In another study, *Fusarium oxysporum* was treated with the various extracts of *Excoecaria agallocha* (different dilutions from different parts of the plant). It was observed that the 20% dilution of stem extract brought about 87.1 percent inhibition of spore germination (Deepa and Padmaja, 2013).

Dwivedi and Dwivedi (2012) studied antifungal activity of some plant extracts against *Fusarium solani* the causal agent of guava wilt. They found that the extract of Clove (*Eugenia caryophyllata*) was most effective against the fungus on 3rd, 5th and 7th day at 50% concentration and conquered the colony growth by 100% compared to control.

Shrestha and Tiwari (2009) assessed the antifungal activity of the crude extracts of six medicinal plants against *Fusarium solani*. The extracts of all the plant species were found to be effective in inhibiting the mycelia growth. The extract of *Allium sativum* completely inhibited the mycelia growth of the fungus at the concentration of 40% and the extracts of *Capsicum annuum* and *Phyllanthusem blica*inhibited the mycelia growth completely at the concentration of 100%.

It was revealed in a bioassay study that different concentrations of *Parthenium hysterophorus* was effective in inhibiting the growth of *Fusarium solani* FCBP-434, the most pathogenic strain of the fungus causing Fusarium wilt in potato (Shafique and Shafique, 2012).

Nasturtium officinale R.Br. (Watercress) belonging to the family Brassicaceae, is an important medicinal herb that grows naturally in flowing streams in most mountainous regions of the world including Iran. This plant has been used by the rural healers as nutritive, anti-inflammatory and antioxidant agent. It is also a vegetable that is consumed raw or cooked in salads, soups and other recipes in European and Turkish cuisine and also used to cure abdominal pain in traditional medicine (Ozen, 2009) and for treatment of diseases such as diabetes and bronchitis (Bahramikia *et al.*, 2009). The extract of watercress contains secondary metabolites such as phenolic and flavonoid compounds (Mazandarani *et al.*, 2013).

Asadi et al. (2012) investigated the effect of watercress extract on immunological and hematological parameters of rainbow trout (*Oncorhynchus mykiss*). The results indicated that oral administration of watercress extract might be useful to improve fish's immune system. The extract of watercress has shown nematicide effect on northern root-knot nematode (NRKN), *Meloidogyne hapla* (Zahradníková and Petříková, 2012). Freitas et al. (2013) found synergistic antibacterial activity effects between watercress extract and antibiotics, indicating the potential of watercress compounds as anti-microbial substances.

In this study the effect of alcoholic extract of watercress on inhibiting the mycelia growth of *F. solani*, the main causal agent of potato dry rot was investigated *in vitro*.

2. Materials and Methods

2.1. Plant materials

The medicinal plant used in the experiment was watercress (*Nasturtium officinale* R.Br.) collected from flowing streams in Lorestan province of Iran. The required amount of watercress was collected in autumn and after washing was air dried in the shade.

2.2. Preparation of plant extracts

The alcoholic plant extract of watercress was prepared using maceration method described by Durling et al. (2007). The extraction was done briefly as follows: 200 g dried watercress was ground and 1000 ml 70% ethanol was added to the resulting powder and mixed well. The mixture was stirred every day for two weeks. After 14 days, the resulting extract was clarified with filter paper. The clarified extract was then allowed to air dry at room temperature.

2.3. Pathogen

The pathogenic fungus was isolated from dry rot affected potato tubers gathered from potato fields in Hamadan province of Iran. The isolation was done by culturing the diseased potato flesh on potato dextrose agar (PDA) medium and subsequent purification of the fungus.

2.4. Preparation of spore suspension of the fungus

Two weeks old purified cultures of the *Fusarium solani* (when mycelia had produced spores) were used for preparing spore suspension. The spore suspension was prepared by adding some sterilized distilled water (~ 1 ml) to each petri dish containing the fungus culture to allow the spores to be suspended in the water. The spore suspension was then collected and the spore suspension was adjusted to 1×10^6 spore per milliliter.

2.5. Assessment of antifungal activity of the extract

Using the paper disc diffusion method (Rasooli *et al.*, 2006), the assessment was done by measuring the growth inhibition zone of the fungus on PDA medium. Different concentrations (300, 400, 500, and 600 mg/ml) of watercress extract were prepared by dissolving the required amounts of dried extract into one milliliter distilled water. To remove any microbial contamination, the extracts were filtrated by using two-micrometer filters (Millipore filter 2). Then some autoclaved filter paper discs (6 mm in diameter) were submerged in any of the prepared concentrations of the watercress extract or in sterilized distilled water (as negative control) and in 0.2 percent fungicide carbendazim+iprodion 52% WP solution (as positive control). The discs were allowed to be saturated with the solutions. The submerged paper discs were then air dried. Half a milliliter of spore suspension of *F. solani* (1×10^6 spore/ml) was transferred to PDA medium and was evenly spread on the surface of the medium. Then one paper disc loaded with each solution was placed in the center of *F. solani* inoculated plate.

The experiment was conducted as a completely randomized design with six treatments and four replicates. The treatments were five concentrations of the watercress extract, as mentioned above and two controls (sterilized water as negative and fungicide solution as positive control). The treated plates were then incubated at 26°C in the dark. The average diameter of the mycelia growth inhibition zone around the paper discs loaded with each treatment was measured 7 days post incubation (before the plates were completely covered with mycelia of the fungus). The growth inhibition percent was calculated using the formula:

IP = dc - dt/dc × 100, where IP was the growth inhibition percent, dc and dt were the diameter of growth inhibition zone in negative control and each of the other treatments, respectively.

2.6. Statistical analysis

The statistical analysis of the data and comparison of the means was done using the SAS software and the Duncan's multiple range test, respectively. Transformation of the data was done as needed.

3. Results and discussion

Statistical analysis indicated that the growth inhibition rates for *F. solani* due to treating with the various given treatments were significantly different (Table 1).

Table 1. Statistical analysis of the data of growth inhibition percent of *F. solani* by different concentrations of Watercress extract

Sources of variance	Degrees of freedom	Sam of squares	Mean of squares	*F*-value
Treatment	5	62.316	12.46	347.7*
Error	18	0.645	0.36	8
Total	23	62.961		

* $P < .001$, CV: 4.63

Comparison of the means of growth inhibition rates resulting from various given treatments divided them into three groups (Table 2). The highest and the lowest growth inhibition zone were those of fungicide and Sterilized distilled water treatments, respectively. Among various concentrations of the watercress extract, the concentration 600 mg/ml inhibited the growth of *F. solani* more than the other concentrations. Moreover, the effect of the watercress extract on the growth inhibition of *F. solani* was dose dependent, that is: the higher the concentration the more inhibition growth of the fungus. However, no significant difference between the growth inhibition rates of *F. solani* was seen between the concentrations 500 mg/ml and 400 mg/ml or between the concentrations 400 mg/ml and 300 mg/ml of extract.

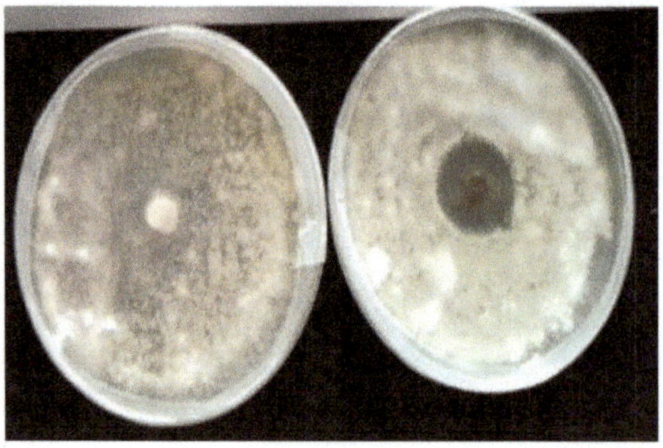

Negative Control treatment: Watercress treatment

Fig.1. *In vitro* growth Inhibition zone of *F. solani on* PDA medium resulting from treatment of the fungus with Watercress extract, negative control (left) and watercress extract (right).

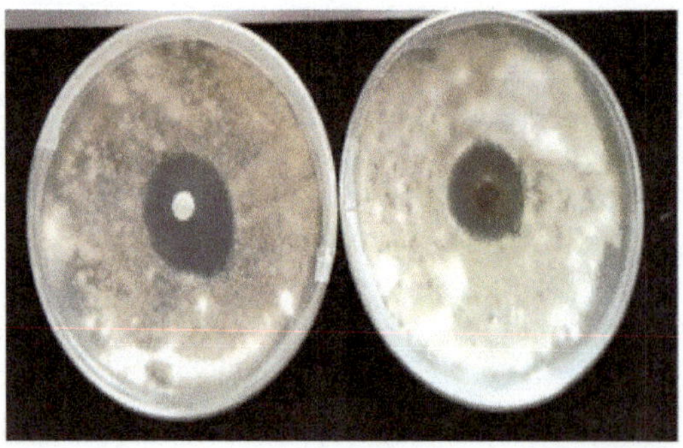

Positive Control treatment: Watercress treatment 600mg/ml

Fig.2. *In vitro* growth Inhibition zone of *F. solani*
On PDA medium resulting from treatment of the fungus with Watercress extract, negative control (left) and Watercress extract (right).

This report indicates that the extract of watercress has anti-pathogenic, in particular antifungal, activity, the fact that has been reported previously (Zahradníková and Petříková, 2012; Freitas *et al.*, 2013). We found that the growth of *F. solani* can be inhibited by the application of the watercress extract as found Ataee-Azimi et al. (2006) by using the extract of *Sorghum bicolor* and Shrestha and Tiwari (2009) by using *Thymus* essence. This preliminary study proved that the watercress extract could be used as an alternative to for the control of *F. solani*, *in vitro*. However, it needs to be applied in virtual condition on the potato.

Table 2. Grouping the means of growth inhibition rates of *F. solani* by the different concentrations of Watercress extract using Duncan's multiple range test

Treatment	Mean of growth inhibition (percent)
Watercress extract 600mg/ml	26.2^{b}
Watercress extract 500mg/ml	19.8^{c}
Watercress extract 400mg/ml	17.6^{cd}
Watercress extract 300mg/ml	16.5^{d}
Fungicide	32.7^{a}
Sterilized distilled water	0^{e}

*The means followed by different superscript letters are significantly different.

4. Conclusion

It was proved that the alcoholic extract of Watercress was capable of bringing about the desired antifungal effect in a concentration dependent manner.

5. References

Al-Mughrabi, K. I. 2010. Biological control of Fusarium dry and other potato tuber diseases using *Pseudomonas fluorescens* and *Enterobacter cloacae. Biological Control.*, 53: 280-284.

Anonymous, 2012. FAOSTAT. http://faostat.fao.org/site/567/DesktopDefault.aspx?PageID=567#ancor

Asadi, M.S., Mirvaghefei, A.R., Nematollahi, M.A., Banaee, M. and Ahmadi, K. 2012. Effects of watercress (*Nasturtium nasturtium*) extract on selected immunological parameters of rainbow trout

(Oncorhynchus mykiss). *Open Veterinary Journal.*, 2: 32-39.

Ataee-Azimi, a., Delnavaz Hashemian, B. and Ghanaee, A.M. 2006. Effect of Watery, alcoholic and phenolic extracts of seed and leaf of *Sorghum bicolor* on *Fusarium solani* and *Fusarium poae*. *Journal of Medicinal Plants.*, 21: 26-31.

Babu, J., Dar, M.A. and Kumar, V . 2008. Bioefficacy of plant extracts to control *Fusarium solani* f.Sp. Melongenae incitant of Brinjal Wilt. *Global Journal of Biotechnology & Biochemistry.*, 3 (2): 56-59.

Bahramikia, S., Ardestani, A. and Yazdanparast, R. 2009. Protective effects of four Iranian, medicinal plants against free radical-mediated protein oxidation. *Food Chemistry.*, 1159(1): 37-42.

Bahraminejad, S., MaerefatzadahKhamenah, M., Abbasi, S., ZareKhafari, A. 2010. In vitro screening of 27 plant species against phytopathogenic fungi. *Modern Technology in Agriculture.*, 4(2): 1-11.

Deepa, M. and Padmaja, C.K. 2013. Effect of the extracts of *Excoecaria agallocha* on spore formation and budding in fungi. *Asian Journal of Plant Science and Research.*, (6): 14-19.

Durling, N.E., Catchpole,O. J., Grey, J.B., Weebby, R.F., Mitchell, K.A., Foo, L.Y., and Perry, N.B. 2007. Extraction of phenolics and essential oil from dried sage (*salvia officinalis*) using ethanol – water mixtures. *Food Chemistry.*, 101: 1417-1424.

Dwivedi, S.K. and Dwivedi, N. 2012. Antifungal activity of some plant extracts against guava wilt pathogen. *International Journal of Environmental Sciences.*, 3(1): 412-420.

El-Kot, G.A.N. 2008.Biological Control of Black Scurf and Dry Rot of Potato. *Egyptian Journal of Phytopathology.*, 36(1-2): 45-56.

Freitas, E., Aires, A., de Santos, R. EA, and Saavedra, M.J. 2013. Antibacterial activity and synergistic effect between watercress extracts, 2-phenylethyl isothiocyanate and antibiotics against 11 isolates of Escherichia coli from clinical and animal source. *Letters in Applied Microbiolgy.*, 57(4): 266-73. doi: 10.1111/lam. 12105.

Gould, M., Nelson, L M., Waterer, D., and Hynes, R. K. 2008. Biocontrol of *Fusarium sambucinum*, dry rot of potato, by *Serratia plymuthica* 5-6. *Biocontrol Science and Technology.*, 18(9/10): 1005-1016.

Jafarpour M., Golparvar, A.R., and Lotfi, A. 2013. Antibacterial activity of essential oils from *Thymus vulgaris*, *Trachyspermum ammi* and *Mentha aquatic* against *Erwinia carotovora* in vitro. *Journal of Herbal Drugs.*, 4(3): 115-118.

Kiran, K., Linguraju, S. and Adiver, S. 2006. Effect of plant extract on *Sclerotiumrolfsii,* the incitant of stem rot of ground nut. *Journal of Mycology and Plant Pathology.,* 36: 77-79

Kirk, W. and Wharton, P. 2008. Fusarium dry rot posing problems in potatoes. Michigan State University Extension, Department of Plant Pathology. http://msue.anr.msu.edu/news/fusarium dry rot posing problems in potatoes

Mangang, H.C. and chhetry, G.K.N. 2012. Antifungal Properties of certain Plant Extracts against *Rhizoctonia Solani* Causing Root Rot of French Bean In Organic Soil of Manipur International *Journal of Scientific and Research Publications.*, 2(5): 1-4.

Marasas, W. F. O., Nelson, P. E. andToussoun, T. A. 1984. *Toxigenic Fusarium Species Identity and Mycotoxicology*. Pennsylvania State University Press 328pp.

Mazandarani, M., Momeji, A., ZarghamiMoghaddam, P. 2013. Evaluation of phytochemical and antioxidant activities from different parts of *Nasturtium officinale* R. Br. in Mazandaran. *Iranian Journal of Plant Physiology.*, 3(2): 659-664.

Murdoch A.W. and Wood, R.K.S. 1972. Control of *Fusarium solani* rot of potato tubers with fungicides. *Annals of Applied Biology.*, 75(1): 53–62.

Nikan, J. and Morowati, M. 2013. Investigation on pesticide residue levels in green-house grown cucumber and their influencing factors in Hamadan province, Iran. Final Report of the research project coded 04-83-16-89102, *Agricultural and natural resources Research Organization.*, 44300,

Ownagh, A., Hasani, A., Mardani, K., and Ebrahimzadeh, S. 2010. Antifungal effects of thyme, agastache and satureja essential oils on *Aspergillus fumigatus, Aspergillus flavus* and *Fusarium solani. Veterinary Research Forum.*, 1(2): 99 – 105.

Ozen, T. 2009. Investigation of antioxidant properties of *Nasturtium officinale* (Watercress) leaf extracts'.

Acta Poloniae Pharmaceutica Drug Research., 66 (2): 187-193.

Rasooli, I., Rezaei M. B., and Allameh, A. 2006. Growth inhibition and morphological alterations of *Aspergillus niger* by essential oils from *Thymus eriocalyx* and *Thymus x-porlock*. *Food Control.*, 17: 359-364.

Rowe, R. C. 1993. *Potato Health Management*. APS Press, 178pp.

Shafique, Sh. and Shafique, S. 2012. Biological Control Potential of *Parthenium hysterophorus* against *Fusarium Solani* – A Cause of Fusarium Wilt in Potato. International Conference on Applied Life Sciences, 10-12 Sep., Turkey.

Sharifi, K., Zare, S., Zamanizadeh, H., and Arjmandian, A. 2009. Fusarium species causing dry rot of potatoes in Ardabil, Tehran and Hamedan Provinces. *Journal of Plant Pests and Diseases.*, 76(2): 93-113.

Shrestha, A. K. and Tiwari, R.D. 2009. Antifungal activity of crude extracts of some medicinal plants against *Fusarium solani* (mart.) sacc. ECOPRINT 16: 75-78, Ecological Society (ECOS), Nepal.

Soheili-Moghadam, B. and Hosseinzadeh, A.M. 2013. Study of *Fusarium* Species causing dry rot of potatoes in Ardabil Province. *International journal of Agronomy and Plant Production.*, 4(6): 1226-1233.

Stevenson, W.R., Loria, R., Franc, G.D. and Weingartner, P.D. 2001. *Compendium of Potato Diseases*. second ed. APS Press, St. Paul, Minnesota, USA, pp. 23–25.

Suhr, K.I. and Nielsen, P.V. 2003. Antifungal activity of essential oils evaluated by two different application techniques against rye bread spoilage fungi. *Journal of Applied Microbiology.*, 94: 665–674.

Viana, E., Malto, J.C. and Font, G. 1996. Optimization of a Matrix Solid-Phase Dispension Method for the Analysis of Pesticide residues in Vegetables. *Journal of Chromatography.*, 754: 437-444.

Zahradníková, H. and Petříková, K. 2012. Nematocide effects of watercress (Nasturtium officinale R. BR.) Acta Universitatis Agriculturaeet Silviculturae Mendelianae Brunensis., 233-236. http://dx.doi.org/10.11118/actaun201361010233.

Effects of IAA and BAP on chemical composition and essential oil content of lemon verbena (*Lippia citriodora* H.B.K.)

Hassan Nourafcan[1], Fatemeh Sefidkon[2*], Ahmad Khalighi[1], Amir Mousavi[3], Mozaffar Sharifi[4]

[1]*Department of Horticulture, College of Agriculture, Tehran Science and Research branch, Islamic Azad University, Tehran, Iran;*

[2]*Research Institute of Forests and Rangelands, Tehran, Iran;*
***Email:** Sefidkon@rifr-ac.ir*

[3]*National Institute of Genetic Engineering and Biotechnology, Tehran, Iran;*

[4]*Department of Plant Sciences, Faculty of Biological Sciences, Tarbiat Modares University, Tehran, Iran;*

ARTICLE INFO

Topic: *Plant Physiology*

Key words:

- ✓ *Essential Oil*
- ✓ *Citral*
- ✓ *Iaa And Bap*
- ✓ *1,8 Cineole*
- ✓ *Lemon Verbena*

ABSTRACT

Background & Aim: The world production and consumption of essential oils and perfumes are increasing very fast. *Lippia citriodora* H.B.K. is an herbal species mainly used as a spice and medicinal plant. Endogenous levels as well exogenous application of plant growth regulators (PGR) could affect essential oil production and chemical compositions.
Experimental: To study the effect of exogenous application of pgr on chemical composition and volatile oil content of lemon verbena (*Lippia citriodora* H.B.K.), an experiment was conducted based on Randomized Complete Block Design (RCBD) with three replications. Experimental treatments included distillated water (positive Control), without treatment (negative Control), indole-3-acetic acid (IAA) ($2mgL^{-1}$), 6-benzyl amino purine (BAP) ($2mgL^{-1}$) and IAA + BAP ($2mgL^{-1}$). The hydro-distillated essential oil was analyzed by GC and GC/MS.
Results: More than 23 volatile components have been characterized as constituents of *L. citriodora* oil. Neral, geranial, 1,8-cineole and limonene were the major compounds of the essential oil from lemon verbena. Neral significantly increased by exogenous application of IAA + BAP ($2mgL^{-1}$), whereas 1,8-cineole significantly increased by IAA ($2mgL^{-1}$).
Recommended applications/industries: Citral (geranial + neral) is a valuable flavor and scent reagent that is used in food and perfume industries. Generally, exogenous application of IAA, IAA+BAP and distilled water can increase medicinal and nutritional values of *L. citriodora*.

1. Introduction

Medicinal plants are well-known natural sources of remedies for the treatment of various diseases since antiquity. According to a report by World Health Organization (WHO), nearly 20000 plant species are currently being used for medicinal purposes (Zare *et al.*, 2011). Lemon verbena, *Lippia citriodora* (Ort.)H.B.K. (Verbenaceae) is an herbal species mainly used as a spice and medicinal plant (Pastorelli *et al.*, 2012; Mosavi, 2012). *L. citriodora*is found at South Africa and some parts of Asia , which is planted in some area for plant essence production (Mohammadi *et al.*, 2013).

Generally, the leaves are being used for flavoring beverages, desserts, fruit salads and jellies and for seasoning food. A decoction made from the leaves and flowers is given as febrifuge, sedative and anti-flatulent. In addition, the herb has antispasmodic and antibacterial and anti-*Candida* (Rao *et al.*, 2013).

Essential oils are a diverse group of natural products that are important sources of aromatic and flavoring chemicals in food, industrial and pharmaceutical products (Charles and Simon, 1990). The essential oil production depends to genetic factors, the developmental stage of plants, environmental factors and techniques of agronomical management. Plant growth regulators (PGR) or plant hormones influence on essential oil production. Endogenous levels as well exogenous application could affect essential oil production and chemical composition. The environmental factors can influence biochemical pathways and physiological processes that alter plant metabolism such as essential oil biosynthesis. Plant Growth Regulators (PGR_S) have been defined as one of the main factors influence plants growth and their primary and secondary metabolites pool. The PGRs have been shown to improve herb yield in basil and coriander and fenugreek (Rohamare *et al.*, 2013). Researchers reported that application of growth regulators (gibberellic acid or indole acetic acid) did not increase herb and oil yields in *Mentha piperita*. Foliar application of mepiquat chloride (MC) under field conditions reduced excessive vegetative growth of plants. It decreased plant height, leaf area and main stem node number (Abbas and El-Saeid, 2012). Essential oil of chamomile was increased by foliar spray of benzyl adenine (Rada *et al.*, 2010).

Another research showed that α-bisabolol oxide A, increased in chamomile with application of 100 ppm IAA (Reda *et al.*, 2010). Growth and essential oil yield of Mentha piperita were improved by the application of polyamines (Youssef *et al.*, 2002). Silva et al., (2005) reported that auxin and cytokinin increased some components of the lemon balm oil. Povh and Ono (2007) showed that application of gibberellic acid influenced the chemical composition of Salvia oil. A report revealed that sodium salt of NAA and IAA increased the essential oil of Mentha piperita (Koseva-kovacheva and Staev, 1978).

From those bibliographic data, we are interested in studying the influence of two plant growth regulators (IAA and BAP) on the yield and chemical composition of essential oils of lemon verbena in order to provide useful information to pharmaceutical or cosmetic industries by changing these compositions.

2. Materials and Methods

2.1. Plant material

2.2. Lemon verbena, *Lippia citriodora* was field-grown at the Medicinal Plant Research Field (Miyaneh, located in East Azerbaijan province, Iran) during summer 2013. The experiment was arranged in Randomized Complete Block Design (RCBD) with three replicates. The plants were sprayed at pre-flowering stage for three times within ten days with distilled water (positive control), without treatment (negative control), indole-3-acetic acid (IAA) ($2mgL^{-1}$), 6-benzyl amino purine (BAP) ($2mgL^{-1}$) and combination of IAA ($2mgl^{-1}$) and BAP ($2mgL^{-1}$) (Sigma-Aldrich). Solutions were sprayed to the point of runoff. At flowering stage (one week after the last application), the aerial parts of *L. citriodora* were harvested. The leaves were dried naturally on laboratory benches at room temperature (23-27°C) until crisp. The dried leaves were subjected to hydro-distillation using an all glass Clevenger-type apparatus, to extract essential oils, The essential oils were separated from the aqueous layer, dried over anhydrous sodium sulfate and stored in sealed vials at low temperature (4°C) before gas chromatography (GC) and gas chromatography-mass spectrometric (GC/MS) analysis (Alavi *et al.*, 2011; Khani *et al.*, 2012; Agah and Najafian, 2012).

2.3. GC and GC/MS analysis

GC analyses were performed using a ultra-fast gas chromatograph (UFGC) (Thermo-UFM). The GC column was PH-5, 10m, 0.1mm (ID), 0.4 (FT), Oven: 60-285 °C/min, Rate: 80 °C/min, Hold time: 3 min, Run Time: 5.8min. Detector: FID, 280 °C, Injector: 280 °C, Carrier Gas: He, 0.5ml/min With Chrom-card software in Research Institute of Forests and Rangelands, Tehran.

GC-MS analyses were done on a Varian 3400 GC-MS system equipped with a DB-5 fused silica column (30 m x 0.25 mm i.d.); Oven temperature was 40°C to 250°C at a rate of 4°C, transfer line temperature 260° C, carrier gas helium with a linear velocity of 31.5 cm/s, split ratio 1/60, Ionization energy 70 eV; scan time 1s and mass range of 40-300 *amu*. The percentages of compounds were calculated by the area normalization method, without considering response factors. The components of the oil were identified by comparison of their mass spectra with those of a computer library or with authentic compounds and confirmed by comparison of their retention indices either with those of authentic compounds or with data published in the literature (Shibamoto, 1987; Adams, 1995). The retention indices were calculated for all volatile constituents using a homologous series of *n*-alkanes

2.3. Statistical analysis

The data were analyzed by using SAS ver. 9.1 statistical software. Means were compared using Duncan's Multiple Range Test (DMRT) at 5% probability level.

3. Results and Discussion

More than 23 volatile components have been characterized as constituents of *L.citriodora* oil. The identified constituents with their RIsare summarized in Table 1.

Essential oils are a diverse group of natural products that are important sources of aromatic and flavoring chemicals in food, industrial and pharmaceutical products. Essential oils are largely composed of terpenes and aromatic polypropanoid compounds derived from the acetate-mevalonic acid and the shikimic acid pathways, respectively. Essential oil composition of plants varies and is due to genetic and environmental factors that influence genetic expression (Charles and Simon, 1990). Citral is a valuable flavor and scent reagent that is used in the food and perfume industries. Previous investigations have reported that citral is synthesized from geraniol or nerol by an alcohol dehydrogenase or alcohol oxidase (Iijima *et al.*, 2006).

The quality and quantity of essential oil isolated from the leaves of *L. citriodora* that were affected by PGRs are shown in Table 3. The analysis of *L. citriodora* essential oil revealed that neral, geranial, limonene and 1,8-cineole were the main components of the oil and each of these compounds is 10 to 25%.

Table 1. Chemical composition of the essential oil from *L.citriodora* identified by GC/MS

Row	Compounds	RI
1	α-Pinene	940
2	Sabinene	976
3	β-Pinene	980
4	Limonene	1039
5	1,8-Cineole	1031
6	γ-Terpinene	1060
7	Terpinolene	1090
8	*cis*Limonene oxide	1138
9	*trans*-Pinocarveol	1141
10	*Cis*-Sabinol	1145
11	Citronellal	1155
12	α-Terpineol	1191
13	Neral	1240
14	Geranial	1269
15	α-Terpinylacetate	1352
16	Geranylacetate	1380
17	β-caryophyllene	1420
18	γ-Elemene	1438
19	α-Humulene	1456
20	Cubenol	1517
21	Spathulenol	1580
22	Globulol	1587
23	*epi*-α-Cadinol	1640

The analysis of variance indicated that all measured compounds except Transpinocarveol and Cissabinol were significantly different at 5% of probability (Table 2).

Table 2. Analysis of variance for volatile oil compositions of *Lippia citriodora* H.B.K. affected by plant growth regulators.

S.O.V.	D.F.	Mean of squares									
		α-Pinene	Sabinene	β-Pinene	Limonene	1,8-Cineole	γ-Terpinene	Terpinolene	*cis*Limonene oxide	Citronellal	α-Terpineol
Block	2	0.002^ns	0.0001^ns	**0.25	0.1 ^ns	**1.004	**0.052	**0.07	**0.035	**0.04	**0.03
Treatment	4	**0.01	*0.01	**0.9	**5.09	**1.1003	**0.044	**0.03	**0.02	**0.02	**0.232
Error	8	0.001	0.002	0.003	0.03	0.035	0.0023	0.0004	0.001	0.0006	0.001
C.V. (%)		4.98	14.05	1.2	1.125	1.26	3.91	1.76	6.2	3.72	1.96

ns: non-significant, * and ** : significant at 5% and 1% of probability levels, respectively.

Table 2 Continued

S.O.V.	D.F.	Mean of squares										
		Neral	Geranial	α-Terpinyl acetate	Geranylacetate	β-caryophyllene	γ-Elemene	α-Humulene	Cubenol	Spathulenol	Globulol	*epi*-α-Cadinol
Block	2	0.036**	0.066**	0.05**	0.064**	0.06**	0.04**	0.03**	0.063**	0.04**	0.025**	0.045**
Treatment	4	6.89**	16**	0.01**	0.01**	0.256**	1.36**	0.012**	0.05**	0.33**	1.178**	0.02**
Error	8	0.0005	0.002	0.00002	0.0002	0.001	0.0006	0.0008	0.001	0.0024	0.001	0.001
C.V. (%)		0.14	0.17	0.49	3.52	1.83	0.46	5.18	2.78	1.3	0.7	5.09

ns: non-significant, * and ** : significant at 5% and 1% of probability levels, respectively.

Furthermore, lesser amounts of the other components include α-pinene, sabinene, *trans*pinocarveol, geranyl acetate, α-humulene and *epi*-α-cadinol were existed in essential oil of the plant. According to research findings, the main components in the essential oils of *L. citriodora* leaves were geranial, neral, limonene, 1,8-cineole, spathulenol, geraniol, β-caryophyllene, nerol and sabinene. The main constituents of the essential oil extracted from fresh leaves of *L. citriodora*, were geranial, neral and limonene. Also, GC/MS analysis of essential oils revealed that 1, 8-Cineole, α-curcumene, geranial, limonene and caryophyllene oxide were the main components of essential oils of *L. citriodora* leaves, respectively (Khani *et al.*, 2012).

Table 3. Effect of foliar sprays plant growth regulators on essential oil components (%) on *Lcitriodora*

Component / Treatment	α-Pinene	Sabinene	β-Pinene	Limonene	1,8-Cineole	γ-Terpinene	Terpinolene
Control	0.55^{b}	0.36^{a}	4.83^{b}	15.23^{b}	14.09^{d}	1.08^{c}	1.23^{b}
Distilled water	0.59^{ab}	0.36^{a}	4.48^{c}	14.23^{d}	14.96^{b}	1.34^{ab}	1.13^{c}
IAA (2mgL^{-1})	0.49^{c}	0.29^{ab}	5.07^{a}	17.04^{a}	15.72^{a}	1.36^{a}	1.35^{a}
BAP (2mgL^{-1})	0.62^{a}	0.25^{b}	4.45^{c}	14.68^{c}	15.12^{b}	1.15^{c}	1.2^{b}
IAA + BAP (2mgL^{-1})	0.48^{c}	0.24^{b}	3.63^{d}	13.63^{e}	14.6^{c}	1.25^{b}	1.1^{c}

Means in each column with the same letters are not significantly different at 5% level of probability DMRT.

Table 3. Continued

Component / Treatment	*Cis*-Limonene oxide	Citronellal	α-Terpineol	Neral	Geranial	α-Terpinylacetate	Geranylacetate
Control	0.5^{bc}	0.71^{a}	1.17^{d}	15.9^{d}	23.34^{d}	0.9^{a}	0.4^{b}
Distilled water	0.52^{b}	0.61^{b}	1.11^{e}	16.95^{b}	26.75^{a}	0.79^{b}	0.3^{c}
IAA (2mgL^{-1})	0.65^{a}	0.55^{c}	1.8^{a}	13.33^{e}	20.93^{e}	0.9^{a}	0.42^{a}
BAP (2mgL^{-1})	0.45^{c}	0.7^{a}	1.25^{c}	16.4^{c}	25.99^{b}	0.8^{b}	0.32^{c}
IAA + BAP (2mgL^{-1})	0.52^{b}	0.7^{a}	1.35^{b}	17^{a}	24.74^{c}	0.8^{b}	0.43^{a}

Means in each column with the same letters are not significantly different at 5% level of probability DMRT.

Table 3. Continued

Component / Treatment	β-Caryophyllene	γ-Elemene	α-Humulene	Cubenol	Spathulenol	Globulol	*epi*-α-Cadinol
Control	1.79^{a}	5.65^{b}	0.55^{ab}	1.12^{a}	4.1^{a}	4.25^{b}	0.62^{a}
Distilled water	1.07^{e}	4.41^{e}	0.45^{c}	0.85^{c}	3.44^{c}	3.85^{d}	0.45^{b}
IAA (2mgL^{-1})	1.7^{b}	5.89^{a}	0.61^{a}	1.01^{b}	3.95^{b}	4.21^{b}	0.6^{a}
BAP (2mgL^{-1})	1.39^{d}	4.6^{d}	0.5^{bc}	0.81^{c}	3.4^{c}	4.04^{c}	0.49^{b}
IAA + BAP (2mgL^{-1})	1.64^{c}	5.57^{c}	0.59^{a}	1^{b}	4.02^{ab}	4.5^{a}	0.6^{a}

Means in each column with the same letter(s) are not significantly different at 5% level of probability using DMRT.

The antimicrobial activity of 1,8-cineole has been reported (Folashade and Omoregie, 2012). The main use of 1,8-cineoleextracted from *Eucalyptus* oils is for the pharmaceutical industry, and citronellaluses for the perfumery and piperitone and α-phellandreneare used for industrial use (Fathi and Sefidkon, 2012). According to the literature, geranial, neral and limonene were the component found to occur in higher quantities in essential oils of the *L. citriodora* (Khani*et al.*, 2012) In this study, neral, geranial, and 1,8-cineole significantly increased by exogenous application of IAA + BAP, distilled water, and by IAA, respectively. Mahmoud (1996) studied the influence of GA_3, IAA and kinetin on yield and chemical composition of essential oil of *O. basilicum*. He reported that the GA leads to the decrease in essential oil yield, while kinetin and IAA increased the yield oil. This change is accompanied by a decrease in levels of the main compound (methyl chavicol) for all treatments. This variation in yield directly to the number of glandular hairs: GA leads to a decrease in the number of these structures, whereas treatment with BAP increases the number of glands in the leaves in several species (*Lavanduladentata, Thymus mastichina* and *Piceaabies*) (Prins *et al.*, 2010). IAA leads to an increase in neither yield of *O. gratissimum* L. essential oils which passes from 0.22% to 0.3%, with no significant change neither in the content nor the main compounds composition of essential oils. These results are the same as those found in the literature (Hazzoumi *et al.*, 2014).

Unexpectedly, in essence performance, were not significantly different between treatments. The reports of Hazzoumi *et al.* (2014) showed that the regarding various medicinal plants as influenced by different plant growth regulators. They stated that application of IAA increases slightly the yield of *O. basilicum* oil; this variation goes with small change in methyl chavicol. The same observation was made on lemon balm (*Melissa officinalis* L.) and thyme (*Thymus vulgaris* L.) (Shukla and Farooqi, 1990; Affonso *et al.*, 2009). Some scientists reported that monoterpenes *O. baslicum* and *Lavendula dentata* are highly influenced by plant growth substance treatments due to the genes regulation, which cause an increase in enzyme numbers related to the metabolic pathways of these compounds They suggested that cytokinins stimulate the metabolism and accumulation of essential oils, specifically monoterpenes in *M .piperita*, and *Salvia officinalis* L. (Kim *et al.*, 2006; Li *et al.*, 2007; Hazzoumi*et al.*, 2014). The application of growth regulators may affect essential oils due to their effects on enzymatic pathways of terpenoid biosynthesis (Amiri*et al.*, 2014).

It is well known that essential oil is derived from mevalonic acid via the isoprene pathway in a manner similar to that for other terpenes. Thus, PGRs that exert their effect at the level of gibberellins metabolism, might increase the accumulation of essential oil in plants. Growth retardants such as phosphone-D and chlormequat chloride (CCC) which influence gibberellins metabolism have been shown to increase terpene formation resulting in increased essential oil content of peppermint and sage (Abbas and El-Saeid, 2012).

4. Conclusion

Essential oils synthesis is basically controlled by genetically processes but their synthesis is strongly affected by environmental parameters. Lemon balm growth and essential oil production were stimulated with exogenously applied plant growth regulators.

5. References

Abbas, S.M. and El-Saeid, H.M. 2012. Effects of some growth regulators on oil yield, growth and hormonal content of lemon grass (*Cymbopogon citrates*). *BotanicaSerbica.*, 36 (2): 97-101.

Adams, R.P. 1995. *Identification of essential oil components by gas chromatography/mass spectroscopy*, Carol Stream, IL: Allured Publishing Co. Pp.230.

Affonso, V.R., Bizzo, H.R., Lage, C.L.S. and Sato, A. 2009. Influence of growth regulators in biomass production and volatile profile of *in vitro* Plantlets of *Thymus vulgaris* L. Journal of Agriculture and Food Chemistry. 57: 6392–6395.

Agah, M. and Najafian, S. 2012.Essential oil content and composition of *Lippia citriodora* as affected by drying method before flowering stages. *European Journal of Experimental Biology.*, 2 (5):1771-1777.

Alavi, L., Barzegar, M., Jabbari, A. and Naghdibadi, H. 2011.The effect of heat treatment on chemical composition and antioxidant property of *Lippia citriodora* essential oil. *Journal of Medicinal Plants.*, 10(39): 65-75.

Amiri, S. Sharafzadeh, S. and Ordookhani, K. 2014. The effect of gibberellic acid and benzyl adenine on growth and essential oils of German chamomile. *Indian Journal of Fundamental and Applied Life Sciences.*, 4(1):186-188.

Charles, D.J. and Simon, J.E. 1990. Comparison of extraction methods for the rapid determination of essential oil content and composition of Basil. *Journal of American Society Horticultural Sciences.*, 115(3): 458-462.

Fathi, E. and Sefidkon, F. 2012. Influence of drying and extraction methods on yield and chemical composition of the essential oil of *Eucalyptus sargentii. Journal of Agriculture and Sciences Technology.,* 14: 1035-1042.

Folashade, K.O. and Omoregie, E.H. 2012. Essential oil of *Lippiamultiflora*Moldenke: A review.*Journal of Applied Pharmaceutical Science*., 2 (1): 15-23.

Hazzoumi, Z., Moustakime, Y. and Joutei, K.A. 2014. Effect of gibberellic acid (GA_3), indole acetic acid (IAA) and benzylaminopurine (BAP) on the synthesis of essential oils and the isomerization of methyl chavicol and *trans*-anethole in *Ocimum gratissimum* L. *Springer Plus*., 3(321): 1-7.

Iijima, Y., Wang, G., Fridman, E. and Pichersky, E. 2006.Analysis of the enzymatic formation of citral in the glands of sweet basil. *Archives of Biochemistry and Biophysics*., 448: 141–149.

Khani, A., Basavand, F. and Rakhshani, E. 2012.Chemical composition and insecticide activity of lemon verbena essential oil. *Journal of Crop Protection.,*1(4): 313-320.

Kim, H.J., Chen, F., Chen, F. and Rajapakse, N.C. 2006. Effect of methyl jasmonate on secondary metabolites of sweet basil (*Ocimum basilicum* L.). Journal of Agriculture and Food Chemistry. 54: 2327–2332.

Li, Z., Wang, X., Chen, F. and Kim, H.J. 2007. Chemical changes and over expressed genes in sweet basil (*Ocimum basilicum* L.) upon methyl jasmonate treatment. Journal of Agriculture and Food Chemistry. 55: 706–713.

Mahmoud, S.E.D. 1996. Response of growth and essential oil content of sweet basil (*Ocimum basilicum* L.) to some natural hormones. International Symposium on Medicinal and Aromatic Plants. ISHS Acta Horticulturae 426.

Mohammadi, M. Tobeh, A., Fakhari, R., Naghdi, H. and Ochi, M. 2013. The quantitative yield of lemon verbena (*Lippia citriodora*) as influenced by different biological Fertilizers.*International Journal of Agronomy and Plant Production*., 4(9): 2126-2129.

Mosavi, A.A. 2012. The optimization of lemon verbena (*Lippia citriodora*) medicinal plant tissue culture. *International Journal of Agronomy and Plant Production*., 3(11): 561-565.

Pastorelli, G. Rossi, R. and Corino, C. 2012. Influence of *Lippia citriodora* verbascoside on growth performance, antioxidant status, and serum immunoglobulins content in piglets. *Czech Journal of Animal Sciences*, 57(7): 312–322.

Prins, C.L., Vieira, I.J.C. and Freitas, B.S.P. 2010. Growth regulators and essential oil production. Journal Plant Physiology. 22: 91–102.

Rada, F., Abd El-Wahed, M.S.A. and Gamal El Din, K.M. 2010.Effect of Indole acetic acid, gibberellic acid and kinetin on vegetative growth, flowering, essential oil pattern on a Chamomile plant (*Chamomile recutita* L. Rausch). *World Journal of Agricultural Sciences*, 6(5): 595-600.

Rao, G.V., Gopalakrishnan, M. and Mukhopadhyay, T. 2013. Secondary metabolites from the leaves of *Lippia citriodora* H.B.K. *Der Pharmacia Lettre*. 5(3): 492-495.

Rohamare, Y., Nikam, T.D. and Dhumal, K.N. 2013.Effect of foliar application of plant growth regulators on growth, yield and essential oil components of Ajwain (*Trachyspermumammi* L.). *International Journal of Seed Spices*., 3(2): 34-41.

Shibamoto, T. 1987. *Retention indices in essential oil analysis.* (eds) Sandra P, Bicchi, C. HuethigVerlag, New York, 259-274.

Shukla, A. and Farooqi, A.H.A. 1990. Utilization of plant growth regulators in aromatic plant production. Current Research Medicinal and Aromatic Plants.12: 152–157.

Zare, Z., Majd, A., NejadSattari, T., Iranbakhsh, A. and Mehrabian, S. 2011. The comparative study of an antimicrobial activity of leaves and flowers methanolic extracts of *Lippia citriodora* H.B.K. (Verbenaceae). *American-Eurasian Journal of Agriculture and Environmental Science*, 10(5): 901-905.

Reda, F., Abd El Wahed, M.S.A. and Gamal El Din, K.M. 2010. Effect of indole acetic acid, gibberellic acid and kinetin on vegetative growth, flowering and essential oil pattern of chamomile plant. World Journal of Agricultural Sciences, 6:595-600.

Youssef, A.A., Aly, M.S., Abou Zied, E.N., Iliey, L. and Titiana, S. 2002. Effect of some growth substances on mass production and volatile oil yield of Mentha piperita. Egyptian Journal of Applied Sciences, 17:610-623.

Povh, J.A. and Ono, E.O. 2007. Efeito do acido giberelico na composicao do oleo essencial de Salvia officinalis L. Public UEPG Biological and Health Sciences, 13:7-10.

Essential oil composition of Pennyroyal (*Mentha pulegium* L.) from Southern Iran

Ali Khalilipour, Mahmood Dejam*

Department of Agriculture, Fasa Branch, Islamic Azad University, Fasa, Iran;

***Email:** mahmooddejam@yahoo.com

ARTICLE INFO

Topic: *Phyochemistry*

Key words:

- Mentha pulegium
- *Volatile constituents*
- *Pulegone*
- *GC-MS*

ABSTRACT

Background & Aim: Essential oil of pennyroyal (*Mentha pulegium* L.) has many applications in food, perfume and pharmaceutical industries. The aim of this study was to determine the content and chemical constituents of pennyroyal essential oil growing wild in Southern Iran.
Experimental: The aerial parts of the plant were collected around Hajiabad, Hormozgan province in 2013. The essential oil of dried aerial parts was extracted by hydro-distillation and analyzed using GC-MS.
Results: The oil yield of pennyroyal aerial parts was 0.6% (v/w). In total, 55 compounds were identified in the essential oil that oxygenated monoterpenes were dominant. The major oil constituents were pulegone (46.18%), piperitenone (19.56%), 1,8-cineole (4.55 %), and piperitenone oxide (4.23%).
Recommended applications/industries: *Mentha pulegium* is a good raw source of pulegone that has been widely used in food and drug industries.

1. Introduction

Mentha species belonging to the Lamiaceae family constitute one of the most popular essential oil crops (Lawrence, 2007). These species show considerable chemical diversity in the essential oil composition. Their essential oils contain a complex mixture of monoterpenoids that are extensively used in pharmaceutical, food, flavor, beverages and allied industries (Zargari, 1996; Lawrence, 2007). Pennyroyal (*Mentha pulegium* L.) is one of the *Mentha* species that grows wildly in humid and damp areas and water banks of south Europe, north Africa and near east countries (Zargari, 1996). *Mentha pulegium* is used as antispasmodic, carminative, diaphoretic, sedative, stimulant, diuretic, antiseptic bronchitis and menstruate and externally for skin diseases in traditional medicine (Zargari, 1996; Akhondzadeh, 2002). Moreover, it has been used as an insect repellent (Mkaddem *et al.*, 2007), spice and flavoring agent and fragrance in cosmetics (Akhondzadeh, 2002). The aerial parts of this plant contain a wide diversity of secondary metabolites such as tannins, resins, pectins, bitter principles and essential oils (Zargari, 1996; Lawrence, 2007). The essential oil of pennyroyal exhibits several biological properties particularly antibacterial (Mahboubi & Haghi, 2008; Derwich *et al.*, 2010; Boukhebti *et al.*, 2011), antifungal (Morteza-Semnani *et al.*, 2011), antioxidant (El-Ghorab, 2006; Teixeria *et al.*, 2012) and insecticidal (Zekri *et al.*, 2013) activities. The chemical composition of *M. pulegium* essential oil has been the subject of many studies (Chalchat *et al.*, 2000; Lorenzo *et al.*, 2002; Aghel *et al.*, 2004; Kokkini *et al.*, 2004; Agnihotri *et al.*, 2005; Stoyanova *et al.*, 2005; Mkaddem *et al.*, 2007; Hassanpouraghdam *et al.*, 2011; Shahmohamadi *et al.*, 2011; Hasniye *et al*,. 2012; Rodrigues *et al.*, 2013; Sardashti & Adhami, 2013) and three chemotypes have been established, pulegune-type, piperitenone/piperitone-type and isomenthone/neoisomenthol-type (Kokkini *et al.*, 2004). Despite various reports from different regions of the world and some studies in north, west and east of Iran, there is no previous report on essential oil composition of *M. pulegium* from southern parts of Iran. Therefore, the aim of present study was chemical analysis of volatile constituents of *M. pulegium* from south of Iran.

2. Materials and Methods

2.1. Plant materials and essential oil extraction

Flowering aerial parts of *M. pulegium* L. were harvested from wild plants growing in a date palm orchard around Hajiabad (Hormozgan province, Iran) with latitude of 28° 19′ N and longitude of 55° 54′ E and 920 m above sea level in spring of 2013. After identification, a voucher specimen (IAUF-92-4) was deposited in the herbarium of Agriculture College of Islamic Azad University, Fasa Branch, Iran. The aerial parts were dried in shade and powdered using a grinder. The volatile oils were isolated by water distillation using a Clevenger type apparatus. Distillation was continued for about 2 h and then the oils were separated from aqueous layer and dried over anhydrous sodium sulfate. This procedure was repeated several times. Finally, the yield of extracted oil was expressed as v/w% of dry weight.

2.2. Essential oil analysis

The composition of essential oil was analyzed by GC and GC/MS. GC analysis was done on an HP7890 A series gas chromatograph (Agilent Technologies) equipped with Flame Ionization Detector (FID) and with a HP-5 silica capillary column (30 m × 0.25 mm ID, film thickness of 0.25 μm). The oven temperature was held at 60 °C for 5 min and then programmed from 60 to 210 °C at a rate of 3 °C /min and from 210 °C to 240 °C at 20 °C /min and held for 8.5 min. The carrier gas was helium at a flow rate of 1 ml/min. Injector and detector temperatures were 280 °C. GC/MS was performed by a HP5975A system (Agilent Technologies). An HP-5 MS capillary column (30 m × 0.25 mm ID, film thickness 0.25 μm) was directly coupled to mass spectrometer. The carrier gas was helium with a flow rate of 1 ml/min. The oven

Table 1. Chemical composition of the essential oil of *Mentha pulegium* L. from southern Iran.

No	Compounds [a]	RI [b]	%
1	Tricyclene	921	0.009
2	α-Thujene	924	0.058
3	α-Pinene	931	1.317
4	Camphene	946	0.365
5	Sabinene	970	0.664
6	β-Pinene	974	1.685
7	Myrcene	988	0.482
8	3-Octanol	992	0.551
9	α-Phellandrene	1003	0.058
10	δ-3-Carene	1009	0.027
11	α-Terpinene	1014	0.122
12	*p*-Cymene	1022	0.328
13	Limonene	1026	2.294
14	1,8-Cineole	1029	**4.552**
15	(Z)-β-Ocimene	1034	0.097
16	€-β-Ocimene	1044	0.031
17	γ-Terpinene	1055	0.405
18	*cis*-Sabinene hydrate	1064	0.062
19	Terpinolene	1086	0.098
20	Linalool	1098	0.173
21	1-Octen-3-yl acetate	1109	0.057
22	3-Octanol acetate	1121	0.183
23	*trans*-Pinocarveol	1136	0.209
24	Camphor	1141	0.108
25	Menthone	1150	0.319
26	*iso*-Menthone	1161	0.848
27	Borneol	1163	0.953
28	α-Terpineol	1189	0.155
29	Myrtenal	1193	0.129
30	Pulegone	1237	**46.178**
31	Piperitone	1252	0.458
32	Bornyl acetate	1283	0.272
33	Thymol	1295	0.184
34	Carvacrol	1303	2.139
35	Piperitenone	1342	**19.558**
36	Piperitenone oxide	1365	**4.230**
37	α-Copaene	1372	0.043
38	β-Bourbonene	1381	0.149
39	4a-α,7-β,7a-α-Nepeta lactone	1397	0.313
40	β-Caryophyllene	1416	2.325
41	α-Humulene	1449	0.353
42	(E)-β-Farnesene	1453	0.213
43	Germacrene D	1476	0.302
44	(E)-β-Ionone	1482	0.041
45	Phenyl ethyl 3-methyl butanoate	1488	0.042
46	Bicyclogermacrene	1492	0.17
47	γ-Cadinene	1509	0.033
48	δ-Cadinene	1519	0.067
49	(E)-γ-Bisabolene	1539	0.043
50	(E)-Nerolidol	1560	0.042
51	Spathulenol	1573	0.451
52	Caryophyllene oxide	1579	2.457
53	Salvial-4(14)-en-1-one	1589	0.037
54	Humulene epoxide II	1604	0.2
55	Dill apiol	1620	0.129

temperature program was the same as GC conditions. The samples were injected manually with a split ratio of 1:50. For GC/MS detection, an electron ionization system with ionization energy of 70 eV and mass range of 50-480 m/z was used.

2.3. Identification and quantification of components

Chemstation software was used for handling of mass spectra and chromatograms. Retention indices were calculated by using retention times of *n*-alkanes (C_9-C_{18}) which were injected at the same chromatographic conditions. The identification of compounds was made by comparison of their mass spectra and relative retention indices either with those given in the literature or with authentic samples (Adams, 2007). For quantification, the relative area percentage obtained for each constituent from GC-FID analysis of the oil was used to calculate the mean values without using correction factors.

3. Results and discussion

In this investigation, the essential oil yield of pennyroyal aerial parts was 0.6 % (v/w) based on dry weight. The essential oil yield in this study is similar to that obtained by Aghel et al. (2004), although higher (Lorenzo *et al.*, 2002; Boukhebti *et al.*, 2011; Hassanpouraghdam *et al.*, 2011; Hasniye *et al.*, 2012; Zeki *et al.*, 2013) and lower (Chalchat *et al.*, 2000; Mahboubi & Haghi, 2008) oil yields have also been reported for wild *M. pulegium*. These differences in oil yield of *M. pulegium* may be due to different geographical origins, climates, growth stages and/or extraction procedures.

Table 2. Main classes and subclasses of *Mentha pulegium* L. volatile oil components from southern Iran

Class and subclass of compound	%
Monoterpenes	88.88
monoterpene hydrocarbons	8.10
oxygenated monoterpenes	80.78
Sesquiterpenes	7.06
sesquiterpene hydrocarbons	3.70
oxygenated sesquiterpenes	3.36
Others	0.83
Total identified	96.77

GC-MS analyses of hydro-distillated essential oil of *M. pulegium* allowed the identification of 55 compounds representing 96.77% of the total oil (Table 1).

The chromatographic analysis of extracted volatile oil of this plant showed a complex mixture consisting mainly of monoterpenes. It was dominated by oxygenated monoterpenes (80.78%), while sesquiterpenes were only present in small percentage (Table 2). The major compounds of pennyroyal essential oil in this study were pulegone (46.18%), piperitenone (19.56%), 1,8-cineole (4.55 %), piperitenone oxide (4.23%), caryophyllene oxide (2.45%), β-caryophyllene (2.33%), limonene (2.29%), carvacrol (2.14%), β-pinene (1.69%) and α-pinene (1.32 %) (Table 1). The most similar composition to the results of present investigation is the report of Stoyanova et al. (2005) from Bulgaria that pulegone (42.9% - 45.4%) and piperitenone (21.7% - 23.1%) were major oil constituents of *M. pulegium*. In addition, similar to the results of this study, pulegone (> 40%) has been the main component of pennyroyal essential oil from Iran (Morteza-Semnani *et al.*, 2011; Shahmohamadi *et al.*, 2011; Sardashti & Adhami, 2013) and other countries (Lorenzo *et al.*, 2002; Agnihotri *et al.*, 2005; El-Ghorab, 2006; Mkaddem *et al.*, 2007; Rodrigues *et al.*, 2013; Zekri *et al.*, 2013), although there are great variation in other oil constituents of *M. pulegium* among these reports. While it has been reported that menthone (15.1% - 38.7%) is one of the major oil components of Iranian *M. pulegium* (Aghel *et al.*, 2004; Hassanpouraghdam *et al.*, 2011; Morteza-Semnani *et al.*, 2011; Shahmohamadi *et al.*, 2011), the amount of this compound was very low (0.32%) in present study. In total, great quantitative and qualitative variations in volatile composition of *M. pulegium* were seen between this and other studies. These variations may be due to the influence of geographical differences, environmental conditions, physiological differences, different extraction and analytical procedures and genetic factors (Kokkini *et al.*, 2004: Hassanpouraghdam *et al.*, 2011). Moreover, since major oil constituents such as pulegone, menthone, isomenthone, piperitone and piperitenone have a common biosynthetic pathway (Davis *et al.*, 2005); therefore, the existence of different chemotypes is a common feature in *Mentha* species and hybrids.

4. Conclusion

The major constituents of *M. pulegium* essential oil from southern Iran were pulegone (46.18 %) and piperitenone (19.56 %). The oil composition in this study was different with most of previous reports. These variations reflect the influence of different geographical origins, climatic conditions, physiological and biochemical states of plants and many other factors.

5. References

Adams, R.P. 2007. *Identification of essential oil components by gas chromatography/mass spectrometry*. 4th ed. Allured Publ., Carol Stream, IL.

Aghel, N., Yamini, Y., Hajiakhoondi, A. and Pourmortazavi, S.M. 2004. Supercritical carbon dioxide extraction of *Mentha pulegium* L. essential oil. *Talanta*., 62: 407-411.

Agnihotri, V.K., Agarwal, S.G., Dhar, P.L., Thappa, R.K., Kapahi, B., Saxena, R.K. and Qazi, G.N. 2005. Essential oil composition of *Mentha pulegium* L. growing wild in the north-western Himalayas, India. *Flavour and Fragrance Journal*., 20: 607-610.

Akhondzadeh, S. 2002. *Encyclopedia of Iranian Medicinal Plants*. Arjmand Publication, Tehran, Iran. (In Persian)

Boukhebti, H., Chaker, A.N., Belhadj, H., Sahli, F., Ramdhani, M., Laouer, H. and Harzallah, D. 2011. Chemical composition and antibacterial activity of *Mentha pulegium* L. and *Mentha spicata* L. essential oils. *Der Pharmacia Letters*., 3: 267-275.

Chalchat, J., Gorunovic, M.S., Maksimovic, Z.A. and Petrovic, S.D. 2000. Essential oil of wild growing *Mentha pulegium* L. from Yugoslavia. *Journal of Essential Oil Research*., 12: 598-600.

Davis, E.M., Ringer, K.L., Mc Conkey, M.E. and Croteau, R. 2005. Monoterpene metabolism: Cloning, expression and characterization of menthone reductase from peppermint. *Plant Physiology*., 37: 873-881.

Derwich, E., Benziane, Z. and Boukir, A. 2010. GC/MS analysis and antibacterial activity of the essential oil of *Mentha pulegium*, *Journal of Agriculture and Biological Sciences*., 6: 191-198.

El-Ghorab, A.H. 2006. The chemical composition of *Mentha pulegium* L. essential oil from Egypt and its antioxidant activity. *Journal of Essential Oil Bearing Plants*., 9: 183-195.

Hasniye, Y., Onar, H.C. and Yusufoglu, A.S. 2012. Chemical composition of the essential oil of *Mentha pulegium* L. from Bodrum, Turkey. *Journal of Essential Oil Bearing Plants*., 15: 1040-1043.

Hassanpouraghdam, M.B., Akhgari, A.B., Aazami, M.A. and Emarat-Pardaz, J. 2011. New menthone type of *Mentha pulegium* L. volatile oil from Northwest Iran. *Czech Journal of Food Sciences*., 29: 285-290.

Kokkini, S., Hanlidou, E., Karousou, R. and Lanaras, T. 2004. Clinal variation of *Mentha pulegium* essential oils along the climatic gradient of Greece. *Journal of Essential Oil Research*, 16: 588-593.

Lawrence, B.M. 2007. *Mints: The Genus* Mentha, CRC Press, Boca Raton, Fl., 170 pp.

Lorenzo, D., Paz, D., Dellacassa, E., Davies, P., Vila, R. and Calgueral, S. 2002. Essential oil of *Mentha pulegium* and *Mentha rotundifolia* from Uruguay. *Brazillian Archives of Biology and Technology*., 45: 519-524.

Mahboubi, M. and Haghi, G. 2008. Antimicrobial activity and chemical composition of *Mentha pulegium* L. essential oil. *Journal of Ethnopharmacology*., 119: 325-327.

Mkaddem, M., Boussaid, M. and Ben Fadhel, N. 2007. Variability of volatiles in Tunisian *Mentha pulegium* L. (Lamiaceae). *Journal of Essential Oil Research*., 19: 211-214.

Morteza-Semnani, K., Saeedi, M. and Akbarzadeh, M. 2011. Chemical composition and antimicrobial activity of essential oil of *Mentha pulegium* L. *Journal of Essential Oil Bearing Plants*., 14: 208-213.

Rodrigues, L., Povoa, O., Teixeira, G., Figueiredo, A.C., Moldao, M. and Monteiro, A. 2013. Trichomes micromorphology and essential oil variation at different developmental stages of cultivated and wild growing *Mentha pulegium* L. populations from Portugal. *Industrial Crops and Products*., 43: 692-700.

Sardashti, A. and Adhami, Y. 2013. Chemical composition of the essential oil of *Mentha pulegium* L. from Taftan area by means of gas chromatography/mass spectrometry (GC/MS). *Journal of Medicinal Plant Research*., 7: 3003-3007.

Shahmohamadi, R., Sariri, R., Rasa, M., Ghafoori, H., Aghamol, M., Nasuti, S. and Tahery, M. 2011. Chemical composition and antimicrobial activity of flowering aerial parts of *Mentha pulegium* from Gilan. *Pharmacology Online*., 3: 651-659.

Stoyanova, A., Georgiev, E., Kula, J. and Majda, T. 2005. Chemical composition of the essential oil of *Mentha pulegium* L. from Bulgaria. *Journal of Essential Oil Research*., 17: 475-476.

Teixeria, B., Marques, A., Ramos, C., Batista, I., Serrano, C., Matos, O., Neng, N.R., Nogueira, J.M.F., Saraiva, J.A. and Nunes, M.L. 2012. European pennyroyal (*Mentha pulegium*) from Portugal: chemical composition of essential oil and antioxidant and antimicrobial properties of extracts and essential oil. *Industrial Crops and Products*., 36: 81-87.

Zargari, A. 1996. *Medicinal Plants*, Tehran University Publication, Iran. (In Persian)

Zekri, N., Amalich, S., Boughdad, A., El Belghiti, M.A. and Zair, T. 2013. Phytochemical study and insecticidal activity of *Mentha pulegium* L. oils from Morocco against *Sitophilus oryzae*. *Mediterranean Journal of Chemistry*., 2: 607-619.

7

Folk Herbal Veterinary Medicines of Zilberchay Watershed of East Azerbaijan (Iran)

Ardavan Ghorbani*, Farzad Mirzaei Aghjeh Qeshlagh, Roghayyeh Valizadeh Yonjalli

University of Mohaghegh Ardabili, Ardabil, Iran;

***Email:** a_ghorbani@uma.ac.ir

ARTICLE INFO

Topic: *Medicinal Plants*

Key words:

- ✓ *Ethnoveterinary*
- ✓ *Herbal Veterinary Medicines*
- ✓ *livestock*
- ✓ *ZilberChay*
- ✓ *East Azerbaijan*

ABSTRACT

Background & Aim: Ethnoveterinary medicinal plants of Iran are not scientifically well known, but they have been using traditionally especially in rural areas. This study was carried out to identify the Folk Herbal Veterinary Medicines (FHVM) of ZilberChay watershed in east Azerbaijan province in northwest of Iran.

Experimental: FHVM plants were identified by collecting plant species from the study area and comparing them with previous studies to identify the plant with FHVM value. Overall, 493 plant species that were belong to 243 genera and 59 families were collected. From those, 42 species belong to 37 genera and 23 families were identified as FHVM.

Results: These plants can be used for treatment of different disease and syndromes in livestock, such as internal parasites, mastitis, burns, skin disease, gastrointestinal tract problems, diarrhea, etc. Results showed that most of the FHVM belong to the families including: Fabaceae (14.29%), Asteraceae (14.29%), Apiaceae (7.14%), Poaceae (7.14%), Rosaceae (7.14%), Cupressaceae (4.76%), Lamiaceae(4.76%) and Moraceae (4.76%). Moreover, results showed that chrotypes of identified FHVM belong to IT (Irano-Toranian) with 49.1%, Plur (Plural) with 27.27%, ES (Euro-Siberian) with 18.18 % and M (Mediterranean) regions with 5.45%, respectively. Furthermore, identified FHVM belong to life forms of He (Hemicryptophytes) with 55%; Ph (Phanerophytes) with 26.19%; Th (Therophytes) with 14.28% and Ch (Chamaephytes) with 4.76%, respectively.

Recommended applications/industries: Identifying FHVM of ZilberChay and their application in treating domestic animals can give us opportunity to increase our knowledge about FHVM and attempt to conserve the area and its plant species.

1. Introduction

Studying of Folk Herbal Veterinary Medicines (FHVM) and traditional methods for health, hygiene and treatment of animal diseases is called Ethnoveterinary (Bahmani *et al.,* 2011). History of the ethnoveterinary refers to the time that humans domesticated the animals. Information of this knowledge, like others is achieved with trial and error (Bahmani *et al.,* 2011). Even in developed countries, veterinary care and animal welfare in rural populations is based on ethnomedical veterinary practices, particularly when access to chemical drugs is difficult or too expensive for the local farmer (Nyamanga *et al.,* 2008). Traditional veterinary knowledge is comprised by a collection of beliefs and practices regarding animal welfare that involves the use of natural resources (plants and animals) and other materials. This knowledge is generally transmitted orally from generation to generation and, as other traditional beliefs, is currently threatened by technological development, sociocultural and environmental changes (McCorkle *et al.,* 1998; Tabuti, 2003). However, within the industrialized and urban society there is an increasing interest in alternative or complementary medicine which, together with other natural therapies, is based on the use of FHVM. Thus, the use of homeopathic and phytotherapeutic remedies in veterinary medicine has gained interest, among other reasons, due to increasing demands on the quality of meat and milk products such as the requirements for producing organic food goods, (Pieroni *et al.*, 2004). FHVM often provides cheaper options than comparable western drugs, and the products are locally available and more easily accessible too (Selvaraju *et al.*, 2011). Based on the facts, there is an interest to identify and increase the application of FHVM in different countries and researchers are identifying and introducing different species of these plants. Some FHVM have been introduced in the studies such as Masika *et al.* (2000); Takar (2004); Fajimi and Taiwo (2005); Ishtiaq *et al.* (2006); Lans *et al.* (2006); Guarrera and Lucia (2007); Lans *et al.* (2007); Pande *et al.* (2007); Lulekal et al. (2008); Davidović *et al.* (2011); Khan (2009); Martínez and Luján (2011); Selvaraju *et al.* (2011); Bahmani *et al.* (2012); Chakraborty and KantiPal (2012); Ul Islam *et al.* (2012); Manoj *et al.* (2012); Laudato and Capasso (2013); Adnan *et al.* (2014); Panda and Dhal (2014); Rajkumari *et al.* (2014); Verma (2014). Iran's flora consists of more than 7500 plant species that most of them are classifying as medical plants (Omid Beigi 1993; 1997). Based on these variations in climate condition and plant flora, application of herbal plants were common in Iran for years and nowadays, these plants are applying for different aims according to the culture and faith of people in each area. Based on above, Iranian researchers in their studies have been introduced FHVM of different regions but number of these studies is not adequate to introduce all of them. For example, Bahmani *et al.* (2010) studied medical plants in treating disease and syndromes in small ruminants in southern areas of Ilam province, west of Iran. They have studied 35 disease and syndrome in small ruminants and 35 FHVM of these areas. This study found that 24 disease and syndrome were treating with identified medicinal plants and 13 disease and syndrome were found without herbal treating. Moreover, they introduced some plants with new remedy effects. Plants such as *Phoenix dactylifera: poisones*; *Triticum* aestivum: mastitis; *Peganum harmala:* Snake bite; *Astragulus golicucanthus, Nerium indicum, Amygdalus lycioides* and *Marsdenia erecta for* respiratory signs of *Oestrus ovis* larva and their ethnoveterinary effects were introduced for the first time. Malek Mohammadi and Mirzavash Azar (2010) have identified medical utilization and domestication of some wild edible plants in west Azerbaijan. Kouhpayeh *et al.* (2011) studied the FHVM in Kerman province in south of Iran. They have stated that 42 plants as FHVM value in this region. Toupchi (2011) have identified FHVM in Arshad Chamani rangelands of East Azerbaijan. Bahmani *et al.* (2012) introduced FHVM used by Kurdish owners of Ilam province. Based on their findings, 46 different plant species were identified as beneficial plants in curing 36 animal diseases and syndromes in this area. Chalechale *et al.* (2013) studied the anthropology and antiparasitic remedies in Kurdish Ethno (veterinary) medicines. They introduced plant species like *Andropogon nardus, Artemisia absinthium*, *Cucurbita verrucosa, Cinchona officinalis, Gossypium herbaceum, Marrubium vulgar* and *Hippophae rhamnoidesas* herbal medicine in Kurdistan province of Iran. However it seems, there is little attempt on the FHVM studies in northwest of Iran, especially in east Azerbaijan and ZilberChay flora. Thus, this study aimed to identify the FHVM of ZilberChay watershed in the east Azerbaijan of Iran to conserve and revive this treasure and apply them as replacement for veterinary chemical drugs.

2. Materials and Methods

2.1. Study area

ZilberChay watershed with 261437 ha is located in 45°·04′,44′′ to 55°,33′,55′′ E and latitude of 38°,18′,09′′ to 37°, 40′,57′′ N in East Azerbaijan, Iran. Elevation of this area varies between 937 to 3207m. Average precipitation in northern and southern slopes varies from 123 to 787 mm. In ZilberChay watershed July is the hottest month of year with the average temperature of 24°C and coldest month is December with the average temperature of -4°C. Due to this climate variation verity of plant species are growing in this area (Ghorbani *et al.*, 2013).

2.2. Data collection and Identification

Plants were collected by considering the affective ecological factors in plants distribution such as elevation, slope, aspect, temperature, precipitation, soil, etc. Mainly, two west-east elevation profiles from low elevation to the highest and 6 north-south profile were applied for collecting plants. Information of each plant (date of collection, number, ecological condition and elevation, etc) was recorded. Samples were transferred to the lab and all collected species were identified using reference flora, such as: Flora Iranica (Rechinger, 1963-1998), Iraq (Townsend and Guest, 1966-1985), Palestine (Zohary, 1966-1972), Turkey (Davis, 1965-1988), East (Boissier, 1867-1888), Soviet union (Komarov, 1934-1954), Iran (Assadi *et al.*, 1988-2013), Colored flora of Iran (Ghahreman, 1979-1992), Iranian *Astragalus* (Maassoumi, 1986-2005), Cromophites of Iran (Ghahreman, 1996), plants of Iran (Mobayen, 1975-1996). Scientific names of species were assigned using International Plant Name Index (IPNI, 2013). For determining life forms, Raunchier (1934)'s classification method was applied. Published article and references, such as Takhtajan (1986), Ghorbani *et al.* (2013), Sokhanvar *et al.* (2013), etc. were used for determining chorology of the identified FHVM species.

3. Results & Discussion

In this study, for identifying FHVM species at ZilberChay watershed, initially 493 plant species that were belong to 243 genera and 59 families were collected. Although there is high disturbance on the watershed, this area is rich from flora of FHVM species perspective. However, because of the lack of references in identifying FHVM species we were unable to record all ethnoveterinary species. Identified FHVM species are presented in Table 1. As can be seen from Table, 42 FHVM species were identified, which were belonging to 23 plant families and 37 genera.

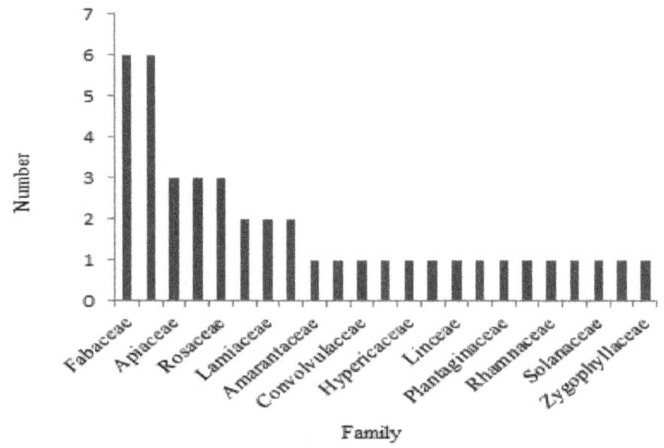

Fig 1. Number of ethnoveterinary medical species families in ZilberChay watershed.

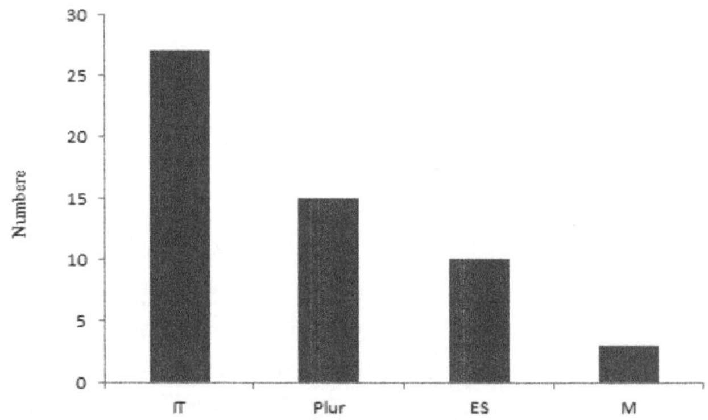

Fig 2. Comparison of chrotypes among ethnoveterinary medical species in ZilberChay watershed.

Main FHVM families are presented in Fig. 1. According to this Figure, the most common FHVM species belonged to the families of Fabaceae, Asteraceae, Apiaceae, Poaceaeand Rosaceae, respectively. These species were used for treating different disease and syndromes like endoparasites, mastitis, burns, bloat, Gastro Intestinal diseases, swelling, skin infection, digestive problem, wounds, Ectoparasites, diarrhea, and some other disease and syndromes in livestock. Identified FHVM species can be used as powder, past, decoction or even mixture of two or more. Moreover, different parts of species such as leaves, flower, roots, bark, fruits, seeds, mucilage, aerial part, bulb and whole plant can be used in the cure of each disease.

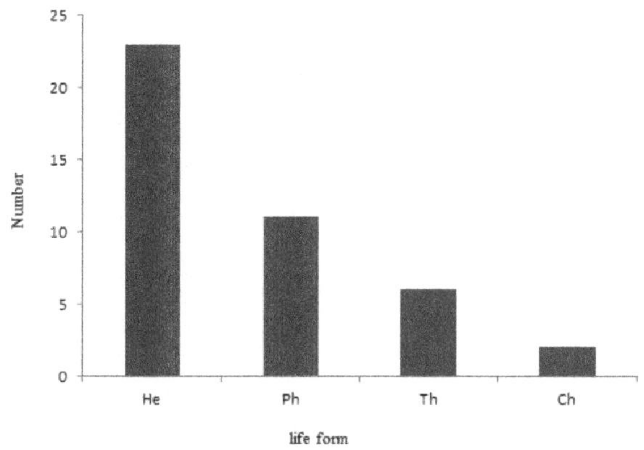

Fig 3. Comparison of life forms number among ethnoveterinary medical species in ZilberChay watershed.

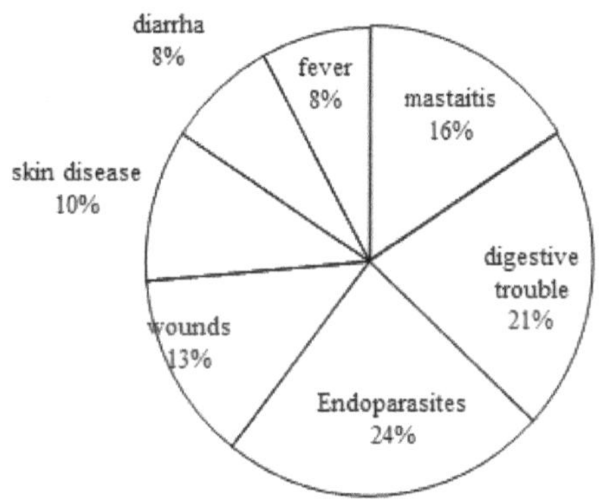

Fig 4. Most common treated disease and syndromes with ethnoveterinary species in ZilberChay watershed

Number of chrotypes among the studied FHVM are compared presented in Fig. 2. These chrotypes included IT (Irano-Toranian) with 49.1 %, Plur (More than 2 chrotypes) with 27.27 %, ES (Euro-Siberian) with 18.18 %M (Mediterranean) with 5.45 %. According to the table, the most common chrotype among the ZilberChay watershed FHVM are belong to Irano-Toranian chrotype.

Comparison of different life forms (i. e. He= Hemicryptophytes with 55%; Ph= Phanerophytes with 26.19 %; Th= Therophytes with 14.28 % and Ch= Chamaephytes with 4.76 %) among the studied plant species of ZilberChay watershed are given in Fig. 3. This figure represents that the most common life form among the FHVM of this area is hemicryptophytes.

Additionally, Fig. 4 shows the most common disease and animal health problems which have been treating with identified FHVM species in the study area. According to the results, endoparasites with 24 percent and skin disease with 16 percent are the most common treated disease by identified FHVM species and the less treated disease with medicinal plants are fever and diarrhea. These FHVM species are distributed on 900 to 3200m asl elevation.

Some of the identified ethnoveterinary species from the study area have already been reported in other studies. For example, Lautado and Capasso (2013) in ethnoveterinary study of useful plants in animal therapy showed that latex of *Achille amillefolium* is useful for fever treatment. Kouhpayeh *et al.* (2011) in the study of ethnoveterinary plants in Kerman province of Iran have reported that therapeutic potential of *Achille awilhelmsii* can cure wounds. Chalechale *et al.* (2013) found that *Amygdalus lycioides* which is growing in Kurdistan province of Iran can be mixed and grounded with the bark of brinjl (egg-plant) in vinegar and used as paste during 10 days to treat ulcerative lesions of leishmaniasis. Khan (2009) has reported that decoction of leaves and thorns of *Cichorium intybus* is used in impaction in cattle, sheep, goats and camels. Pande *et al.* (2007) and Ul Islam *et al.* (2012) have demonstrated the application of *Cynodon dactylon* to treat mastitis, gastric troubles, internal injury, food poisoning, wounds and as tonic, antiseptic and analgesic. Kouhpayeh *et al.* (2011) have also found that the leaves of *Gundelia tournefortii* is using against scabies in sheep and goat by local people of Kerman province in Iran. Laudat and Capasso (2013) and Lans *et al.* (2007) found that *Juniperus communis* affords in treating skin diseases, Ectoparasites, Endoparasites and liver fluke. Ul Islam *et al.* (2012) and Lans *et al.* (2007) respectively reported *Morus alba* and *Salix alba* as ethnoveterinary plants in mastitis. Some of herbal plants are being used by local people for curing indigestion like *Punicagranatum* and *Triticum aestivum* in the study of Pande *et al.* (2007). Some plants are useful for treating mineral elements deficiencies like *Urtica dioica* for treating zinc deficiencies and *Medicago sativa*in selenium deficiency (Lans *et al.*, 2007).

Table 1. List of ethnoveterinary species of ZilberChay watershed in northwest of Iran. IT= Irano-Toranian; M= Mediterranean; Plur= More than 2 chorotypes; ES= Euro-Siberian; Th= Therophytes; He= Hemicryptophytes; Ch= Chamaephytes; Ph= Phanerophytes.

No.	Family& Scientific name	Elevation	Chrotype	Life forms	Application
	1. Amarantaceae				
1	*Amaranthus viridis* L.	2000-3000	IT	Th	Emollient
	1. Apiaceae				
2	*Carum carvi* L.	2000-3200	IT	He	Ectoparasites, Digestive &Gastric troubles, Skin diseases, Fever, Dehydration, Mouth infection
3	*Daucus carota* L.	900-2000	IT	He	Endoparasites
4	*Prangosferulacea* (L.) Lindley.	900-2200	IT,M	He	Treatment of thick and louse (Ruminants)
	2. Asteraceae				
5	*Achillea millefolium* L.	1500-2000	Plur	He	Fever, Mastitis, Wounds, Sternal abscess
6	*Achillea wilhelmsii* C.Koch	1500-3200	Plur	Ch	Wound relief in cattle, sheep and camel
7	*Arctium lappa* L.	900-2000	IT,ES	He	Mastitis
8	*Cichorium intybus* L.	900-2000	Plur	He	Endoparasites
9	*Gundelia tournefortii* L.	1500-2000	IT,M	He	Scabies in sheep &goat
10	*Taraxacum officinalis* Webber.	1500-2500	IT	He	Gastrointestinal diseases
	3. Brassicaceae				
11	*Sisymbrium officinale* L.	900-2500	IT	Th	Febrifuge, Expectorant
	4. Convolvulaceae				
12	*Convolvulus arvensis* L.	1000-2000	Plur	He	Purgative
	5. Cupressaceae				
13	*Juniperus communis* L.	1500-3200	Plur	Ph	Skin diseases, Ectoparasites, Endoparasites, Liver fluke
14	*Juniperus excels* M. B.	1500-3200	IT	Ph	Topical pain of motion organs in camel
	6. Elaeagnaceae				
15	*HippophaerhamnoidesL.*	900-1500	IT	Ph	Gastrointestinal endoparasites
	7. Fabaceae				
16	*Alhagi camelorum* Fisch.	900-2500	IT	He	Impaction in cattle, sheep, goats and camels
17	*Glycyrrhiza glabra* L.	900-2000	IT,ES	He	Reducing pain and swell in strains bruise, Stomach swell in horse
18	*Lotus corniculatus* L.	900-2000	M,IT	Th	Endoparasites
19	*Medicago sativa* L.	900-2000	Plur	He	Growth and enhancing camel and weak &young sheep, Selenium deficiency, Nutrition after calving
20	*Melilotus officinalis* (L.) Desr.	900-2000	Plur	He	Increase the milk production in ruminants
21	*Trifolium repens* L.	1200-2300	ES, IT	He	Nervous disease
	8. Hypericaceae				
22	*Hypericum perforatum* L.	1500-3200	Plur	Ch	Wounds, Proud flesh
	9. Juglandaceae				
23	*Juglance regia* L.	900-2000	ES,IT	Ph	Rape leaf and fruit for worm excretion
	10. Lamiaceae				
24	*Mentha longifolia* L.	1500-2500	Plur	He	As (stomachic) and (febrifuge)Commonly
25	*Prunella vulgaris* L.	900-2000	Plur	He	Wounds
	11. Linceae				
26	*Linumus itatissimum* L.	900-2500	Plur	He	Mastitis, tonic
	12. Malvaceae				

27	*Malva neglecta* Wallr.	900-1500	IT, ES	He	Digestive problem , For food poisoning, As fodder, But excess amount cause loose motion
	13. Moraceae				
28	*Morus alba* L.	900-1500	ES, IT	Ph	Leaves are used as fodder. In excess amount cause loose motion. It is also laxative and tonic, mastitis
29	*Morusnigra*L.	900-1500	IT	Ph	The leaves are used as fodder for sheep, goats and cows. These are also tonic and laxative
	14. Plantaginaceae				
30	*Plantago major L.*	900-2000	IT	He	Hits or Inflammations
	15. Poaceae				
31	*Cynodon dactylon* (L.) Press.	900-2500	Plur	He	As fodder for veterinaries. As tonic, antiseptic and analgesic, wounds for blood clouting, relieving pain mastitis, gastric troubles, internal injury, sprains, bone fracture, food poisoning, sunstroke, broken horn, clotting of blood
32	*Hordeum vulgar* L.	900-2000	IT	Th	Anemia, Post calving care, Itching, Haematuria, Strength, Density, Skin disease, Heat stroke, Cough, Regulate fertility, Lactation
33	*Triticum aestivum* Lamk.	900-1200	IT	Th	Bloat in goats, Skin infection, Stomachache, Indigestion, Anemia, Throat infection, Ricket, Remove serility, scabies, Tympany, Gas problem of goat
	16. Punicaceae				
34	*Punica granatum* L.	1200-2200	IT, ES	Ph	Diarrhea, fever, Dehydration, Indigestion, Gastric troubles, Tonic, Internal parasite, Burn, Paralysis, Flatulence, Tympany
	17. Rhamnaceae				
35	*Rhamnus virgata* Roxb.	2000-3000	IT	Ph	Swelling
	18. Rosaceae				
36	*Amygdalus lycioides* Spach.	1500-2500	IT	Ph	Ulcerative lesions of leishmaniasis
37	*Rosa canina* L.	900-2500	IT, ES	Ph	Inflammation
38	*Sanguisorba minor* Scop.	1500-3200	IT, ES	He	Joint troubles in camel
	19. Salicaceae				
39	*Salix alba* L.	900-1500	ES,IT	Ph	Eye disease, Diarrhea, Scours, Mastitis, Pain, Unknown illness
	20. Solanaceae				
40	*Datura stramonium* L.	900-1500	Plur	Th	Burns, Infected wounds, Parasite in cattle &sheep
	21. Ulmaceae				
41	*Urtica dioica* L.	900-3200	Plur	He	Endoparasites, Diarrhea, Pre-show protection, Zinc deficiency
	22. Zygophyllaceae				
42	*Peganum harmala* L.	900-1700	Plur	He	Snake bite(in all species)

Some of the identified ethnoveterinary plants are good against parasaites. Species such as *Carum carvi* and *Juniperus communis* for Ectoparasites, *Cichorium intybus*, *Daucus carota*, *Punica granatum* and *Urticadioica* in treating endoparasites and *Hippophae rhamnoides*is using for gastrointestinal endoparasites (Lans *et al*., 2007; Kouhpayeh *et al*., 2011; Chalechale *et al*., 2013; Lautado and Capasso, 2013). Moreover, in different studies some of the ethnoveterinary plants are reported for applying in specific disease, syndromes or problems. Plants such as *Peganum harmala* for snake bite (Bahmani *et al*., 2012); *Trifolium repens* for nervous disease (Pande *et al*., 2012); *Salix alba* for eye disease (Martínez and Luján, 2011); *Gundelia tournefortii* for scabies in sheep and goat (Kouhpayeh *et al.,* 2011); *Juniperus communis* for skin diseases (Lautado and Capasso, 2013).

4. Conclusion

Forty two ethnoveterinary plant species with their medical effects were identified in ZilberChay watershed as the results of this study. Traditional knowledge of medical plants varies according to the culture and faith of different tribes all around the world, but because of the lack of previous studies, most of the ethnoveterinary plants are still unknown. Thus, there is a need to widespread study of ethnoveterinary medical plants and documentation of traditional knowledge of using them in treating domestic animals for conservation of medicinal flora and regional biodiversity that is particularly threatened around the world especially in Iran and east Azerbaijan.

5. References

Adnan, M., Ullah, I., Tariq, A., Murad, V., Azizullah, A., Khan, A.L. and Ali, N. 2014. Ethnomedicine use in the war affected region of North West Pakistan. *Journal of Ethnobiology &* Ethnomedical, 10: 1-16.

Assadi, M. (Ed.) 1988-2013. *Flora of Iran*. Vols. 1-70. Research Institute of Forests and Rangelands, Tehran, Iran.

Bahmani, M., Avijgan, M., Hosseini, S.R., Najaf zadeh Varzi, H. and Mehrzadi, S. 2010. Application of Medical plants of Southern areas of Ilam province in treating disease and syndromes of small ruminants. *Journal of Herbal Drugs*, 2: 51-60.

Bahmani, M., Rafieian-Kopaei, M., Avijgan, M., Golshahi, H., Eftekhari, Z. and Haji Gholizadeh, Gh. 2012. Ethnobotanical Studies of Medicinal Plants Used by Kurdish Owner's in South Range of Ilam Province, West of Iran. *American-Eurasian Journal of Agriculture & Environment Science,* 12: 1527-1532.

Boissier, P.E. 1867-1888. *Flora Orientalis*. vols. 1-5. Genevaeet Basileae. H. Georg, Geneva.

Chakraborty, S. and Kanti Pal, S. 2012. Plants for Cattle Health: A Review of Ethno-Veterinary Herbs in Veterinary Health Care. *Annals Ayurvedic Medicine*, 1: 44-152.

Chalechale, A., Karimi, I., Zavareh, S. and Karimi, A. 2013. Brief Anthropology and Antiparasitic remedies in Kurdish ethno (Veterinary) Medicine: A neglected treasure trove. *World's Veterinary* Journal, 3: 29-32.

Davidović, V., Joksimović-Todorović, M., Maksimović, Z., Hristov, S., Stanković, B. and Relić, R. 2009. A Review of Plants used in Ethnoveterinary Medicine. *Macedonian Journal of Animal Science,* 1: 377–382.

Davis, P.H. 1965-1988. *Flora of Turkey and the East Aegean*. vols. 1- 8. Edinburgh University Press, Scotland.

Ghahreman, A. 1996. *General code of the families and genera of the flora of Iran*. Research Institute of Forests and Rangelands, Tehran.

Ghahreman, A. 1979-1992. *Colorful flora of Iran*. Research Institute of Forests and Rangelands, Tehran

Ghorbani, A., Ahmad Abadi, S. and ElyasiBrojeni, H. 2013a. Ecological characteristics of medicinal plants in rangeland ecosystems of ZilbarChay watershed of East Azerbaijan, *Journal of Plant Ecosystem & Conservation,* 1: 65-86.

Hossaini, (Reza) S.A., Abarsaji, Gh. and Hossaini, (Habib) S.A. 2009. Medicinal plants of Golestan province. *Iranian Journal of Medicinal and Aromatic Plants*, 24: 498-472.

IPNI, 2012. The International Plant Names Index. Available on internet at: http://www.ipni.org.

Ishtiaq, M., Khan, Ch.M.A. and Hanif, V. 2006. Ethnoveterinary medical uses of plants from Samahni valley dist. Bhimber, (Azad Kashmir) Pakistan. *Asian Journal of Plant Science,* 59:390-396.

Khan, M. F. 2009. Ethno-Veterinary Medicinal Usage of Flora of Greater Cholistan Desert (Pakistan).*Pakistan Veterinary Journal,* 29: 75-80.

Komarov, V.L. (Ed.) 1934-1954. *Flora of USSR*. vols. 1-30. Izdatel'stvoAkademiNauk SSSR Leningrad (English translation from Russian, Jerusalem, 1968-1977).

Kouhpayeh, A., Ghasemipibaloti, A., Yazdanpanahravi, M.M., PourMohseninasab, E. and Arjmand, D. 2011. Ethnoveterinary study of medical plants of Kerman province. *Journal of Herbal Drugs*, 2: 211-216.

Lans, Ch., Turner, N., Brauer, G., Lourenco, G. and Georges, K. 2006. Ethnoveterinary medicines used for horses in Trinidad and in British Columbia, Canada. *Journal of Ethnobiology & Ethnomedical,* 2: 31-51.

Lans, C., Turner, N., Khan, T., Brauer, G. and Boepple, B. 2007. Ethnoveterinary medicines used for ruminants in British Columbia, Canada. *Journal of Ethnobiology & Ethnomedical*, 3: 1-22.

Laudato, M. and Capasso, R. 2013. Useful plants for animal therapy. *OA Alternative Medicine*, 1: 1-6.

Lulekal, E., Kelbessa, E., Bekele, T. and Yineger, H. 2007. An ethnobotanical study of medicinal plants in Mana Angetu District, southeastern Ethiopia. *Journal of Ethnobiology & Ethnomedical*. 4: 1-10.

Malek Mohammadi, L. and Mirzavash Azar, S. 2012. Gathering, identification, medicinal utilization and domestication of some wild edible plants in Ghasemloo valley, West Azerbaijan, Iran. *Journal of Rangeland Sc*ience, 2: 521-539.

Manjo, Y., Anupama, Y. and Ekta, G. 2012. Ethnoveterinary practices in Rajistan, India (A review). *International Researcch Journal of Biology Science,* 1: 80-82.

Martínez, G. J. and Luján, M. C. 2011. Medicinal plants used for traditional veterinary in the Sierras de Córdoba (Argentina): An ethnobotanical comparison with human medicinal uses. *Journal of Ethnobiology & Ethnomedical,* 7: 1-18

Masika, P. J., Van Averbeke, W. and Sonandi, A. 2000. Use of herbal remedies by small-scale farmers to treat livestock diseases in central Eastern Cape Province, South Africa. *Journal of South African Veterinary Association,* 71: 87–91.

Maassoumi, A. A. 1986-2005. *The genus Astragalus in Iran*. vols. 1-4. Research Institute of Forests and Rangelands, Tehran, Iran.

McCorkle, C. and Martin, M. 1998. Parallels an d potentials in animal and human ethnomedical technique. *Agricalture and Human Values*, 15:139-144.

Mobayen, S. 1975-1996. *Flora of Iran*: *vascular plants*. Vols. 1-4. Tehran University Press, Tehran, Iran.

Moradi, A., Asri, Y. and Sobh-Zahedi, Sh. 2013. An introduction of flora, life form, chorotype and habitat of plants around Sepidroud dam, Iran. *Taxonomy & Biosy*stem, 15: 95-112.

Moreki, J. C. 2012. Use of Ethnoveterinary Medicine in Family Poultry Health Management in Botswana-a Review. *Journal of Veterinary Advance,* 2: 254-260.

Nyamanga, P.A., Suda, C. and Aagaard-Hansen, J. 2008. The socio-cultural context and practical implications of ethnoveterinary medical pluralism in western Kenya. *Agriculture &. Human Values*, 25: 513-527.

Omid Beigi, R. 1993. *Production of medicinal plants*. 1th ed. Tehran University. Iran. P.139.

Omid Beigi, R. 1997. *Approach the Production And Processing Plants*. Tarahan Publisher, Tehran, Iran.

Panda, S.S. and Dhal, N.K. 2014. Plants used in Ethno-Veterinary Medicine by native people of Nawarangpur District, Odisha, India. *World Journal of Pharmacy & Pharmaceutical Science*, 3: 787-798.

Pande, P.C., Tiwari, L. and Pande, H.C. 2007. Ethnoveterinary plants of Uttaranchal- a review. *Indian Journal of Traditional Knowledge,* 6: 444-458.

Parsa, A. 1943-1950. *Flora of Iran*. vols. 1-5, Tehran University Press, Tehran, Iran.

Pieroni, A., Howard, P., Volpato, G. and Santoro, R.F. 2004. Natural remedies and nutraceuticalused in ethnoveterinary practices in Inland Southern Italy. *Veterinary Research Community,* 28: 55-80.

Rajkumari, R., Nirmala, R.K., Singh, P.K., Kumar, A.D., Dutta, B.k. and Pinokiyo, A. 2014. Ethnoveeterinary plants used by the Chiru tribes of Manipur, northeast India. *Indian Journal of Traditional Knowledge,* 13: 368-376.

Raunkiaer, C. 1934. *The life form of plant and statistical plant geography*. Clarendon Press, Oxford.

Rechinger, K. H. (Ed) 1963–1998. *Flora Iranica*, vols. 1-180. Akademische Druck-u. Verlagsanstalt, Graz, Austria.

Selvaraju, A., Ayyanar, M., Rathinakumar, S.S. and Sekar, T. 2011. Plants used in ethno-veterinary medicine by Malayalitribals in Salem district of Tamil Nadu, India. *Medicinal Plants*. 3: 1-7.

Sokhanvar, F., Ejtehadi, H., Vaezi, J., Memariani, F., Joharchi, M.R. and Ranjbar, Z. 2013. Flora, life form and chorology of plants of the Helali protected area in Khorasan-e Razavi province. *Taxonomy & Biosy*stem, 16: 85-100.

Tabuti, J.R.S. 2003. Ethnoveterinary medicines for cattle (Bosindicus) in Bulamogi County, Uganda: plant species and mode of use. *Journal of Ethnopharmacology,* 88: 279-286.

Takhar, H.K. 2004. Folk herbal Veterinary medicines of southern Rajasthan. *Indian Journal of Traditional Knowledge,* 3: 407-411.

Takhtajan, A. 1986. *Floristic regions of the world.* University of California Press, Berkley.

Toupchi, Zh. 2011. Identification of medicinal plants in Arshadchamani rangelands of East Azerbaijan. *Journal of Rangeland Sci*ence, 1: 103-110.

Townsend, C.C. and Guest, E. 1966-1985. *Flora of Iraq*. vols. 1-9. Ministry of Agriculture and Agrarian Reform, Baghdad.

Ul Islam, M., Anwar, Z., Tabassum, S., Ahmed Khan, S., Chand Zeb, A., Abrar, M., Khattak, Kh.U. and Khattak, J.Z.Kh. 2012. Plants of ethno-veterinary uses of Tunglai Mountain Baffa Mansehra, Pakistan. *International Journal of Animal Veterinary Advance,* 4: 221-224.

Verma, R.K. 2014. An ethnobotanical study of plants used for the treatment of livestock diseases in Tikamgarh District of Bundelkhand, Central India. *Asian Pacific Journal Tropical Biomedicine,* 4: 460-467.

Zohary, M. 1966-1972. *Flora Palaestina.* Jerusalem Academic Press, Israel.

Neuroprotective role of vitamin E, green tea extract, and *spirulina* in rats treated with cadmium chloride

Amir Ali Shahbazfar[1]*, Seyyed Jamal Emami[1], Reza Asadpour[2]

[1]*Department of Pathobiology, Faculty of Veterinary Medicine, University of Tabriz, Tabriz-Iran;*
***Email: amirali.shahbazfar@gmail.com**

[2]*Department of Clinical Sciences, Faculty of Veterinary Medicine, University of Tabriz, Tabriz-Iran;*

ARTICLE INFO

***Topic:** Medicinal Plants*

Key words:

- *Cadmium chloride*
- *Green tea*
- *Oxidative stress*
- *Vitamin* E
- Spirulina

ABSTRACT

Background & Aim: Spirulina (*Spirulina plantesis*) and Tea (*Camellia sinensis*) has a long history of use in folk medicine. Recently, They have been widely studied for their potential antioxidant properties. The present study investigated neuroprotective effect of Spirulina and green tea extract against Cadmium [Cd]-induced brain lesions and to compare these effects with neuroprotective effect of Vitamin E.

Experimental: The rats were randomly divided into 5 groups and were treated with the following treatment for a period of 4 weeks. Control, $CdCl_2$ alone, Vitamin E with $CdCl_2$, Green tea extract with $CdCl_2$, Spirulina solution with $CdCl_2$. On the 29th day, animals were sacrificed humanely and their brains were placed in formalin. Hippocampus, caudate putamen, corpus callosum, cerebellum, and cerebrum were studied by light microscopy.

Results: Neuronophagia, satellitosis of oligodendrocytes, hyperemia, hemorrhage, neuronal necrosis, central chromatolysis, neuronal atrophy, laminar necrosis, and status spongiosus were the observed changes. Thickness of granular layer and molecular layer of cerebellum and size/diametr of purkenje cells reduced when cadmium used alone at $P<0.05$. A thicker and different molecular layer and almost normal purkenje cells were observed when Spirulina was combined with cadmium at $P<0.05$. Likewise,spirulina significantly decreased the number of cadmium-induced necrotic cells in hippocampus and cerebral cortex but not in caudate putamen at $P<0.05$. Spirulina showed the most protective effect on brain tissue in comparison with vitamin E and green tea extract. Green tea extract had the weakest effect. The hippocampus was the most affected area of the brain among the others in this survey.

Recommended applications/industries: The results shows Spirullina as excellent antioxidant source indicating its use possibly in combination with vitamin E and other antioxidant agent in order to prevent adverse effects of free radicals.

1. Introduction

Cadmium (Cd) is one of the potent environmental and occupational metallic toxicants, widely dispersed in the environment (Méndez-Armenta and Ríos, 2007). Cd toxicity as an industrial pollutant, a food contaminant, and as one of the major components in cigarette smoke has been proven (Manca *et al.*, 1991). In nonsmokers, food is the most important route of Cd entrance into the body (Donma and Metin Donma, 2005). Because of its great involvement in cancer, Cd has been classified as a category 1 carcinogen by the International Agency for Research on Cancer and the USA's National Toxicology Program (Waisberg et al., 2003). It damages a variety of organs, including the liver, kidney, lung and testis (El-Refaiy and Eissa, 2012), as well as brain (Mendez-Armenta *et al.*, 2001; Nishimura *et al.,* 2011). Acute exposure to Cd produces hepatic, pulmonary, and testicular injury, while chronic exposure results in renal and bone injury and cancer (Klaassen *et al.*, 1999). Cadmium is able to enter the brain parenchyma and cause neurological alterations (Nishimura *et al.,* 2011). It is more toxic to young animals due to the immaturity of the blood brain barrier (Wong and Klaassen, 1982).

A well-known effect of Cd both *in vitro* and *in vivo* is the generation of free radicals in cells (Méndez-Armenta and Ríos, 2007), followed by oxidative stress (El-Refaiy and Eissa, 2012). It induces lipid peroxidation (LPO) in all tissues, mainly in the lung and brain (Manca *et al.,* 1991). Brain tissue is highly susceptible to LPO due to its high rate of oxygen utilization, its abundant supply of polyunsaturated fatty acids, and a high content of transition metals like copper and iron in several regions (Calabrese *et al.,* 2000). Another mechanism through which cadmium induces oxidative stress is by inhibiting enzymatic and non-enzymatic antioxidants in various tissues (Shagirtha *et al.*, 2011).

Spirulina [Spirulina platensis], is a microscopic and filamentous blue-green alga used as food it is considered as a rich source of some macro- and micronutrients including amino acids, chlorophyll, gamma-linolenic acid, carotenoids, and vitamins (Belay, 2002). It has an antioxidant effect that might be associated with phycocyanin, a phycobiliprotein found at high concentration in *Spirulina* (Pinero Estrada *et al.*, 2011). *Spirulina* protects the liver from the toxic effects caused by Cd (Amin *et al.*, 2006).

Tea (*Camellia sinensis*) is one of the most common drinks around the world (Graham, 1992). In recent years, green tea has been widely studied for its contribution in preventing hypercholesterolemia, cancer, atherosclerosis, coronary artery diseases and inflammation (Sharangi, 2009). Green tea is an excellent source of polyphenols known as green tea catechins. The important catechins of green tea are (−)-epicatechin, (−)-epicatechin-3-gallate, (−)-epigallocatechin, and (−)-epigallocatechin- 3-gallate (Babu et al., 2006). They are able to enter the brain (Abd El Mohsen *et al.,* 2002), contributing to antioxidant effect by scavengering free radicals (Sharangi, 2011). Green tea extract intake in rats increased total antioxidant statue index and decreased lipid peroxidation products in the liver (Skrzydlewska *et al.,* 2002).

Present study is designed to investigate the neuroprotective effects of Spirulina and green tea extract against Cd, and to compare these effects with those of vitamin E, as a major non-enzymatic antioxidant present in the lipid structures of cells (Wagner *et al.,* 1996).

2. Materials and Methods

2.1. Chemicals and reagents

Vitamin E in the form of α-tocopherol (95.5%), cadmium in the form of cadmium chloride hydrate (98%) ($CdCl_2$), and *Spirulina* (algal lyophilized cells) were purchased from Sigma-Aldrich Corporation, Milwaukee,WI, USA. Green tea was purchased from a traditional herbal shop.

2.2. Animals

Thirty healthy weanling albino Wistar rats, each weighing 40-50 g, were obtained from the animal house at the Faculty of Veterinary Medicine, University of Tabriz. They were kept under constant temperature of 23 °C with a 12h light/dark cycle, and fed a standard pellet diet and water ad libitum. After one week of acclimatization, the animals were divided into five groups of six and were treated with the following treatment for a period of 4 weeks.

Group I: Untreated control rats, **GroupII**: $CdCl_2$ [50 ppm mixed with diet]**, Group III**: Vitamin E [intraperitoneal, 100 mg/kg body weight [b.w.] weekly]

+ $CdCl_2$ [50 ppm mixed with diet], **Group IV**: Spirulina solution [500 mg/kg b.w., in 5 cc water by gavage weekly] + $CdCl_2$ [50 ppm mixed with diet], **Group V**: Green tea alcoholic extract [1.5% w/v] [dissolved in drinking water] + $CdCl_2$ [50 ppm mixed with diet]

2.3. Preparations of green tea extract

In order to prepare decaffeinated tea extract, green tea leaves were first soaked in hot distilled water [1:5 w/v] for 15 min. The supernatant was then removed from the hot water by ethyl acetate in equal volume. Then, by maceration method, the remaining part from tea leaves was extracted with 70% ethanol. The extract was filtered and the solvent was evaporated in a rotary evaporator under reduced pressure at 40°C. The resulting extract was frozen at -20°C until use.

2.4. Histopathology

Experiments were performed according to the guidelines established in the National Institutes of Health Guide for the Care and Use of Laboratory Animals. At the end of exposure [29th day], the animals were sacrificed by ether anesthesia. Each rat's entire brain was removed and fixed immediately in 10% neutral buffered formalin. To reach the cortex, corpus callosum, and caudate putamen, one slice was taken involving these regions. A similar action was performed for excision of the hippocampus. Half of the cerebellum was removed by a sagittal incision (Fig1).

All the landmarks were chosen from the book, "The Rat Brain in Stereotaxic Coordinates" (Paxinos and Watson, 2007). After routine histological procedures, paraffin blocks were sectioned into 5-µm thick sections, stained with hematoxylin and eosin and examined under light microscope. For histopathological and histomorphometric studies, the following parameters were examined.

I. Thickness of the cerebellar cortex molecular layer [ML] and granular layer [GL] using a microscope with a graticule attached to the eyepiece.

II. Mean diameter / size of the Purkinje cell using the same microscope.

III. Number of necrotic neurons in cerebral cortex, hippocampus and caudate putamen.

IV. Histopathological changes.

Necrotic neurons were identified microscopically by chromatolysis, atrophied, pyknotic nuclei, and loss of nucleus. The means and the standard deviation of each of the parameters measured were determined. All data are reported as the mean ± S.E.M. To compare the values acquired after treatment among all groups, one-way analysis of variance [ANOVA] was used followed by Tukey post hoc test using SPSS software version 11.5. Differences were considered significant at $p < 0.05$.

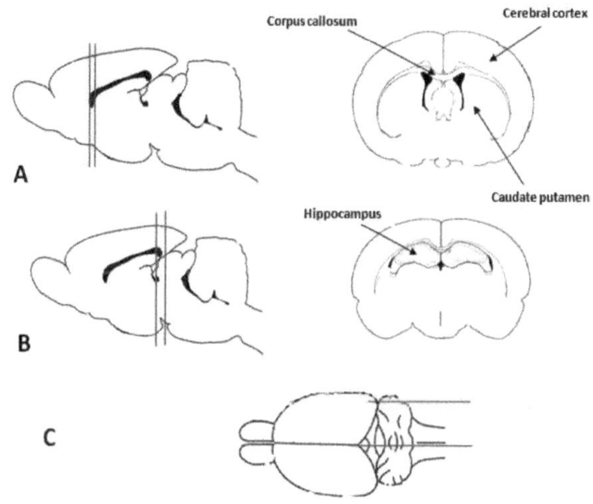

Fig 1. Incision lines and cross sections of the rat brain for specimens taking. **(A)**. Incision lines and cross section of the rat brain for receiving to Caudate putamen;Corpus callosum and cerebral cortex. **(B)**. Incision lines and cross section of the rat brain for receiving to hippocampus. **(C)**. Incision lines on the rat brain for receiving to cerebellar nuclei and cortex.

3. Results and discussion

No death was observed throughout the 4-week period of the experiment. Under light microscopy, the control group showed no lesions. In other groups, lesions with varying severity were observed. The hippocampus was found the most vulnerable region to Cd toxicity with major neurodegenerative changes. The other regions were the cerebral cortex, cerebellar nuclei, caudate putamen, cerebellar cortex, and corpus callosum respectively. In the Cd treated group changes in the cerebellum consisted of scattered necrosis in the Purkinje layer with hyperemia in the granular layer. Cerebellar nuclei showed neuronal necrosis with neuronophagia, satellitosis of oligodendrocytes, and hyperemia. In the hippocampus, observed lesions were neuronal necrosis with predominant pyknotic nuclei and loss of nucleus in some neurons, central chromatolysis, oligodendrocyte satellitosis, capillary hyperemia, hyperchromatic neurons, and atrophied neurons with detachment from surrounding neuropil, neuronophagia, and vacuolization. Infiltration of macrophages and lymphocytes to perivascular spaces was observed with lymphocytes predominating. Caudate putamen showed mild hemorrhage in Virchow-Robin spaces [VRS]. Neuronal necrosis, gemistocytic astrocytes, neuronophagia, and hyperemia were obvious too. In the corpus callosum, axonal swelling, hyperemia, and mild hemorrhage were observed. In some regions, status spongiosus was evident as well. Oligodendrocyte satellitosis, gemistocytes, macrophages and lymphocytes infiltration to perivascular spaces, distinct laminar necrosis of the neurons in external pyramidal layer, severe hyperemia, gliosis, and neuronal vacuolization were observed in cerebral cortex. White matter showed axonal degeneration, interstitial edema, and edema in VRS (Fig 2).

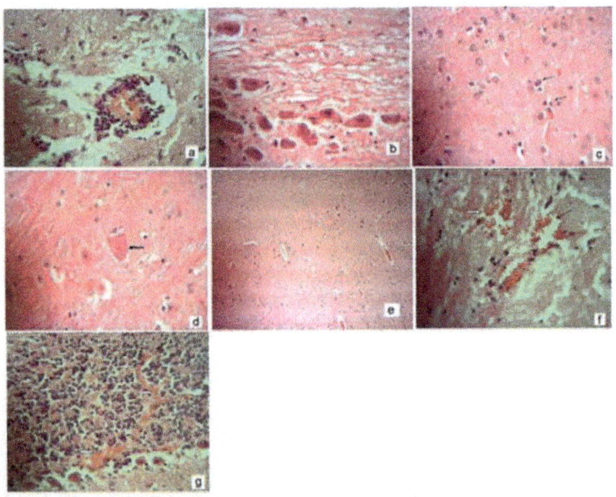

Fig 2. Histopathological findings of brain tissue. **(a).** Perivascular cuffing with mononuclears in hippocampus.H&E staining.×800. **(b).** Neuronal necrosis in one cerebellar nucleus.H&E staining.×800. **(c).** Oligodendriocytessatellitosis in cerebral cortex.H&E staining.×800. **(d).** Central chromatolysis and vacuolation in a neuron of caudate putamen.H&E staining. ×800. **(e).** Marked laminar necrosis in external pyramidal layer of cerebral cortex.H&E staining. ×200. **(f).** Hyperemia and mild hemorrhage in corpus callosum.H&E staining. ×800. **(g).** Necrosis in purkinje and hyperemia in granular layer of cerebellum.H&E staining. ×800.

Co-administration of *Spirulina* with Cd reduced the degenerative changes to a remarkable level in comparison with the Cd treated group. Hemorrhage and laminar necrosis were absent, although scattered neural necrosis did exist. Furthermore, other changes like edema, satellitosis, neuronal necrosis, and slight gliosis were present. In simultaneous administration of vitamin E with Cd, histopathological lesions were slighter than those observed in the group treated with Cd alone. The cortex showed only scattered neural necrosis. The group that received green tea extract with Cd showed slighter lesions compared with the Cd treated group. The kind of the lesions was similar with the other groups. Laminar necrosis with hemorrhage observed in the cerebral cortex. Changes were more severe than in the vitamin E treated group.

Histomorphometric studies showed that Cd reduced the thickness of GL and ML of cerebellum [148.0±2.5 μm and 173.0±8.0 μm, respectively] as compared with control group [166.0±4.30 μm and 215.0±5.3 μm, respectively]. A thicker and markedly different ML was observed when *Spirulina* combined with Cd. The mean diameter of the Purkinje cell was significantly reduced in the cadmium as well as in the cadmium and vitamin E and cadmium and green tea extract groups compared with the control group. These were statically significant at $p<0.05$. Spirullina significantly impeded this effect at $p<0.05$ (Table 1). Likewise, number of cadmium-induced necrotic cells in cortex, hippocampus significantly reduced when *Spirulina* combined with Cd (Table 2). The difference between green tea extract and Vitamin E groups with Cd group alone was not significant at $p<0.05$.

The most prominent change detected from light microscopy of the five brain regions was neuronal degeneration and necrosis, characterized mainly by chromatolysis, neuronal atrophy, pyknotic nuclei, and finally loss of nucleus. It can be attributed mainly to the oxidative stress caused by Cd. Cadmium exposure increases reactive oxygen species, leading to lipid and protein peroxidation, changes to intercellular stability, damage to deoxyribonucleic acid (DNA) and membranes and consequently inducing cell death (Stohs *et al*., 2001; Waisberg *et al.,* 1999). Likewise, Cd is able to reduce the activity and level of antioxidant enzymes like superoxide dismutase (SOD) and concentration of reduced glutathione (GSH) (El-Sokkary and Awadalla, 2011). SOD and GSH are potent antioxidant agents and their depletion indicates oxidative stress (Manca *et al.,* 1991). There are relatively low levels of antioxidants such as GSH, vitamin E, catalase and SOD in the brain (Calabrese *et al.*, 2000). Cd causes morphological changes in neurons by sustained increase in intracellular Ca^{2+} concentratin (Yoshida, 2001).

Table 1. Mean thickness of cellebelar layers and mean diameter of purkenje cells (mean ±SEM) in micrometer (μm).

	Group I	Group II	Group III	Group IV	Group V
Granular layer	166.0±4.30	148.0±2.5*	158.0±4.6	160.0±3.5	148.0±2.5*
Molecular layer	215.0±5.3	173.0±8.0*	195.0±5.0	210.0±3.7§	181.0±6.7*†
Purkenje cells	25.6±1.5*	18.8±1.2*	20.4±1.02*	25.0±1.3§	19.4±0.6 *†

*: statically significant difference from control group, §: statically significant difference from group II, †: statically significant difference from group III, ($p<0.05$)

Table 2. Mean number of cadmium- induced necrotic cells (mean±SEM)

	Group I	Group II	Group III	Group IV	Group V
Cortex	0.0±0.0	1.8±0.3*	1.2±0.3	0.2±0.2§	1.6±0.2*†
Hippocampus	0.0±0.0	2.4±0.4*	1.8±0.3*	0.6±0.2§	1.8±0.3*
Caudate putamen	0.2±0.2	1.8±0.3*	1.4±0.2	0.8±0.3	1.6±0.4*

*: statically significant difference from control group, §: statically significant difference from group II, †: statically significant difference from group III, ($p<0.05$).

Our findings are in agreement with a previous study which reported morphological changes such as hyperchromatic cells, necrosis, interstitial edema, and alteration of Purkinje cells in the brain of rats exposed to Cd (Mendez-Armenta *et al.*, 2001). In young rats, Cd produced slight damage to the endothelium of some blood vessels in a necrotic area with hemorrhage and infiltration of macrophages and lymphocytes into the perivascular space (Wong and Klaassen, 1982). Infiltration of macrophages and lymphocytes and hemorrhage were observed in our examination.

In order to prevent long-term Cd exposure toxicity, both endogenous antioxidants synthesized in tissues and exogenous antioxidants in the diet are needed. In the current study, introducing different co-treatment supplementations such as vitamin E, *Spirulina*, and green tea extract into the diet resulted in reduction of histopathological changes in the brain. Vitamin E, as an effective liposoluble antioxidant, is proven to interact with free radicals and prevents lipid peroxidation (Silva *et al.*, 2005). In the vitamin E treated group, histopathological changes were significantly reduced. Laminar necrosis in the cortex was diminished to scattered necrosis in some regions. It is speculated that vitamin E impedes oxidative stress initiated by free radicals in the cells, which lead to cell necrosis. It is speculated that vitamin E impedes oxidative stress initiated by free radicals in the cells, which lead to cell necrosis.

We also observed that green tea extract slightly mitigated histopathological changes in several brain regions. This can be attributed to the antioxidants that exist in green tea extract. Green tea co-administered with lead increased the activity of SOD and concentration of GSH and ameliorated histopathological changes induced by lead in the three regions of brain in treated rats (Khalaf *et al.*, 2012).

Besides phycocaine, *Spirulina* is found to be a good source of flavonoids, vitamin C, vitamin E and GSH (Jeyaprakash and Chinnaswamy, 2005). Furthermore, Zn^{2+} found in *Spirulina* is a potent antagonist against Cd neurotoxicity (Valko *et al.*, 2005). In rats exposed to lead, *Spirulina* was effective against oxidative damage caused by lead (Upasani and Balaraman, 2001).

Spirulina protected brain tissue better than the other materials of our research. Green tea extract was least effective among the others tested. This can be attributed to the several antioxidant components that exist in *Spirulina*. In addition, metals like Cu and Zn in *Spirulina* can serve as cofactors for the SOD enzyme and consequently antioxidant status will increase. In one study, an alcohol extract of *Spirulina* displayed better antioxidant property in the inhibition of LPO (65%) in comparison with α-tocopherol (35%) and β-carotene (48%) (Belay, 2002). Hippocampus lesions were more intense than those of other regions. It implies that Cd exerts its toxicity mainly in hippocampus. In a recent study of rats exposed to Cd, the greatest concentration of Cd was observed in the hippocampus region (Mendez-Armenta *et al.*, 2001). Another study revealed that the hippocampus is the region most affected after cadmium intoxication (Kaoud *et al.*, 2010).

4. Conclusion

Spirulina protected brain tissue better than the other materials of our research. Green tea extract was least effective among the others tested. The hippocampus was the most affected area of the brain among the others. Those other regions were the cerebral cortex, cerebellar nuclei, caudate putamen, cerebellar cortex, and corpus callosum respectively.

5. References

Abd El Mohsen, M.M., Kuhnle, G., Rechner, A.R., Schroeter, H., Rose, S., Jenner, P. and Rice-Evans, C.A. 2002. Uptake and metabolism of epicatechin and its access to the brain after oral ingestion. *Free Radical Biology andMedicine*., 33: 1693–1702.

Amin, A., Hamza, A.A., Daoud, S. and Hamza, W. 2006. Spirulina protects against cadmium-induced hepatotoxicity in rats. *American Journal of Pharmacology and Toxicology*., 1: 21-26.

Babu, P.V., Sabitha, K.E. and Shyamaladevi, C.S. 2006. Green tea impedes dyslipidemia, lipid peroxidation, protein glycation and ameliorates Ca2+-ATPase and Na+/K+-ATPase activity in the heart of streptozotocin-diabetic rats. *Chemico-Biological Interactions*., 162: 157–64.

Belay, A. 2002. The potential application of Spirulina [Arthrospira] as a nutritional and therapeutic supplement in health management. *The journal of american nutraceutical association*., 5: 27–48.

Calabrese, V., Bates, T.E. and Stella, A.M. 2000. NO synthase and NO-dependent signal pathways in brain aging and neurodegenerative disorders, the role of oxidant/antioxidant balance. *Neurochemimestry Research*., 25: 1315–41.

Donma, O. and Metin Donma, M. 2005. Cadmium, lead and phytochemicals. *Medical Hypotheses*., 65: 699–702.

El-Refaiy, A.I. and Eissa, FI. 2012. Protective effects of ascorbic acid and zinc against cadmium-induced histopathological, histochemical and cytogenetic changes in rats. *Comunicata Scientiae*., 3: 162–80.

El-Sokkary, G.H., and Awadalla, E.A. 2011. The protective role of vitamin C against cerebral and pulmonary damage induced by cadmium chloride in male adult albino rat. *Open Neuroendocrinology Journal*., 4: 1–8.

Graham, H.N. 1992. Green tea composition, consumption, and polyphenol chemistry. *Preventive Medicine*., 21: 334–50.

Jeyaprakash, K. and Chinnaswamy, P. 2005. Effect of spirulina and Liv-52 on cadmium induced toxicity in albino rats. *Indian journal of Experimental Biology*., 43:773-81.

Kaoud, H.A., Kamel, M.M., Abdel-Razek, A.H., Kamel, G.M. and Ahmed, K.A. 2010. Neurobehavioural, neurochemical and neuromorphological effects of cadmium in male rats. *Journal of American Science*., 202: 54-63.

Khalaf, A.A., Moselhy, W.A. and Abdel-Hamed, M.I. 2012. The protective effect of green tea extract on lead induced oxidative and DNA damage on rat brain. *Neurotoxicology*., 33:280–89.

Klaassen, C.D., Liu, J. and Choudhuri, S. 1999. Metallothionein, an intracellular protein to protect against cadmium toxicity. *Annual Review in Pharmacology and Toxicology*., 39: 267–94.

Manca, D., Ricard A.C., Trottier B. and Chevalier, G. 1991. Studies on lipid peroxidation in rat tissues following administration of low and moderate doses of cadmium chloride. *Toxicology*., 67: 303–23.

Méndez-Armenta, M. and Ríos, C., 2007. Cadmium neurotoxicity. *Environmental Toxicology and Pharmacology*., 23: 350–8.

Mendez-Armenta, M., Barroso-Moguel, R., Villeda-Hernandez, J., Nava-Ruíz, C. and Ríos, C. 2001.

Histopathological alterations in the brain regions of rats after perinatal combined treatment with cadmium and dexamethasone. *Toxicology.*, 161: 189–99.

Nishimura, Y., Yamaguchi, J.Y., Kanada, A., Horimoto, K., Kanemaru, K., Satoh, M. and Oyama, Y. 2006. Increase in intracellular Cd[2^+] concentration of rat cerebellar granule neurons incubated with cadmium chloride, Cadmium cytotoxicity under external Ca[2+]-free condition. *Toxicology In Vitro.*, 20: 211–16.

Paxinos, G., and Watson, C. 2007. The rat brain in stereotaxic coordinates. Academic Press, Sydney, Australia

Pinero Estrada, J.E., Bermejo Bescos, P. and Villar del Fresno, A.M. 2001. Antioxidant activity of different fractions of Spirulina platensis protean extract. *Farmaco.*, 56: 497–500.

Shagirtha, K., Muthumani, M. and Prabu, SM. 2011. Melatonin abrogates cadmium induced oxidative stress related neurotoxicity in rats. *European Review for Medical and Pharmacological Science.*, 15: 1039–50.

Sharangi, A.B. 2009. Medicinal and therapeutic potentialities of tea [Camellia sinensis L.] – A review. *Food Research International.*, 43:529-31.

Silva, M.G., Castro, A.A., Ramos, E.A., Peixoto, E., Miranda, F.Jr., Pitta Gde, B., Costa Rde, F. and Juliano, Y. 2005. Histological and biochemical serum effects of alpha-tocopherol on ischemia/reperfusion-related injuries induced in the pelvic limb of rats. *Acta cirúrgica brasileira.*, 20: 375–81.

Skrzydlewska, E., Ostrowska, J., Farbiszewski, R. and Michalak, K. 2002. Protective effect of green tea against lipid peroxidation in the rat liver, blood serum and the brain. *Phytomedicine.*, 9: 232–238.

Stohs, S.J., Bagchi, D., Hassoun, E. and Bagchi, M. 1999. Oxidative mechanisms in the toxicity of chromium and cadmium ions. *Journal of environmental pathology, toxicology and oncology.*, 19: 201–13.

Upasani, C.D and Balaraman, R. 2001. Effect of vitamin E, vitamin C and spirulina on the levels of membrane bound enzymes and lipids in some organs of rats exposed to lead. *Indian Journal of Pharmacology.*, 33:185–91.

Valko, M., Morris, H. and Cronin, M.T. 2005. Metals, toxicity and oxidative stress. *Current Medicinal Chemistry.*, 12: 1161–1208.

Wagner, B.A., Buettner, G.R. and Burns, C.P. 1996. Vitamin E slows the rate of free radical-mediated lipid peroxidation in cells. *Archives of biochemistry and biophysics.*, 334: 261–67.

Waisberg, M., Joseph, P., Hale, B. and Beyersmann, D. 2003. Molecular and cellular mechanisms of cadmium carcinogenesis. *Toxicology.*, 192: 95–117.

Wong, K.L. and Klaassen, C.D. 1982. Neurotoxic effects of cadmium in young rats. *Toxicology and AppliedPharmacology.*, 63: 330–37.

Yoshida, S. 2001. Re-evaluation of acute neurotoxic effects of Cd 2+on mesencephalic trigeminal neurons of the adult rat. *Brain Research.*, 892: 102–10.

Essential oil composition of *Marrubium vulgare* L. from Iran

Ahmad Reza Golparvar[1*], **Amin Hadipanah**[2], **Ali Mehras Mehrabi**[3], **Arezoo Armin**[1]

[1]*Department of Agronomy and Plant Breeding, College of Agriculture, Isfahan (Khorasgan) Branch, Islamic Azad University, Isfahan, Iran;*
[*]**Email: *dragolparvar@gmail.com***

[2]*Department of Horticultural, Science and Research Branch, Islamic Azad University, Tehran, Iran;*

[3]*Department of Plant Breeding, Kermanshah Branch, Islamic Azad University, Kermanshah, Iran;*

ARTICLE INFO

Topic: *Phytochemistry*

Key words:

- ✓ Marrubuim vulgare *L.*
- ✓ *Chemical constitutes*
- ✓ *GC/MS*

ABSTRACT

Background & Aim: White horehound (*Marrubium vulgare* L.) is a perennial medicinal plant of the family Lamiaceae. The aim of this study was to identify of the chemical components of white horehound collected from Isfahan.

Experimental: The aerial parts of *M. vulgare* were collected from (Kamu Mountain) Isfahan province central of Iran, during 2014. The essential oils of samples were obtained by hydro-distillation, and analyzed using gas chromatography–mass spectrometry (GC–MS).

Results & Discussion: Results of GC/MS indicated that 44 compounds were identified in the essential oil from the aerial parts of *M. vulgare*. The major constituents of the essential oil were β-caryophyllene (32.19%), (E)-β-farnesene (11.39%), 1,8-cineole (8.17%), and α-pinene (6.64%). A comparison of our results with different reports, differences in the volatile composition of the plants could be attributed to genetic (genus, species, and ecotype), chemotype, distinct environmental and climatic conditions, seasonal sampling periods, geographic origins, plant populations, vegetative plant phases, and extraction and quantification methods.

Industrial and practical recommendations: The biosynthesis of secondary metabolites, although controlled genetically, is strongly affected by the environmental influences of a particular growing region.

1. Introduction

It is a major constituent of many species of the genus *Marrubium* (Lamiaceae) and includes about 97 species found along the Mediterranean, Asia, America, and Australia and also in temperate regions. In Iran, nine of them are endemic. The plant is a perennial, C3, herbaceous plant, stems usually branched to form a rounded bushy plant (100 cm) tall. The leaves arranged opposite along stem, leaf blades broadly ovate, oval, in axils of upper leaves; flowers sessile and crowded in dense whorls. The flowers are white. Chromosome number of *M. vulgare* is polyploid (2n=34) (Mozaffarian, 2008). Extensive pharmacological studies have demonstrated that marrubiin displays a suite of activities including antinociceptive (De Jesus *et al.,* 2000), antioxidant, antigen toxic, cardioprotective (Mnonopi *et al.,* 2011), vasorelaxant (El Bardai*et al.,* 2003), gastro protective, antispasmodic (Paula de Olivera *et al.,* 2011), immunomodulating (Karioti *et* *al.,* 2003), antioedematogenic (Hellen *et al.,* 2006), analgesic (Meyre-Silva *et al.,* 2005), and antidiabetic properties (Mnonopi *et al.,* 2012). The chemical composition of plants is known to be influenced by several external factors including climate, as some compounds may be accumulated at a particular period to respond to environmental changes (Abedi *et al.,* 2015; Golparvar *et al.,* 2015).

Khanavi *et al.* (2006) showed that the major component of *M.* vulgare from other region of Iran were β-bisabolene (25.4%), β-caryophyllene (11.6%), germacrene D (9.7%) and *E*-β-farnesene (8.3%). Asadipour *et al.* (2005) found that caryophyllene oxide (18.7%), β-caryophyllene (12.8%) and germacrene D (10.0%) were the major compounds of *M. vulgare* collected from another region of Iran. Hamedeyazdan *et al.* (2013) reported that the major constituents of the *Marrubium persicum* essential oil were m-tolualdehyde (19.2%) followed by acetophenone (14.6%), germacrene D (10.5%), β-caryophyllene (7.4%), β-farnesene (6.2%), and α-pinene (4.6%). In studies (Kadri *et al.,* 2011) indicated the major constituents obtained of *M.* vulgare the essential oil were γ-eudesmol (11.93%), β-citronellol (9.90%), citronellyl formate (9.50%) and germacrene D (9.37%). The aim of this study was to identify of the chemical components of (*Marrubium vulgare* L.) from Iran.

2. Materials and Methods

2.1. Plant material

The aerial parts of the plant samples of (*Marrubium vulgare* L.) were collected from (Kamu Mountain) Isfahan province. Kamu is a city in Qamsar district, Kashan County, Isfahan province, in center Iran (33°, 36′ N and 51°, 14′ E), during 2014. The samples of the plants were identified by regional floras and authors with floristic and taxonomic references, and voucher specimens were deposited at the Herbarium of Agriculture Researches Islamic Azad University, Isfahan (Khorasgan), Iran.

2.2. Essential oil extraction

The essential oils were extracted from 100 g of ground tissue in 1 L of water contained in a 2 L flask and heated by heating jacket at 100 °C for 3 h in a Clevenger-type apparatus, according to procedures outlined in the British Pharmacopoeia. The collected essential oil was dried over anhydrous sodium sulfate and stored at 4°C ± 1°C until analyzed.

2.3. GC/MS analysis

Compositions of the essential oils were determined by GC–MS. The GC/MS analysis was carried out with an Agilent 5975 GC-MSD system. HP-5MS column (30 m x 0.25 mm, 0.25 μm film thickness) was used with helium as carrier gas with flow rate of 1.0 mL/min. The oven temperature was kept 20°C at 50°C for 4 min and programmed to 280°C at a rate of 5°C /min, and kept 20°C constant at 280°C for 5 min, at split mode. The injector temperature was at 20°C at 280°C. Transfer 20 line temperatures 280°C. MS were taken at 70 eV. Mass range was from *m/z* 35 to 450. Retention indices were calculated for all components using a homologous series of *n*-alkanes (C_5-C_{24}) injected under conditions used with the oil samples. Identification of the essential oil components was accomplished based on comparison of retention times with those of authentic standards and by comparison of their mass spectral fragmentation patterns (WILLEY/ChemStation data system) (Adams, 2007).

3. Results and discussion

The chemical constituents identified by GC-MS, are presented in Table 1. GC–MS analysis resulted in identification of 44 constituents of the oil composition. Their sum constituted the bulk of the oils and ranged from 99.89% oil. The results indicated that the major components were β-caryophyllene (32.19%), (E)-β-farnesene (11.39%), 1,8-cineole (8.17%) and α-pinene (6.64%) (Fig 1).

The biosynthesis of secondary metabolites, although controlled genetically, is strongly affected by the environmental influences of a particular growing region, and also by the agronomic conditions, harvesting time and the type of processing. In addition, for maximum oil production, long days and high light intensities are required during the maturation period (Salehi *et al.,* 2014). Monoterpenes are a large and diverse class of volatile C_{10} isoprenoids that are the major constituents of many plant essential oils and resins. These natural products play important chemo-ecological roles in the interactions of plants with their environments (Hallahan, 2000). Previous works from different countries showed that yields of *M. vulgare* dried aerial parts EO varied depending on many factors such as climatic, seasonal and geographic conditions; it's about 0.07% for Slovakia (Nagy and Svjdlenka, 1998), 0.08% for Iran (Khanavi *et al.,* 2006).

Table 2. Chemical composition of essential oils of *Marrubium vulgare* L.

Row	Compound	RI	%
1	*trans*-2-Hexanal	823	0.77
2	Heptanal	901	4.26
3	α-Thujene	931	0.22
4	α-Pinene	937	6.64
5	Camphene	945	0.36
6	Benzaldeyde	965	0.19
7	p-Cymene	1025	4.76
8	1,8-Cineole	1035	8.17
9	γ-Terpinene	1063	2.62
10	linalool	1092	0.43
11	γ-Terpineol	1189	1.39
12	Decanal	1209	0.95
13	Carvone	1219	0.64
14	Piperitone	1225	2.11
15	Eugenol	1355	2.91
16	α-Copaene	1378	0.51
17	β-Cubebene	1382	1.08
18	β-Caryophyllene	1417	32.19
19	Geranyl linalool	1439	2.58
20	(E)-β-Farnesene	1443	11.39
21	α-Humulene	1454	1.59
22	Alloaromadendrene	1474	0.97
23	Germacrene D	1479	0.41
24	β-Ionone	1482	1.16
25	ß-Guaiene	1491	0.92
26	α-Farnesene	1499	0.31
27	α-Muurolene	1503	0.23
28	β-Bisabolene	1507	0.81
29	*trans*–calamenene	1510	0.64
30	δ–Cadinene	1526	0.36
31	α-Calacorene	1529	0.37
32	Spathulenol	1573	0.24
33	Caryophyllene oxide	1579	4.06
34	Viridiflorol	1592	0.28
35	1,10-di-*epi*-cubenol	1616	0.17
36	*Epi*-α-cadinol	1643	0.25
37	β-Eudesmol	1652	0.19
38	α-Cadinol	1657	0.27
39	β-Cubebene	1674	0.18
40	Citronellylbutanoate	1682	0.39
41	α-Bisabolol	1691	0.19
42	Geranyltiglate	1712	0.18
43	Benzyl benzoate	1762	1.08
44	Cyclononasiloxane	2195	0.47
	Total		99.89

RI: Retention indices determined on HP-5MS capillary column.

Said-Al Ahl *et al.* (2015) reported that the major constituents of the *Marrubium vulgare* essential oil cultivated in Egypt were carvacrol (36.28%), β-phellandrene (15.49%), carvyl acetate (11.52%), transcaryophyllene (4.06%), linalool (3.86%), α-terpinene (3.83%), β-pinene (3.53%), trans-sabinene hydrate (3.29%), β-thujone (2.93%), 1-octen-3-ol (2.48%), 1,8-cineol (1.49%), α-Pinene (1.44%) and borneol (1.12%). Zawislak, (2012) reports that the main components of the oil of *Marrubiumvulgare* L. were E-caryophyllene (25.91–32.06%), germacrene D (20.23–31.14%) and δ-amorphene (8.38–10.22%), while in the oil of *Marrubium incanum* Desr. the following compounds were germacrene D (32.46–37.87%), E-caryophyllene (22.49–30.79%) and α-cadinol (14.36–17.87%). Morteza-Semnani and Saeedi (2004) reported that the major constituents of the essential oil of *Marrubium astracanicum* from Iran were β-bisabolene (20.4%), 8-cadinene (19.1%) and isocaryophyllene (14.1%).

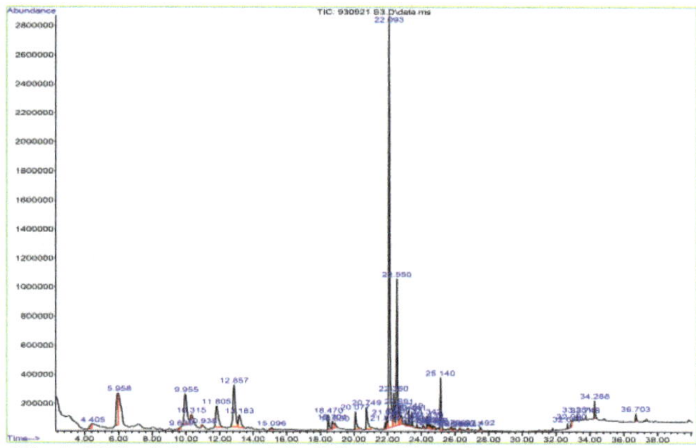

Fig 1. TIC of the essential oil from *Marrubium vulgare* L.

About the chemical composition of *M. vulgare*from different parts of the world, Saleh and Glombitza (1989) reported tricyclene, β-pinene, bisabolol, β-elemone and isomenthon-8-thiol as the main compounds of *M. vulgare*. From Libya, EL-Hawary *et al.* (2013) reported the main components of the oil of *M. vulgare*werecarvacrol, E-β-farnesene and thymol. In Algeria,Abadiand Hassani (2013) reported the main components of the oil of *M. vulgare*were 4,8,12,16-tetramethyl heptadecan-4-olid (16.97 %), germacrene D-4-ol (9.61%), α- pinene (9.37 %), phytol (4.87%), dehydro-sabina ketone (4.12 %), piperitone (3.27%), δ-cadinene (3.13%), 1-octen-3-ol (2.35%) and benzaldehyde (2.31%).

In Tunisian, Hamdaoui *et al.* (2013) reported the main components of the oil of *M. vulgare*were β-bisabolene (28.3%), (*E*)-β-farnesene (7.4%) and β-caryophyllene (7.8%). In Egypt, Salama *et al.* (2012) reported the main components of the oil of *M. vulgare* were thymol and γ-cadineneas. Nagy and Svajdlenka (1998) found that the main constituent of *M. vulgare* from Slovakia were β-caryophyllene (45.8%) and germacrene-D (14.4%). Weel *et al.* (1999) reported that (Z)-β-farnesene, β-caryophyllene, (E)-2-hexenal, α-humulene and germacrene-D were the main components of *M. vulgare* growing in Lithuania.

4. Conclusions

In conclusion, the results obtained in the study indicated that the major components of the oil of *Marrubium vulgare* L. collected from (Kamu Mountain) Isfahan provincewere β-caryophyllene, (E)-β-farnesene, 1,8-cineole and α-pinene. A comparison of our results with different reports, differences in the volatile composition of the plants could be attributed to genetic (genus, species, and ecotype), chemotype, distinct environmental and climatic conditions, seasonal sampling periods, geographic origins, plant populations, vegetative plant phases, and extraction and quantification methods.

5. Acknowledgement

This research project has been supported by Islamic Azad University, Isfahan (Khorasgan) branch, Isfahan, Iran.

6. References

Abadi, A. and Hassani, A. 2013. Essential oil composition and antioxidant activity of *Marrubium vulgare* L. growing wild in Eastern Algeria. *International Letters of Chemistry, Physics and Astronomy.*, 9(1): 17-24.

Abedi, R., Golparvar, A.R. and Hadipanah, A. 2015. Identification of the essential oils composition from four ecotypes of *Menthalongifolia* (L.) Huds. growing wild in Isfahan province, Iran. *Journal of BioScience and Biotechnology.*, 4(2): 117-121.

Adams, R.P. 2007. Identification of Essential Oil Components by Gas Chromatography/Mass Spectrometery, 4th edition (Allured Publishing Corporation, Carol Stream, IL) 456.

Asadipour, A., Mehrabani, M., Nazeri, V. and Tabarraii, M. 2005. Composition of the essential oil of *Marrubium vulgare* L. *Ulum-i-Daroei.*, 2: 77-82.

De Jesus, R.A.P., Cechinel-Filho, V., Oliveira, A.E. and Schlemper, V. 2000. Analysis of the antinociceptive properties of marrubiin isolated from *Marrubium vulgare*. *Phytomedicine.*, 7: 111–115.

El Bardai, S., Morel, N., Wibo, M., Fabre, N., Llabres, G., Lyoussi, B. and Quetin-Leclercq, J. 2003. The vasorelaxant activity of marrubenol and marrubiin from *Marrubium vulgare*. *Planta Med.*, 69: 75–77.

EL-Hawary, S., EL-Shabrawy, A., Ezzat, S. and ELShibany, F. 2013. Gas chromatography-mass spectrometry analysis, hepatoprotective and antioxidant activities of the essential oils of four Libyan herbs. *Journal of Medicinal Plants Research.*, 7(24): 1746-1753.

Golparvar, A.R., Hadipanah, A. andMehrabi, A.M. 2015. Diversity in chemical composition from two ecotypes of (*MenthaLongifolia* L.) and (*Menthaspicata* L.) in Iran climatic conditions. *Journal of Biodiversity and Environmental Sciences.*, 6(4): 26-33.

Hallahan, D.L. 2000. Monoterpenoid biosynthesis in glandular trichomes of labiate plants. *Advance Botanical Research.*, 31: 77-120.

Hamdaoui, B., AidiWannes, W., Marrakchi, M., Ben Brahim, N. and Marzouk, B. 2013. Essential Oil Composition of Two Tunisian Horehound Species: *Marrubium vulgare* L. and *Marrubium aschersonii* Magnus. *Journal of Essential Oil Bearing Plants.*, 16(5): 608–612.

Hamedeyazdan, S., Fathiazad, F. and Asnaashari, S. 2013. Chemical Composition of the Essential Oil from *Marrubium persicum* C. A. Mey. (Lamiaceae). *Pharmaceutical sciences.*, 19(2): 35-38.

Hellen, K., Stulzer, H.K., Tagliari, M.P., Zampirolo, J.A., Cechinel-Filho, V. and Schlemper, V. 2006. Antioedematogenic effect of marrubiin obtained from *Marrubium vulgare*. *J. Ethnopharmacol.*, 108: 379–384.

Kadri, A., Zarai, Z., Bekir, A., Gharsallah, N., Damak, M. and Gdoura, R. 2011. Chemical composition and antioxidant activity of *Marrubium vulgare* L.

essential oil from Tunisia. *African Journal of Biotechnology.,* 10(19): 3908-3914.

Karioti, A., Skopeliti, M., Tsitsilonis, O., Heilmann, J. and Skaltsa, H. 2007. Cytotoxicity and immunomodulating characteristics of labdanediterpenes from *Marrubium cylleneum* and *Marrubiumvelutinum. Phytochemistry*., 68, 1587–1594.

Khanavi, M., Ghasemian, L., Motlagh, E.H., Hadjiakhoondi, A. and Shafiee, A. 2006. Chemical composition of the essential oils of *Marrubium parvi florum* Fisch. & C. A. Mey. And *Marrubium vulgare*L. from Iran. *Flav. Fragr. J.,* 20: 324-326.

Meyre-Silva, C., Yunes, R.A., Schlemper, V., Campos-Buzzi, F. and Cechinel-Filho, V. 2005. Analgesic potential of marrubiin derivatives, a bioactive diterpene present in *Marrubium vulgare* (Lamiaceae). *Farmaco*., 60: 321–326.

Mnonopi, N., Levendal, R.A., Davies-Coleman, R.T. and Frost, C.L. 2011. The cardioprotective effects of marrubiin, a diterpenoid found in *Leonotis leonurus* extracts. *J. Ethnopharmacol.,* 138: 67–75.

Mnonopi, N., Levendal, R.A., Mzilikezi, N. and Frost, C.L. 2012. Marrubiin, a constituent of *Leonotus leonurus*, alleviates diabetic symptoms. *Phytomedicine.,* 19: 488–493.

Morteza-Semnani, K. and Saeedi, M. 2004. The Essential Oil Composition *of Marrubium astracanicum* Jacq. From Iran. *J. Essent. Oil Bearing Plants.,* 7: 239-242.

Mozaffarian, V. 2008. A pictorial dictionary of botany botanical taxonomy Latin-English-French-Germany-Persian. Germany: Koeltz Scientific Books. 522.

Nagy, M. and Svajdlenka, E. 1998. Comparison of Essential Oils from *Marrubium vulgare* L. and *M. peregrinum* L. *J. Essent. Oil Res.*, 10:585-587.

Paula de Olivera, A., Santin, J.R., Lemos, M., Klein, L.C.J., Couto, A.G., Bittencourt, C.M.S., Cechinel, F. and Valdir, F.A. 2011. Gastroprotective activity of methanol extract and marrubiin obtained from leaves of *Marrubium vulgare L.* (Lamiaceae). *J. Pharm. Pharmacol*., 63: 1230–1237.

Said-Al Ahl, H.A.H., Gendy, A.S.H., Mahmoud, A.A. and Mohamed, H.F.Y. 2015. Essential Oil Composition of *Marrubiumvulgare* L. Cultivated in Egypt. *International Journal of Plant Research.,* 1 (4): 138-141.

Salama, M.M., Taher, E. E. and El-Bahy, M.M. 2012. Molluscicidal and mosquitocidal activities of the essential oils of *Thymus capitatus* HOFF. ET LINK. And *Marrubium vulgare* L. Rev. *Inst. Med. Trop. Sao Paulo.,* 54(5): 281-286.

Saleh, M.M. and Glombitza, K.W. 1989. Volatile Oil of *Marrubium vulgare* and its Anti-schistosomal Activity. *Planta Med.,* 55:105-108.

Salehi, S., Golparvar, A.R. and Hadipanah, A. 2014. Effect of harvest time on yield and quality of *Thymus vulgaris* L. essential oil in Isfahan province, Iran. *Agriculturae Conspectus Scientificus.,* 79(2): 115-118.

Weel, K.C.G., Venskutonis, P.R., Pukalskas, A., Gruzdiene, D. and Linssen, J.P.H. 1999. Antioxidant activity of horehound (*Marrubium vulgare*) grown in Lithuania. *Fett/Lipid.,* 101(10): 395-400.

Zawislak, G. 2012. Chemical composition of essential oils of *Marrubium vulgare* L. and *Marrubium incanum* Desr. grown in Poland. *Chemija.,* 23(2): 136–140.

10

Effects of Jasmonic acid on essential oil yield and chemical compositions of two Iranian landraces of basil (*Ocimum basilicum*) under reduced irrigation

Fatemeh Malekpoor[1*], Azam Salimi[1], Abdollah Ghasemi Pirbalouti[2,3]

[1]*Department of Plant Biology, Faculty of Biology Science, Kharazmi University, 15719-14911, Tehran, Iran;*

[*]**Email:** fmalekpoor87@yahoo.com or std_fmalekpoor@khu.ac.ir

[2]*Medicinal Plants Department, Shahrekord Branch, Islamic Azad University, Shahrekord, 88146, Iran;*

[3]*Medicinal Plants Program, College of Natural Sciences, Massachusetts University, Amherst, 01003, MA, USA;*

ARTICLE INFO

Topic: *Physiology of Medicinal Plants*

Key words:

- ✓ Ocimum basilicum *L.*
- ✓ *Jasmonic acid*
- ✓ *Secondary metabolites*
- ✓ *Reduced irrigation*

ABSTRACT

Background & Aim: Sweet basil (*Ocimum basilicum)*, a plant that is extensively cultivated in some countries, is used to enhance the flavour of salads, sauces, pasta, confectioneries and other products as both a fresh and dried herb. The effect of foliar application of Jasmonic acid and reduced irrigation on essential oil yield and chemical components of two Iranian landrace of basil (*Ocimum basilicum*) were investigated.

Experimental: Treatments comprised control, 0.0, 200, and 400 μL Jasmonic acid applied to plants under normal irrigation and stressed conditions (30 and 60% F.C) based on a completely randomized design with three replications. The essential oils from the aerial parts of basil were analyzed by GC-FID and GC/MS.

Results & Discussion: Results indicated that the different levels of Jasmonic acid and irrigation had significant effects on oil yield and some main components of the essential oil. The highest value of oil content was obtained from application of 400 μL JA. Percentage of some chemical constituents in the essential oil extracted from the plants under stress was higher than non-stressed plants. Foliar application of Jasmonic acid significantly improved methyl chavicol in the oils, but reduced Germacrene- D, α-Cadinol and δ-Cadinene amounts.

Industrial and practical recommendations: Since, essential oil of basil, particularly methyl chavicol component, have many application in pharmaceutical and perfumery industry and has health benefits such as antiviral, antibacterial and antispasmodic activity, we can use Jasmonic acid elicitor to enhance the therapeutic properties of basil and also essential oil content and methyl chavicol of plant.

1. Introduction

Ocimum basilicum L. belongs to the family Lamiaceae is an herb that is extensively cultivated in some countries. Arial parts, especially leaves of sweet basil are widely used to enhance the flavour of foods such as salads, pasta, tomato products, vegetables, pizza, meat, soups, marine foods, confectioneries and other products (Ghasemi Pirbalouti, 2014). Traditionally basil has been used as a medicinal plant in the treatment of headaches, coughs, diarrhea, constipation, warts, worms, and kidney malfunctions (Ghasemi Pirbalouti, 2014; Simon *et al.,* 1984). In Iranian traditional medicine, the aerial parts of the plant are perceived as a carminative, galactogogue, stomachic, and antispasmodic (Sajjadi, 2006). Moreover, basil possesses a range of biological properties, including action as an insect repellent and nematocide (Deshpande and Tipnis, 1997), having antibacterial (Hussain *et al.,* 2008), antiviral (Chiang *et al.,* 2005), antifungal activity (Hussain *et al.,* 2008), and antioxidant properties (Kwee and Niemeyer, 2011). Methyl chavicol, methyl cinnamate, methyl eugenol, citral, and linalool are generally the main chemotypes in sweet basil. Investigations (Sajjadi, 2006) on the chemical composition of the essential oil of basil, have demonstrated considerable variability.

In recent years, scientists have been looking for new alternatives to conventional methods for plant protection, and simultaneously for improvements in health properties and bioactive compound content. One of these methods is elicitation, which is induction of natural plant resistance mechanisms using biotic or abiotic factors. Elicitation can be an important strategy towards obtaining improved production of plant secondary metabolites *in vivo* (Hussain *et al.,* 2012). There are several commercially available chemical compounds that could be used as elicitors to modify plant secondary metabolites and subsequently the bioactivity of medicinal plants (Ghasemi Pirbalouti, *et al.,* 2014).

It has been reported that plant hormonal chemicals such as jasmonic acid (JA) and methyl jasmonate (MeJA), can used as elicitors (Rabea *et al.,* 2003). Endogenous JA is a signaling compound that modulates various physiological processes in plants (Wasternack and Parthier, 1997). Therefore, exogenous JA has been used to induce useful secondary metabolites such as alkaloids, terpenoids, and phenolics in some plants such as *Nicotina* species, *Hyoscyamus muticus*, Norway spruce stems, and some plant cell cultures (Halitschke *et al.,* 2000; Keina *et al.,* 2001; Martin *et al.,* 2002). The increased amounts of secondary metabolites increase not only plants' disease resistance but also their market values regarding the increased health benefits. Moreover, environmental factors such as moisture deficit are known to play an important role in the synthesis of secondary metabolites in plants (Ghasemi Pirbalouti *et al.,* 2015). A lot of researches (Khalid, 2006; Bettaieb, *et al*., 2009; Ghasemi Pirbalouti *et al.,* 2013) showed the effect of water stress on secondary metabolites such as essential oils in different plant species. The present study was performed to evaluate the effect of various concentrations of Jasmonic acid on essential oil yield and essential oil composition two landraces of basil (*Ocimum basilicum* L.) under water deficit.

2. Materials and Methods

2.1. Plant material and experimental site description

Plastic pots were filled with clay loam at a pH of 7.23, containing 0.8% organic matter comprised of 0.01% total N, 11.20 mg/kg available phosphorus, 694 mg/kg available potassium, and a saline value measured at E.C.: 1.35 dS/m.

Two Iranian landraces of sweet basil (*Ocimum basilicum* L.) seeds were obtained the Pakan Seed Company, Isfahan, Iran. In May 2014, pots transferred to the filed in Shahrekord (latitude 32° 20′ N, longitude 50° 51′ E, altitude 2061 m above sea level), southwestern Iran.

Type of study area climate by Emberger's climatology method is cold and semiarid and semi humid with temperate summer and very cold winter by Karimi's climatology method (IRIMO, 2012). In this study, no inorganic fertilizer and systemic pesticide was used during the entire experiment, and weed control was done manually.

2.2. Experimental design and treatments

Treatments included three irrigation regimes, viz., I_1 (unstressed or control), I_2 (irrigation in 70% field capacity when 30% of maximum total available soil water was depleted in the upper 30 cm of the soil profile), I_3 (irrigation in 40% field capacity when 60% of maximum total available soil water was depleted in the upper 30 cm of the soil profile) and three Jasmonic acid treatments (0.0, 200 and 400 μl) sprayed thrice at 10-12 leaves, before flowering, and two weeks later. Jasmonic acid was dissolved in ethanol 80%, diluted in distilled water with various concentrations. These solutions were sprayed at dew point (approximately 100 ml per plant) with a hand sprayer (untreated control plants were sprayed with an equivalent volume of distilled water). The aerial parts of basil were collected after third spray of Jasmonic acid in July 2014.

2.3. Essential oil isolation

Dried plant material (100 g) was powdered and subjected to hydro–distillation for three hours using a Clevenger–type apparatus (British Pharmacopoeia, 1988). The essential oils were dried with anhydrous sodium sulphate and kept in amber vials at 4 °C prior to use.

2.4. Identification of the oil constituents

Composition of the essential oils was determined by gas chromatography (GC) and mass spectrophotometry (GC/MS). The GC analysis was done on an Agilent Technologies 7890 GC (Agilent Technologies, Santa Clara, CA) equipped with a single injector and a flame ionization detector (FID). A polar HP Innowax column and an apolar HP-5 capillary column (30 m x 0.25 mm, 0.25 µm film thicknesses) coated with 5% phenyl, 95% methyl polysiloxane were used. The flow of the carrier gas (N2) was 0.8 ml/min. Initial column temperature was 60°C and programmed to increase at 4°C/min to 280°C. The injector temperature was set at 280 and 300°C. Split injection was conducted with a ratio split of 1:40. Essential oil samples of 0.1 µL were injected neat (directly).

GC-MS analyses of aromatic oil samples were performed on an Agilent Technologies 7890 gas chromatograph coupled to Agilent 5975 C mass selective detector (MSD) and quadrupole EI mass analyzer (Agilent Technologies, Palo Alto, CA, USA). A HP–5MS 5% column (coated with methyl silicone) (30 m x 0.25 mm, 0.25 µm film thicknesses) was used as the stationary phase. Helium was used as the carrier gas at 0.8 mL/min flow rate. The temperature was programmed from 60 to 280°C at 4°C/min ramp rate. The injector and the GC-MS interface temperatures were maintained at 290°C and 300°C, respectively. Mass spectra were recorded at 70 eV. Mass range was from *m/z* 50-550. The ion source and the detector temperatures were maintained at 250 and 150°C, respectively.

Oil constituents were identified based on their retention indices (determined with reference to homologous series of C5-C24 *n*-alkanes), by comparison of their mass spectra with those reported in the literature (Adams, 2007) and stored in NIST 08 (National Institute of Standards and Technology) and Willey (ChemStation data system) libraries. The peak area percentages were computed from HP-5 column without the use of FID response factors.

2.5. Statistical analysis

Simple and interaction effects of experimental factors were derived from two-way analysis of variance (ANOVA) based on the GLM procedure of the SAS statistical package (SAS/STAT® v.9.2. SAS Institute Inc., Cary, NC).

The assumptions of variance analysis were tested by ensuring that the residuals were random and homogenous, with a normal distribution about a zero mean. The significance of differences among treatment means was tested using Duncan's multiple range test (DMRT) at $p \leq 0.05$.

3. Results and discussion

3.1. Essential oil yield

All essential oils extracted from the aerial parts of two landraces of basil under different treatments were clear and yellow liquid. An analysis of variance indicated that different irrigation regimes had a significant effect on oil yield of basil ($p \leq 0.01$) (Table 1). The highest oil yield was obtained from mild drought stress treatment (I_3) with 0.82 ml/100 g dry material (Table 1). Our results indicated that Jasmonic acid at 400 µl produced maximum oil content (0.53 ml/100 g) (Table 1). It has been demonstrated that signal molecules such as Jasmonic acid are very potential elicitors for induction of plant secondary metabolites (Zhao *et al.,* 2005). Recent years, the applications of signal components as elicitors have evolved an effective strategy for the production of target secondary metabolites in plant. Foliar application of Jasmonic acid on oil content of basil was influenced ($p \leq 0.01$) by irrigation regime (Table 2). The highest oil yield (0.89 ml/100 g) was achieved by foliar spray of 400 µL Jasmonic acid under reduced irrigation or mild stress drought (I3 × J4) (Table 2). The lowest oil content was obtained when Jasmonic acid was applied under normal irrigation (Table 2).

There was significant jasmonic acid × landrace interaction effect on oil content (Table 3). In this study, landrace × irrigation had significant effects on oil content ($p \leq 0.01$) (Table 4).

Table 1. The effects of irrigation regime, jasmonic acid and landrace on the essential oil from basil

Treatments	Oil yield (ml/100 g)	1,8-Cineole	Linalool	Methyl chavicol	Nerol	Neral	Geranial	β-Caryophyllene	α-Humulene	Germacrene-D	δ-Cadinene	Caryophyllene oxide	α-Cadinol
Irrigation													
I1 (control)	0.183c	1.120b	4.39	33.24a	1.44b	6.30	7.10	4.82	3.12ab	2.98a	1.79a	1.854b	5.92a
I2 (60% FC)	0.488b	1.349a	4.41	34.71ab	1.77a	5.93	6.93	4.55	2.88b	2.66b	1.59b	1.79b	4.79b
I3 (30% FC)	**0.822a**	1.478a	4.62	35.67a	1.51b	5.74	6.82	4.99	3.16a	2.43b	1.41c	2.24a	5.42a
ANOVA	$p \leq 0.01$	$p \leq 0.01$	*ns*	$p \leq 0.05$	$p \leq 0.01$	*ns*	*ns*	*ns*	$p \leq 0.05$	$p \leq 0.01$	$p \leq 0.01$	$p \leq 0.01$	$p \leq 0.01$
Jasmonic acid													
J1 (control)	0.471c	1.317a	4.44a	34.55ab	1.63ab	6.39a	7.36a	0.49ab	0.99a	4.98a	3.35a	2.70ab	1.68ab
J2 (ethanol)	0.467d	1.316a	4.23a	32.91b	1.51b	5.81ab	6.65a	0.50a	1.09a	5.15a	3.18ab	2.89a	1.78a
J3 (200)	0.518b	1.251a	4.48a	34.41ab	1.79a	6.26ab	7.27a	0.44b	0.99a	4.88a	2.98bc	2.66ab	1.54bc
J4 (400)	**0.535a**	1.378a	4.74a	36.29a	1.28c	5.50b	6.51a	0.45ab	0.98a	4.14b	2.71c	2.51b	1.39c
ANOVA	$P \leq 0.01$	*ns*	*ns*	$P \leq 0.05$	$P \leq 0.01$	*ns*	*ns*	*ns*	*ns*	$P \leq 0.01$	$P \leq 0.01$	*ns*	$P \leq 0.01$
Landraces													
S1 (Green)	0.71a	0.321b	1.50b	28.10b	2.84a	10.83a	12.64a	6.86a	3.79a	2.65	0.32b	2.85a	2.12b
S2 (Purple)	0.285b	2.31a	7.45a	40.98a	0.27b	1.14b	1.25b	2.71b	2.33b	2.73	2.87a	1.06b	8.64a
ANOVA	$p \leq 0.01$	$p \leq 0.01$	$p \leq 0.01$	$p \leq 0.01$	$p \leq 0.01$	$p \leq 0.01$	$p \leq 0.01$	$p \leq 0.01$	$p \leq 0.01$	*ns*	$p \leq 0.01$	$p \leq 0.01$	$p \leq 0.01$

ns: non-significant

Table 2. The interaction effects of irrigation regime × jasmonic acid on the essential oil from basil

Interaction effect	Oil yield	1,8-Cineole	Linalool	Methyl chavicol	Nerol	Neral	Geranial	β-Caryophyllene	α-Humulene	Germacrene-D	δ-Cadinene	Caryophyllene oxide	α-Cadinol
I1 × J1	0.175i	1.00cd	3.84c	29.34e	1.46cd	6.28ab	6.88ab	5.56a	3.52a	3.47a	2.31a	2.15ab	7.28a
I1 × J2	0.175i	1.22bc	4.72abc	34.63bcd	1.42cde	6.33ab	7.11ab	5.03ab	3.30abc	2.86bc	1.76bc	1.94a-d	6.02b
I1 × J3	0.179i	0.80d	3.94bc	35.21bcd	1.44cde	6.35ab	7.24ab	4.77abc	3.05abcde	2.96b	1.52cdef	1.84bcde	4.94bcd
I1 × J4	0.204h	1.44ab	5.06a	33.79bcd	1.44cd	6.23ab	7.16ab	3.94cd	2.61ef	2.63bcd	1.58cde	1.43e	5.44bc
I2 × J1	0.450g	1.42ab	4.36abc	32.09de	1.70abc	5.64ab	6.59ab	4.62bcd	2.80-f	2.70bcd	1.60cd	1.56cde	4.81cd
I2 × J2	0.462f	1.19bc	3.88bc	32.12de	1.87ab	6.76a	7.90a	4.82abc	3.35abc	2.88bc	1.76bc	2.04abc	4.95bcd
I2 × J3	0.525d	1.33abc	4.69abc	34.85bcd	1.95ab	6.09ab	7.24ab	4.91ab	2.89c-f	2.55bcd	1.53cdef	2.08ab	5.31bc
I2 × J4	0.513e	1.44ab	4.70abc	39.80a	1.32de	5.21b	5.99b	3.85d	2.51f	2.52bcd	1.32ef	1.50de	4.08d
I3 × J1	0.775c	1.51ab	4.49abc	37.30ab	1.36cde	5.50ab	6.47ab	5.28ab	3.22a-d	2.51bcd	1.43def	2.40a	5.56bc
I3 × J2	0.775c	1.53ab	4.73abc	36.91abc	1.61bcd	6.07ab	7.07ab	5.08ab	3.42ab	2.37d	1.38def	2.26a	5.37bc
I3 × J3	0.850b	1.60a	4.81ab	33.15cde	1.99a	6.32ab	7.32ab	4.96ab	3.01b-e	2.47cd	1.57cde	1.96a-d	5.46bc
I3 × J4	**0.888a**	1.25bc	4.45abc	35.29bcd	1.08e	5.05b	6.39ab	4.65bcd	3.01b-e	2.38d	1.26f	2.36a	5.31bc
ANOVA	$p \leq 0.01$	$p \leq 0.01$	*ns*	$p \leq 0.01$	$p \leq 0.05$	*ns*	*ns*	*ns*	*ns*	*ns*	$p \leq 0.05$	$p \leq 0.05$	$p \leq 0.05$

Table 3. The interaction effects of jasmonic acid × landrace on the essential oil from basil.

Interaction effect	Oil yield	1,8-Cineole	Linalool	Methyl chavicol	Nerol	Neral	Geranial	β-Caryophyllene	α-Humulene	Germacrene-D	δ-Cadinene	Caryophyllene oxide	α-Cadinol
J1 × S1	0.683c	0.25b	1.20c	28.92d	2.74b	10.46a	12.07a	7.33a	3.96a	2.81ab	0.33d	2.94a	2.22c
J1 × S2	0.250g	2.38a	7.26a	36.90c	0.27d	1.15b	1.23b	2.98c	2.40d	2.98a	3.24a	1.14bc	9.54a
J2 × S1	0.683c	0.24b	1.24c	28.37d	2.94b	11.46a	13.26a	7.08a	3.82ab	2.79ab	0.31d	2.80a	2.12c
J2 × S2	0.258f	2.39a	7.65a	40.73b	0.32d	1.31b	1.46b	2.87cd	2.89c	2.62ab	3.05a	1.36b	8.77ab
J3× S1	0.733b	0.31b	1.55bc	28.95d	3.26a	10.99a	12.87a	6.93a	3.80ab	2.50b	0.32d	2.93a	2.11c
J3 × S2	0.303e	2.19a	7.40a	39.86bc	0.33d	1.52b	1.67b	2.83cd	2.17de	2.81ab	2.75b	0.99bc	8.36b
J4× S1	**0.742a**	0.47b	2.00b	26.15d	2.42c	10.41a	12.37a	6.11b	3.56b	2.51b	0.31d	2.74a	2.01c
J4 × S2	0.328d	2.27a	7.47a	46.43a	0.14d	0.59b	0.65b	2.17d	1.85e	2.50b	2.46c	0.78c	7.87b
ANOVA	$p \leq 0.01$	*ns*	*ns*	$p \leq 0.01$	$p \leq 0.05$	*ns*	*ns*	*ns*	$p \leq 0.05$	*ns*	$p \leq 0.01$	*ns*	*ns*

Table 4. The interaction effects of irrigation regime × landrace on the essential oil from basil.

Interaction effect	Oil yield	1,8-Cineole	Linalool	Methyl chavicol	Nerol	Neral	Geranial	β-Caryophyllene	α-Humulene	Germacrene-D	δ-Cadinene	Caryophyllene oxide	α-Cadinol
I1 × S1	0.225d	0.37d	1.72c	27.71cd	2.72b	11.35a	12.98a	6.65b	3.71b	2.75b	0.31d	2.67b	2.22cd
I1 × S2	0.142e	1.86c	7.05b	38.77b	0.16c	1.25b	1.22b	3.00c	2.54c	3.21a	3.28a	1.01c	9.62a
I2 × S1	0.750b	0.29d	1.52c	30.37c	3.06a	10.49a	12.22a	6.33b	3.45b	2.73b	0.35d	2.37b	1.54d
I2 × S2	0.225d	2.40b	7.29b	39.05b	0.36c	1.36e	1.63b	2.77c	2.32cd	2.60bc	2.83b	1.22c	8.04b
I3 × S1	**1.15a**	0.29d	1.25c	26.21d	2.74b	10.65a	12.72a	7.61a	4.20a	2.48bc	0.30d	3.52a	2.59c
I3 × S2	0.488c	2.66a	1.99a	45.12a	0.28c	0.82b	0.91b	2.37c	2.13d	2.38c	2.52c	0.96c	8.26b
ANOVA	$p \leq 0.01$	$p \leq 0.01$	$p \leq 0.01$	$p \leq 0.01$	*ns*	*ns*	*ns*	$p \leq 0.01$	$p \leq 0.01$	$p \leq 0.05$	$p \leq 0.01$	$p \leq 0.01$	$p \leq 0.05$

Table 5. The interaction effects of irrigation regime × .jasmonic acid × landrace on the essential oil from basil.

Interaction effect	Oil yield	1,8-Cineole	Linalool	Methyl chavicol	Nerol	Neral	Geranial	β-Caryophyllene	α-Humulene	Germacrene-D	δ-Cadinene	Caryophyllene oxide	α-Cadinol
I1 × J1 × S1	0.225k	0.34h	1.32fg	23.70jk	2.74cde	11.28abc	12.65a-d	7.71ab	4.13ab	3.19abc	0.33g	2.98bcd	1.92fgh
I1 × J1 × S2	0.125n	1.67fg	6.35de	34.99de	0.17gh	1.28de	1.12e	3.40gh	2.91efg	3.75a	4.30a	1.33gh	12.63a
I1 × J2 × S1	0.225k	0.40h	1.63fg	27.23g-j	2.64cde	11.48ab	13.07a-d	7.07a-d	3.85a-d	2.89b-f	0.31g	2.79cde	2.12gh
I1 × J2 × S2	0.125n	2.04ef	7.80abc	42.03bc	0.20gh	1.18de	1.15e	3.00g-j	2.77fgh	2.83b-f	3.21bc	1.09hi	9.93b
I1 × J3 × S1	0.0200l	0.21h	1.95fg	33.15def	2.60de	10.34abc	12.04a-d	5.78ef	3.42c-f	2.61c-f	0.32g	2.57c-f	2.87g
I1 × J3 × S2	0.158m	1.39g	5.92e	37.28cd	0.27gh	2.37d	2.44e	3.76g	2.69ghi	3.31ab	2.72de	1.11hi	7.01e
I1 × J4 × S1	0.250j	0.52h	1.98fg	26.78h-k	2.88bcd	12.32a	14.16ab	6.05def	3.44c-f	2.32def	0.29g	2.33def	1.98fgh
I1 × J4 × S2	0.158m	2.35cde	8.13ab	40.79bc	0.01h	0.15e	0.16e	1.82j	1.77k	2.95b-e	2.88cd	0.53i	8.89bcd
I2 × J1 × S1	0.700f	0.15h	1.11fg	32.80de	3.13bc	10.26abc	11.91a-d	6.44c-f	3.42c-f	2.81b-f	0.33g	2.08f	1.73fgh
I2 × J1 × S2	0.200l	2.68a-d	7.62a-d	31.38e-h	0.28gh	10.03de	1.26e	2.79g-j	2.17h-k	2.60c-f	2.88cd	1.04hi	7.89cde
I2 × J2 × S1	0.700f	0.12h	0.99g	29.51e-i	3.31ab	11.73ab	13.64abc	6.52b-f	3.46b-e	2.96bcd	0.31g	2.10ef	1.56gh
I2 × J2 × S2	0.225g	2.26de	6.77cde	34.72de	0.43gh	1.78de	2.15e	3.11ghi	3.23d-g	2.80b-f	3.49b	1.98fg	8.33b-e
I2 × J3 × S1	0.850d	0.42h	1.58ab	38.83f-j	3.34ab	10.25abc	12.21a-d	7.04a-e	3.71a-d	2.39def	0.37g	3.12abc	2.09fgh
I2 × J3 × S2	0.200l	2.25de	7.79abc	40.88bc	0.56g	1.93de	2.27e	2.77g-j	2.07ijk	2.71b-f	2.69de	1.03hi	8.53b-e
I2 × J4 × S1	0.750e	0.47h	2.41f	30.36e-i	2.47de	9.71bc	11.13d	5.30f	3.22d-g	2.76b	0.38g	2.18ef	0.77h
I2 × J4 × S2	0.275i	2.41b-e	6.99b-e	49.23a	0.16gh	0.71de	0.85e	2.40hij	1.80k	2.28ef	2.25f	0.81hi	7.39de
I3 × J1 × S1	1.125c	0.24h	1.16fg	30.27e-i	2.36ef	9.85bc	11.64cd	7.83a	4.32a	2.42def	0.33g	3.76a	3.02fg
I3 × J1 × S2	0.425h	2.79abc	7.82abc	44.34ab	0.36gh	1.15de	1.31e	2.73g-j	2.12h-k	2.59c-f	2.53def	1.04hi	8.09cde
I3 × J2 × S1	1.125c	0.20h	1.10g	28.38f-j	2.87bcd	11.17abc	13.06a-d	7.65abc	4.17a	2.51c-f	0.31g	3.52ab	2.67fg
I3 × J2 × S2	0.425h	2.86ab	8.36a	45.44ab	0.35gh	0.97de	1.09e	2.50g-j	2.66g-j	2.23f	2.45ef	0.99hi	8.06cde
I3 × J3 × S1	1.150b	0.29h	1.12fg	24.87ijk	3.82a	12.38a	14.35a	7.96a	4.28a	2.52cdef	0.28g	3.09abc	1.37gh
I3 × J3 × S2	0.550g	2.92a	8.49a	41.44bc	0.17gh	0.26de	0.30e	1.95ij	1.74k	2.42def	2.86cd	0.82hi	9.54bc
I3 × J4 × S1	**1.225a**	0.43h	1.61fg	21.32k	1.92f	9.19c	11.84bcd	6.99a-e	4.03abc	2.46def	0.27g	3.72a	3.28f
I3 × J4 × S2	0.550g	2.06ef	7.29a-d	**49.27a**	0.24gh	0.91de	0.94e	2.30hij	1.99jk	2.29def	2.24f	0.99hi	7.34de
ANOVA	$p \leq 0.01$	$p \leq 0.05$	$p \leq 0.05$	$p \leq 0.01$	$p \leq 0.01$	$p \leq 0.05$	$p \leq 0.01$	*ns*	*ns*	*ns*	$p \leq 0.01$	$p \leq 0.05$	$p \leq 0.01$

The highest oil yield was observed in the green landrace of basil under reduced irrigation or mild stress drought (Table 4). In this study, jasmonic acid × irrigation × landrace had significant effects ($p \leq 0.01$) on oil yield (Table 5). The highest oil yield (1.22 ml / 100 g dry weight) was achieved by foliar spray of jasmonic at 400 µl under reduced irrigation in the green landrace of basil (Table 5).

Similarly, Simon *et al.* (1992) reported that water stress increased essential oil accumulation via higher density of oil glands due to the reduction in leaf area. Moreover, Shokrani *et al.* (2012) reported an increase in essential oil content and yield in basil with increasing water stress severity and higher yield of essential oil obtained from mild water stress. In general, moisture deficit increases the essential oil content of more medicinal and aromatic plants, because in case of stress, more metabolites are produced in the plants and substances prevent from oxidization in the cells. Essential oil helps to plant that easier adopt to the environmental stress conditions. In addition, stress induced alterations in oil accumulation are considered to be mainly due to its effect on plant growth and differentiation, due to the fact that plants produce high terpene concentrations under water deficit conditions due to a low allocation of carbon to the growth, suggesting a trade-off between growth and defense (Turtola *et al.,* 2003). Probably, improvement in oil yield by exogenous application of Jasmonic acid might be due to the increase in cycle growth, nutrients uptake or changes in leaf oil gland population and monoterpenes biosynthesis (Ghasemi Pirbalouti *et al.*, 2014). Boonlertnirun *et al.* (2008) found that foliar application of elicitor had a significant effect on the growth, and yield of drought-stressed rice plants compared to control plants.

3.2. Chemical compositions of oil

The chemical constituents of the essential oil identified by GC-FID and GC/MS. Tables 1-5 show the effect of different treatments on the chemical composition of essential oil extracted from two landraces of basil. The major components in the essential oil were methyl chavicol, gernial, neral, and β-caryophyllene (Table 1). Our results demonstrated that the essential oils obtained from the landraces of basil contained phenylpropanoids (methyl chavicol), oxygenated monoterpenes (linalool, gernial, and neral), sesquiterpenes hydrocarbons (β-caryophyllene), and oxygenated sesquiterpenes (α-cadinol), confirming earlier reports that major chemical groups obtained from the aerial parts of basil were phenylpropanoids and oxygenated monoterpenes (Sajjadi, 2006; Ghasemi Pirbalouti *et al.*, 2013; Ghasemi Pirbalouti, 2014).

An analysis of variance indicated that the different factors had a significant effect on some major constituents of the essential oil from basil. Results also indicated that there were significant differences between Jasmonic acid, and landraces treatments in term methyl chavicol (Table 1). Results of mean comparison revealed that amount of methyl chavicol, as a main compound in the basil oil, not considerably affected by drought levels (Table 1). Different levels of the foliar application of Jasmonic acid had significant effects on the major constitutes of the essential oils (Table 1). This demonstrated that Jasmonic acid at 400 µL produced the highest levels of methyl chavicol (36.29%), linalool (4.74%), and 1,8-Cineole (1.37%), but at 200µL produced the highest levels of nerol (1.79%), geraniol (0.94%) (Table 1).

Results of interaction effects of irrigation × Jasmonic acid indicated that the highest contents of some main components were obtained from the application of Jasmonic acid under reduced irrigation (Table 2). Our results further indicated that foliar application of Jasmonic acid reduced the effect of water deficit stress on amounts of linalool, methyl chavicol, and geranial, the major compounds in the essential oil from the landraces of basil (Table 2). Jasmonic acid may play an important signaling role in the activation of various plant defense responses, such as the biosynthesis of special secondary metabolites.

In present research, the ANOVA showed that interaction effects of landrace × jasmonic acid had significant effects on the major constitutes of basil essential oils (Table 3). In addition, interaction effects of irrigation × landrace had significant effects on many volatile constituents (Table 4). Morevere, interaction effects of jasmonic acid × irrigation × landrace had significant effects on many volatile constituents (Table 5). The maximum amount of methyl chavicol (49.27%) was obtained by 400 µl jasmonic acid in the purple landrace under mild drought stress.

4. Conclusions

In this research, effects of foliar application of jasmonic acid and drought stress on yield and chemical composition of essential oils of two landraces of basil have evaluated. The investigation showed two landraces of basil are sensitive to the application of elicitors such as jasmonic acid and water deficit. The results revealed that essential oil yield two landraces of basil increased with application of elicitors under drought stress. Not only oil ratio but also oil composition was affected since some components were increased and other components were decreased. Finally, it could be concluded that foliar application of jasmonic acid and deficit irrigation, as a possible technique, can be used to increase volatile oil ratio in basil cultivation. This study provides the basis for further research on improving the quality and pro-health functional value of two landraces of basil using elicitors.

5. References

Adams, R.P. 2007. Identification of essential oil components by gas chromatog-raphy/quadrupole mass spectroscopy. Allured Publishing Corporation, CarolStream, IL, USA.

Bettaieb, I., Zakhama, N., Wannes, W.A., Kchouk, M. E., Marzouk, B. 2009. Water deficit effects on *Salvia officinalis* fatty acids and essential oils composition. *Scientia Horticulturae,* 120: 271–275.

Boonlertnirun, S., Boonraung, C., Suvanasara, R. 2008. Application of chitosan in Rice production. *International Journal of Minerals, Metallurgy, and Materials,* 18: 47–52.

British Pharmacopoeia, 1988. British Pharmacopoeia, vol. 2. HMSO, London, pp.137–138.

Chiang, L.C., Ng, L.T., Cheng, P.W., Chiang, W., Lin, C.C. 2005. Antiviral activities of extracts and selected pure constituents of *Ocimum basilicum. Clinical and Experimental Pharmacology and Physiology*, 32(10): 811–816.

Deshpande, R.S., Tipnis, H.P. 1997. Insecticidal activity of *Ocimum basilicum* L. *Pesticides*, 11, 1–12.

Ghasemi Pirbalouti, A., Samani, M.R., Hashemi, M., Zeinali, H. 2013. Salicylic acid affects growth, essential oil and chemical compositions of thyme (*Thymus daenensis* Celak.) under reduced irrigation. *Plant Growth Regulation*, 72: 289–301.

Ghasemi Pirbalouti, A. 2014. Diversity in chemical composition and yield of essential oil from two Iranian landraces of sweet basil. *Genetika*, 46: 419–426.

Ghasemi Pirbalouti, A., Sajjadi, S.E., Parang, K. 2014. A review (research and patents) on jasmonic acid and its derivatives. *Archiv der Pharmazie*, 347: 229–239.

Ghasemi Pirbalouti, A., Ghahfarokhi, B., Ghahfarokhi, S.A.M., Malekpoor, F. 2015. Chemical composition of essential oils from the aerial parts and underground parts of Iranian valerian collected from different natural habitats. *Industrial Crops and Products,* 63: 147–151.

Halitschke, R., Kessler, A., Kahl, J., Lornez, A., Baldwin, I.T. 2000. Ecophysiological comparison of direct and indirect defenses in Nicotiana attenuata. *Oecologia*, 124: 408–417.

Hussain, A.I., Anwar, F., Hussain Sherazi, S.T., Przybylski, R. 2008. Chemical composition, antioxidant and antimicrobial activities of basil (*Ocimum basilicum*) essential oils depends on seasonal variations. *Food Chemistry*, 108(3): 986–995.

Hussain, S., Fareed, S., Ansari, S., Rahman, A., Ahmad, I.Z., Saeed, M. 2012. Current approaches toward production of secondary plant metabolites. *Journal of Pharmacy and Bioallied Sciences*, 4: 10–20.

IRIMO, 2012. (Islamic Republic of Iran Meteorological Organization). Climatology methods. http://www.irimo.ir.

Keina, M., Oldham, N., Baldwin, I.T. 2001. Rapid HPLC screening of jasmonate-induced increases in tobacco alkaloids, phenolics, and diterpene glycosides in *Nicotiana attenuate*. *Journal of Agricultural and Food Chemistry*, 49: 3553–3558.

Khalid, K.A. 2006. Influence of water stress on growth, essential oil and chemical composition of herbs (*Ocimum sp.*). *International Agrophysics*, 20: 289–296.

Kwee, E.M., Niemeyer, E.D. 2011. Variations in phenolic composition and antioxidant properties among 15 basil (*Ocimum basilicum* L.) cultivars. *Food Chemistry*, 128(4): 1044–1050.

Martin, D., Tholl, D., Gershenzon, J., Bohlmann, J. 2002. Methyl jasmonate induces traumatic resin ducts, terpenoid resin biosysthesis, and terpenoid accumulation in developing xylem of Norway spruce stems. Plant Physiology, 129: 1003-1018.

Rabea, E.I., Badawy, M.E., Stevens, C., Smagghe, G., Steurbaut, W. 2003. Chitosan as antimicrobial agent: applications and mode of action. *Biomacromolecules*, 4: 1457–1465.

Sajjadi, S.E. 2006. Analysis of the essential oils of two cultivated basil *(Ocimum basilicum* L.) From Iran. *DARU Journal of Pharmaceutical Sciences,* 14: 128–130.

Shokrani, F., Pirzad, A., Zardoshti, M., Darvishzadeh, R. 2012. Effect of biological nitrogen on the yield of dried flower and essential oil of *Calendula officinalis* L. under end season water deficit condition. *International Research Journal of Applied and Basic Sciences,* 3: 24–34.

Simon, J.E., Reiss-Bubenheim, D., Joly, R.J., Charles, D.J. 1992. Water stress-induced alterations in essential oil content and composition of sweet basil. *Journal of Essential Oil Research,* 4: 71–75.

Simon, J.E., Chadwick, A.F., Craker, L.E. 1984. Herbs: an indexed bibliography, 1971-1980. The scientific literature on selected herbs, and aromatic and medicinal plants of the temperate zone. Archon Books: Hamden, CT.

Turtola, S., Manninen, A.M., Rikala, R., Kainulainen, P. 2003. Drought stress alters the concentration of wood terpenoids in Scots pine and Norway spruce seedlings. *Journal of Chemical Ecology,* 29: 1981–1985.

Wasternack, C., Parthier, B. 1997. Jasmonate-signaled plant gene expression. *Trends Plant Science*, 2: 1360-1385.

Zhao, J., Davis, L.C., Verpoorte, R. 2005. Elicitor signal transduction leading to production of plant secondary metabolites. *Biotechnology Advances,* 23: 283–333.

11

The effects of hydro-alcohol extract of follower of marshmallow *(Althaea officinalis* L.) on some biochemical and hematological parameters in common carp (*Cyprinus carpio* L.)

Fahimeh Fallahpour[1], Mahdi Banaee[2*], Narges Javadzade[1]

[1]*Department of Fisheries, Khuzestan Science and research Branch, Islamic Azad University, Ahvaz, Iran;*
[2]*Aquaculture Department, Natural Resources and Environmental Faculty, Behbahan Khatam Alanbia University of Technology, Iran;*
[*]**Email: *Mahdibanaee@yahoo.com* (*banaee@bkatu.ac.ir*)**

ARTICLE INFO

Topic: *Medicinal Plants*

Key words:

- ✓ *Common carp*
- ✓ *Marshmallow extract*
- ✓ *Blood cells*
- ✓ *Blood biochemical parameters*

ABSTRACT

Background & Aim: Marshmallow (*Althaea officinalis*) is one of the most popular medicinal plants used in traditional medicine with antibacterial and antioxidant properties. This study was conducted to evaluate the effects of marshmallow extract (*Althaea officinalis* L.) administration on hematological and biochemical parameters in common carp.

Experimental: 150 carp (weighing 37.65 ± 4.40 g) were fed with diets containing 0.0 (control diet), 2.5, 5, and 10 g marshmallow extract for 60 days. Then, the hematological and blood biochemical parameters were measured on days 30 and 60 of the experiment.

Results & Discussion: No significant difference was found ($p>0.05$) in red blood cell (RBC), hemoglobin (Hb), hematocrit (Hct), mean corpuscular volume (MCV), and mean corpuscular hemoglobin concentration (MCH), number of neutrophils, basophils, and eosinophil in fish fed with different concentrations of marshmallow extract on day 60. Administration of marshmallow extract (5 g) significantly increased ($p<0.05$) white blood cells (WBC) and lymphocytes on day 60. On the other hand, administration with 5 and 10 g of marshmallow extract decreased monocytes ($p<0.05$) on day 30. Administrations of *A. officinalis* extract to the fishes for 60 days did not have any significant effect on alanine aminotransferase (ALT), alkaline phosphatase (ALP) and creatine phosphokinase (CPK) activities and creatinine levels. Plasma aspartate aminotransferase (AST), lactate dehydrogenase (LDH) activities and total protein and albumin were significantly high in fishes that fed *A. officinalis* at doses of 10 g/kg ($P < 0.05$) compare to the control group. Plasma cholesterol and triglyceride levels in the treated group were also significantly decreased at the 5 and 10 g/kg dose levels of *A. officinalis* extract. The significant changes was observed in hematological and biochemical parameters in fish fed with 10 g of marshmallow extract may be attributed to cytotoxicity, however 2.5 and 5 g of extract did not have adverse effects on the hematological and biochemical parameters of common carp in this study.

Industrial and practical recommendations: According to the results, it was concluded that preclinical administration of certain concentrations of marshmallow extract (2.5 and 5 g) was beneficial for carp.

1. Introduction

Recent developments in pharmacology and pharmacotherapy in veterinary, especially in aquaculture indicate dramatic changes, so that diseases that were once fatal in aquatic animals are now easily preventable and treatable, thanks to new medicines. In recent decades, many attempts have been directed toward introducing more effective drugs with less severe side effects. Natural resources including medicinal plants, with their good reputation in traditional medicine are one of the ways to develop new drugs with fewer side effects (Banaee, 2010; Asadi *et al.,* 2012).

Using medicinal plants in aquaculture industry goes back to last few decades. However, preclinical evaluation of herbal compounds and the influence of plant derivatives on the health of aquatic animals have not gained much attention and many researchers deal with clinical evaluation of medicinal plants and their effects on the prevention and treatment of diseases (Yin *et al.,* 2006; Divyagnaneswari *et al.,* 2007; Ardó *et al.,* 2008; Yin *et al.,* 2009). That is why in some cases, administration of medicinal plants has not been effective enough in control and treatment of diseases. In fact, prior to conducting any clinical tests and based on the principles of pharmacology, new drugs should be evaluated in terms of immunogenicity and toxicity. In a preclinical stage, usually depending on a drug application, the drug is examined to estimate its toxicity, sub-acute and chronic toxicity, and its effects on blood cells, biochemical and physiological factors and other biological aspects such as mutagenicity and probable side effects on target species or biologically similar species. Hematological and biochemical tests are of great importance in preclinical assessment of new drugs. By conducting biochemical studies, we may predict pharmaceutical effects of a drug on target organs and gain fairly comprehensive information on the physiological state of cells and tissues when changes in tissues are not readily observable, for instance in liver. Such information can be beneficial in evaluating pharmacological and toxicological properties of drugs to determine their nontoxic doses (Banaee *et al.,* 2011, Nafisi Bahabadi *et al.,* 2014). Hematology techniques, including red blood cells count, hemoglobin concentration, hematocrit measurement, mean corpuscular volume (MCV), mean corpuscular hemoglobin concentration (MCH), changes in mean corpuscular hemoglobin concentration (MCHC), and white blood cells and differential count provide valuable information on the health status of fish (Ahmadi *et al.,* 2012).

Marshmallow (*Althaea officinalis*) is one of the most popular medicinal plants used in traditional medicine with antibacterial (Sartoratto *et al.,* 2004; Burt *et al.,* 2005; Astani *et al.,* 2010; Bilia *et al.,* 2014; Kubiça *et al.,* 2014; Abbaszadeh *et al.,* 2014) and antioxidant properties (Jun *et al.,* 2014; Puri *et al.,* 2014; Ramos *et al.,* 2014) because of having mucilage, various polysaccharides, antioxidants, flavonoids, terpenes, terpenoids, plant sterols, saturated and unsaturated fatty acids, and phenolic and volatile compounds (Elmastas *et al.,* 2004; Wynn and Fougére, 2007; Sadighara *et al.,* 2012; Tešević *et al.,* 2012). Therefore, marshmallow can be used as a medicinal plant in veterinary medicine, particularly in aquaculture. So, to gather information on the probable effects of marshmallow extract on certain physiological aspects of fish, this study investigated preclinical and dietary administration of marshmallow extract at different concentrations on blood cells and some of the blood biochemical parameters in common carp (*Cyprinus carpio*) to determine potential adverse effects of this plant, if any, on fish.

2. Materials and Methods

2.1. Fish

One hundred eighty common carps (with the average weight and length of 37.65 ± 4.40 g and 14.15 ± 0.8 cm) were purchased from a private farm (Carp Farm, Shush, Khuzestan province, Iran) and then were transferred to the aquaculture laboratory of Aquaculture Department at Behbahan Khatam Alanbia University of Technology. Then, 15 fish were randomly distributed in 12 closed water-recirculating systems (2000 L). Fish were acclimated to the experimental conditions for 2 weeks (24 ± 2° C; pH: 7.4 ± 0.2; 16 L/8D; 40% water exchange rate/day). During acclimation, the fish were fed a commercial diet by Beyza Feed Mill, Shiraz, Iran twice a day and no more than 2% of their body weight (Table 1).

2.2. Marshmallow (Althaea officinalis) extract preparation

The powder of dried flower *A. officinalis* was mixed with distillated water and ethanol (1:1), and put on the shaker for 24 hours at room temperature. The resulting hydroalcoholic extract was filtered through Whatman filter paper and evaporated to dryness on a rotary evaporator until it became creamy, and was then dried in an oven (50 °C) to finally 7gave 8 g (8 % of initial amount) dried powder. The concentration used in the experiment was based on the dry weight of the extract.

2.3. Fish diet preparation

The formulated fish food was prepared in the laboratory using powder of commercial food obtained from Beyza Feed Mill, Shiraz, Iran. To enrich the normal diet, the 2.5, 5 and 10 g of *A. officinalis* extracts were mixed with 1 kg powder feed. Each supplemented diet was mixed with distilled water (1mL/g) until obtaining a homogenous mixture. This mixture was passed through a meat grinder, producing extruded string shapes, which were dried in an oven at 55°C for 12 h and then broken to produce pellets approximately 10 mm long. The pellets were packed and stored at -20°C in a freezer until be used. The control diet was prepared by the same process, although no supplement was added.

2.4. The final experiment

The final experiment was done in a completely randomized design with 3 treatments and a control sample. The fish were fed twice a day with commercial diet (no more than 2% of their body weight) enriched with 2.5, 5 and 10 g of the hydro-alcoholic extract of marshmallow. After 30 and 60 days, 9 fish were captured randomly from each group and then anesthetized with clove powder solution (200 mg/L). Then, the fish blood was collected from their tail stem, and stored in sterilized glass vials at 4 °C containing the anticoagulant heparin. The blood was centrifuged for 15 min at 6000 g, 4 °C. Plasma samples were immediately stored at -21 °C until biochemical analysis.

2.5. Haematological parameters

2.5.1. WBC and RBC. The blood was immediately used to determine the number of red blood cells (RBC) and white blood cells (WBC) by means of a haemocytometer slide (Improved Neubauer type) at a magnification of x 400. Thus, blood was diluted to with diluting fluid including sodium citrate, Crystal violet dissolved in Ringer solution, brilliant blue dissolved in Ringer solution at pH 7.2 (Vázquez and Guerrero, 2007; Banaee *et al.,* 2008).

2.5.2. Haematocrit (Hct). Haematocrit (Hct) was determined by the microhematocrit method described by Vázquez and Guerrero (2007).

2.5.3. Haemoglobin (Hb). Haemoglobin (Hb) concentration was calculated by using the cyanohaemoglobin method (Vázquez and Guerrero, 2007). Briefly, 20 µl of whole blood was mixed with 5 ml of Drabkin's solution (Zist-chemistry Kit Co., Iran) in a test tube before allowing standing for at least 15 min at room temperature. The absorbance (A) was measured at 540 nm. The haemoglobin concentration of the blood sample was calculated from a curve prepared from known standards.

2.5.4. RBC indices. The mean corpuscular volume (MCV), the mean corpuscular hemoglobin (MCH) and the mean corpuscular hemoglobin concentration (MCHC) index were calculated according to following formula:

$$MCH = \frac{Hb\times10}{RBC};\ MCV = \frac{Hct\times10}{RBC};\ MCHC = \frac{Hb\times100}{Hct}$$

2.6. White blood cell differentiation

To differentiate white blood cell type, blood films of samples were prepared on clean microscope slides before fixation for 5 min in 96% methanol and left to air dry. The slides were stained with Giemsa's stain for 20 min according to Vázquez and Guerrero (2007) and Banaee *et al.* (2008) and examined at a magnification of x 400.

2.7. Biochemical parameters

Measuring the biochemical parameters was done using the kits supplied by Pars Azmoon Company and a UV/ VIS spectrophotometer (model UNISCO 2100). Total protein was measured by the Biuret reaction at 540 nm. The albumin assay is based on the dye-binding properties of plasma albumin with a bromocresol green. An increase in the blue-green color was measured at 630 nm. The plasma globulin based on the ratio of albumin versus total protein (Johnson *et al.,* 1999). Plasma glucose was measured by the glucose-oxidase method at 500 nm (Sacks, 1999). Plasma cholesterol levels by the CHOD-PAP enzymatic method at 510 nm, triglyceride levels by GPO-PAP enzymatic method at 546 nm (Rifai *et al.,* 1999) and creatinine by the JAFFE method and at 510 nm (Foster-Swanson *et al.,* 1994). The activity of aspartate aminotransferase (AST) and alanine aminotransferase (ALT) in plasma was measured by NADPH consumption and its conversion to NAD^+ at 340 nm, lactate dehydrogenase (LDH) in plasma was measured based on the conversion of pyruvate to lactate at 340 nm, alkaline phosphatase (ALP) based on converting nitro phenol phosphate into nitrophenol and phosphate at 405 nm, creatinine phosphokinase (CK) based on the conversion of creatinine phosphate into creatinine at 340 nm and based on optical density (OD) absorption and the formula presented in the kits' manual (Moss and Henderson, 1999). All biochemical parameters were measured according to the instructions provided in the kit's manual.

2.8. Data analysis

Significant difference in the biochemical parameters of specimens treated with the different concentrations of *A. officinalis* extracts was statistically analyzed by one-way ANOVA in SPSS (IBM, Release 19) software. All data were examined for normality (Kolmogorov-Smirnov test). The mean evaluation was done using Duncan's test at a confidence level of 95%. Data were presented as the mean ± SD.

3. Results and discussion

No fish died during the experiment. The fish readily accepted all diets in the first few minutes, which minimized leaching marshmallow extract from the feed into the water.

Table 1. Composition of commercial diet.

Nutrients	Value
Gross energy (Kcal/Kg)	3500
Crude protein (%)	35-37
Crude lipid (%)	9-11
Crude fiber (%)	5%
Moisture (%)	<10
Ash (%)	<10
TVN (mg/100gr)	<45

TVN: Total volatile nitrogen

The findings of this study indicate that marshmallow administration has no effects on the number of red blood cells (RBC count), hemoglobin (Hb), hematocrit (Htc), mean corpuscular volume (MCV) and mean content of hemoglobin per red cell (MCH) during the experiment (Table 2). However, using certain immune stimulating compounds may alter red blood cell indices by affecting the performance of hematopoietic organs such as thymus, spleen, and anterior kidney (Ahmadi *et al.*, 2012). For instance, administration of garlic has a great effect on stimulating the immune system (Sahu *et al.*, 2007; Ndong and Fall, 2007; Nya and Austin, 2009a) and increases hemoglobin, hematocrit, and white blood cells count as well as thrombocytes in Nile tilapia (Shalaby *et al.*, 2006). Also, a significant increase was found in hemoglobin as well as red and white blood cells count in *labeo rohita* that were fed diets enriched with mango kernel powder and garlic compared with the control group (Sahu *et al.*, 2007). Moreover, a significant increase was reported in the number of red blood cells, hematocrit, leukocyte and thrombocyte count in fish fed with garlic (Martins *et al.*, 2002). Feeding flanders with a mixture of herbs including *Medicata fermentata*, *Crataegi fructus*, *Artemisia capillaries* and *Cnidium officinale* increased hemoglobin and hematocrit (Ji *et al.*, 2007). Although there was not any significant difference in MCHC value between the treated groups and control at day 30, the MCHC value was higher in fish fed for 60 days with 2.5 g marshmallow extract compare to groups fed with control group.

Fish fed with 2.5 g marshmallow extract revealed lower numbers of WBC than control group at day 60. The increase in the number of white blood cells (WBC) on day 60 in fish fed with 5 g marshmallow extract may be attributed to the effects of this extract on the lymphoid tissue of fish and on the reproduction and proliferation of white blood cells. The increase in white blood cells is important in strengthening the immune system of fish. A significant increase was reported in red blood cells count, hematocrit, leukocyte and thrombocyte of fish after being fed with garlic (Martins *et al.*, 2002). In a similar experiment, increased number of leukocytes was found in hybrid tilapia (Ndong and Fall, 2007).

Differential leucocyte counts for fish fed marshmallow extract for 60 days have been presented in Table 3. A significant increase in the lymphocyte of fish fed with 0.5 and 10 g marshmallow extract may indicate the influence of this plant on the increased synthesis of lymphocytes in lymphoid tissues such as the anterior kidney and spleen. This might be effective in strengthening cellular immunity and increasing the efficiency of acquired immunity (Secombes *et al.*, 2005). Conversely, the dose of 5 and 10 g extract led to the lowest significant number of monocytes ($p<0.05$). There were no significant difference in the neutrophil, basophile and eosinophil counts between treated fish and control group.

However, administration of 0.5 and 10 g marshmallow extract significantly decreased monocytes on day 30. Moreover, the results indicate that using marshmallow extract in diet of fish had no effects on the number of neutrophils, basophils, and eosinophils. Feeding Pacu (*Piaractus mesopotamicus*) with vitamin supplements (E, C) had no effects on the number of leukocytes, monocytes and neutrophils (Garcia *et al.,* 2007). However, using ginger and garlic in diets given to rainbow trout made significant changes in the number of lymphocytes, monocytes, and neutrophils (Nya and Austin, 2009a; 2009b). Rainbow trout immersion in glucan solution increased neutrophils and activated their non-specific immune responses (Gannam and Schrock, 1999).

As shown in Table 4 administrations of *A. officinalis* extract to the fishes for 60 days did not have any significant effect on ALT, ALP and CPK activities. Although, no significant changes were observed in AST activity on day 30, plasma AST were significantly high in fishes that fed *A. officinalis* at doses of 10 g/kg ($P < 0.05$) compare to the AST activity in the control group on day 60. Plasma LDH activity in the treated group were also significantly increased at the 10 g/kg dose level on day 60 ($p < 0.05$). However, no significant changes were observed in LDH activity on day 30.

Aspartate aminotransferase (AST) and alanine aminotransferase (ALT) are two of the most important liver enzymes which help transfer amine groups from alpha amino acids to alpha-keto acids. These enzymes play an important role in the final stages of protein breakdown to produce ATP and increased activity of these enzymes has no role in using amino acids in the oxidation process or glycogenesis (Murray *et al.,* 2012). Increased hepatic AST on day 60 of the experiment in fish fed with diets containing 10 g marshmallow extract may illustrate increased rate of protein breakdown in liver to provide enough energy to deal with the cytotoxic effects caused by the presence of phytochemical compounds, such as furfural, in marshmallow extract. After being oxidized by liver, furfural turns into a toxic material, pyromucic acid (Veličković *et al.,* 2011). Therefore, furfural may indirectly cause oxidative stress and damage liver cells in fish. Increased AST and ALT was observed in tilapia (Soltan *et al.*, 2008) and rainbow trout fed with a mixture of herbs and yarrow 1%, respectively (Nafisi Bahabadi *et al.,* 2014). This could be due to the liver dysfunction which is in turn caused by anti-nutritional compounds in plants (Soltan *et al.*, 2008). However, administration of silymarin to rainbow trout (Banaee *et al.,* 2011) or using garlic and onion extract in catfish diet (Al-Salahy, 2002) decreased AST and ALT activities. Alkaline phosphatase (ALP) is an enzyme found in the epithelium of the bile ducts and liver cells. Alkaline phosphatase in liver functions in glycogen metabolism and can deactivate phosphorylase enzymes, hence activating glycogen synthesis in liver. Therefore, inhibiting the activity of this enzyme in liver is associated with glycogen breakdown to supply the energy required under stressful conditions, decreasing phosphorylation or preventing oxidative phosphorylation in the respiratory chain (Murray *et al.*, 2012). The plasma ALP activity did not change significantly compares to the control fishes.

Lactate dehydrogenase (LDH) is one of the glycolytic chief enzymes in liver which is substantially found in other tissues too. The level of this enzyme alters in hypoxia and severe damages to organs. Pathological damages to the liver and blood hypoxic conditions may prevent oxidative phosphorylation in the mitochondria which in turn reduces ATP production. Therefore, inhibiting oxidative phosphorylation is followed by fatal consequences. In such circumstances reoxidation of NADH with oxygen is not possible via the respiratory chain. During a biochemical reaction catalyzed by lactate dehydrogenase, pyruvate is converted to lactate by NADH. Thus by reoxidation of NADH by lactate, glycolysis continues in the absence of oxygen (Murray *et al.,* 2012).). Increased plasma LDH on day 60 in fish fed 10 g of marshmallow extract may suggest a cellular toxicity caused by phytochemical compounds in this plant (Ebrahimi, 2005). Decreased LDH was reported in rainbow trout treated with silymarin and marrow (Nafisi Bahabadi *et al.*, 2014; Banaee *et al.,* 2011).

Creatine phosphokinase (CPK) activity appears almost completely unaffected by the *A. officinalis* extract; apparently, no changes were observed when compared with that of the control. The effects of marshmallow extract on the activity of hepatic enzymes is comparable to the effects of other herbs such as *Curcuma longa* (Abdelwahab *et al.,* 2012), and *Cyperus rotundus* (Suresh Kumar and Mishra, 2005). Absence of alterations in the level of hepatic enzymes in fish fed with different concentrations of marshmallow extract could be attributed to the influence of flavonoids and antioxidants on the physiological function of cell membrane in liver tissue, increasing the antioxidant capacity of cells and improving the cell membrane stability (Sadighara *et al.*, 2012).

Table 2. Changes in the haematological parameters of fish fed different concentrations of marshmallow extract.

Hematology Parameters	Treatments	Experimental course	
		30th day	60th day
RBC (10^6 cells)	Control	1.74±0.64[a]	1.50±0.38[a]
	2.5 g MAR	1.43±0.50[a]	1.60±0.37[a]
	5 g MAR	1.28±0.39[a]	1.32±0.39[a]
	10 g MAR	1.25±0.55[a]	1.42±0.59[a]
WBC (10^4 cells)	Control	11.13±3.16[ab]	10.61±2.47[a]
	2.5 g MAR	10.51±6.07[ab]	14.18±4.58[ab]
	5 g MAR	7.73±2.67[a]	14.84±4.54[b]
	10 g MAR	12.38±4.98[b]	12.85±2.59[ab]
Hct (%)	Control	33.23±8.44[a]	35.69±6.63[ab]
	2.5 g MAR	27.73±4.72[a]	32.29±3.58[a]
	5 g MAR	29.09±6.39[a]	38.48±5.03[b]
	10 g MAR	32.18±1.60[a]	33.62±2.78[a]
Hb (g/100 mL)	Control	7.53±1.61[a]	6.64±2.09[a]
	2.5 g MAR	6.96±1.89[a]	8.00±2.69[a]
	5 g MAR	7.74±1.77[a]	6.55±1.57[a]
	10 g MAR	7.05±1.32[a]	6.88±1.52[a]
MCV (10^{-4} mm^3)	Control	2.17±1.04[a]	2.57±0.91[a]
	2.5 g MAR	2.26±1.17[a]	2.19±0.80[a]
	5 g MAR	2.43±0.78[a]	3.09±0.79[a]
	10 g MAR	3.03±1.30[a]	2.89±1.54[a]
MCH (10^{-5} pg)	Control	5.11±2.78[a]	4.63±1.48[a]
	2.5 g MAR	5.34±1.97[a]	5.27±2.15[a]
	5 g MAR	6.56±2.47[a]	5.41±2.20[a]
	10 g MAR	6.53±2.57[a]	5.80±3.04[a]
MCHC (%)	Control	23.30±4.59[a]	18.59±4.45[a]
	2.5 g MAR	25.91±8.37[a]	25.42±10.09[b]
	5 g MAR	28.02±9.73[a]	17.40±4.84[a]
	10 g MAR	22.03±4.63[a]	20.78±5.69[ab]

Effects of different concentrations of *Althaea officinalis* extract as supplement (0, 0.25, 0.5 and 1 % per 1 kg food) on haematological parameters determined in common carp after 30 and 60 days. Effects of different concentrations of *Althaea officinalis* extract on haematological parameters were analyzed using a one-way ANOVA. Significant differences between treatment and control groups were represented by alphabets ($p<0.05$). Values represent mean ± S.D.

Table 3. Changes in the white blood cell differentiation of fish fed different concentrations of marshmallow extract.

WBC differentiation	Treatment	Experimental course	
		30th day	60th day
Lymphocyte	Control	66.07±1.08[a]	66.24±1.07[a]
	2.5 g MAR	67.61±1.08[a]	69.02±1.07[ab]
	5 g MAR	71.90±1.05[b]	71.90±1.05[b]
	10 g MAR	72.81±1.08[b]	73.57±1.07[b]
Neutrophils	Control	19.30±1.23[a]	20.05±1.23[a]
	2.5 g MAR	16.44±1.28[a]	17.42±1.28[a]
	5 g MAR	17.92±1.22[a]	17.29±1.20[a]
	10 g MAR	16.76±1.18[a]	16.85±1.16[a]

Monocyte	Control	11.48±1.45[b]	10.88±1.42[ab]
	2.5 g MAR	13.43±1.32[b]	11.64±1.29[b]
	5 g MAR	8.13±1.27[a]	9.07±1.20[a]
	10 g MAR	8.25±1.48[a]	8.25±1.41[a]
Basophils	Control	1.13±1.45[a]	1.08±1.26[a]
	2.5 g MAR	1.07±1.24[a]	1.07±1.24[a]
	5 g MAR	1.08±1.26[a]	1.08±1.26[a]
	10 g MAR	0.11±0.47[a]	0.11±0.47[a]
Eosinophil	Control	1.82±1.62[a]	1.82±1.92[a]
	2.5 g MAR	1.37±1.81[a]	1.37±1.81[a]
	5 g MAR	1.58±1.83[a]	1.32±1.54[a]
	10 g MAR	1.54±1.73[a]	1.29±1.75[a]

Effects of different concentrations of *Althaea officinalis* extract as supplement (0, 0.25, 0.5 and 1 % per 1 kg food) on white blood cell differentiation determined in common carp after 30 and 60 days. Effects of different concentrations of *Althaea officinalis* extract on white blood cell differentiation were analyzed using a one-way ANOVA. Significant differences between treatment and control groups were represented by alphabets (p<0.05). Values represent mean ± S.D.

Table 4. Changes in the plasma enzyme activities of fish fed different concentrations of marshmallow extract.

Biochemical Parameters	Treatments	Experimental course	
		30th day	60th day
AST (U/L)	Control	49±16[a]	44±10[a]
	2.5 g MAR	48±4[a]	47±17[a]
	5 g MAR	46±9[a]	57±13[ab]
	10 g MAR	44±10[a]	62±13[b]
ALT (U/L)	Control	14±3[a]	14±4[a]
	2.5 g MAR	13±1[a]	11±3[a]
	5 g MAR	14±4[a]	11±2[a]
	10 g MAR	16±3[a]	12±4[a]
LDH (U/L)	Control	198±46[a]	225±35[a]
	2.5 g MAR	232±72[a]	201±40[a]
	5 g MAR	243±120[a]	203±49[a]
	10 g MAR	261±111[a]	314±23[b]
ALP (U/L)	Control	67±17[a]	57±14[ab]
	2.5 g MAR	48±22[a]	61±19[ab]
	5 g MAR	56±30[a]	50±22[a]
	10 g MAR	55±22[a]	72±16[b]
CPK (U/L)	Control	856±179[a]	1090±318[a]
	2.5 g MAR	1093±422[a]	1060±284[a]
	5 g MAR	1103±360[a]	1200±227[a]
	10 g MAR	934±286[a]	951±237[a]

Effects of different concentrations of *Althaea officinalis* extract as supplement (0, 0.25, 0.5 and 1 % per 1 kg food) on the plasma enzyme activities determined in common carp after 30 and 60 days. Effects of different concentrations of *Althaea officinalis* extract on the plasma enzyme activities were analyzed using a one-way ANOVA. Significant differences between treatment and control groups were represented by alphabets (p<0.05). Values represent mean ± S.D.

Table 5. Changes in the some biochemical parameters of fish fed different concentrations of marshmallow extract.

Biochemical Parameters	Treatments	Experimental course	
		30th day	60th day
Glucose (mg/dL)	Control	61.57±11[a]	67.33±12.40[ab]
	2.5 g MAR	62.08±15[a]	58.57±9.83[a]
	5 g MAR	60.81±7.30[a]	73.47±19.50[ab]
	10 g MAR	72.43±20[a]	84.69±21[b]
Protein (g/dL)	Control	3.22±0.81[ab]	3.66±0.77[a]
	2.5 g MAR	2.69±0.60[a]	5.08±0.75[c]
	5 g MAR	3.43±0.55[ab]	4.11±1.03[ab]
	10 g MAR	3.33±0.52[ab]	4.65±0.50[bc]
Albumin (g/dL)	Control	2.12±0.26[b]	1.87±0.70[a]
	2.5 g MAR	1.35±0.23[a]	2.01±0.91[a]
	5 g MAR	1.76±0.30[b]	2.58±0.31[ab]
	10 g MAR	2.08±0.56[b]	2.89±0.86[b]
Globulins (g/dL)	Control	1.10±0.62[a]	1.79±1.26[a]
	2.5 g MAR	1.34±0.48[a]	3.07±1.03[b]
	5 g MAR	1.67±0.70[a]	1.53±1.18[a]
	10 g MAR	1.25±0.52[a]	1.76±0.90[a]
Cholesterol (mg/dL)	Control	70.53±13.17[b]	79.29±13[ab]
	2.5 g MAR	69.20±21.37[ab]	71.45±10.56[a]
	5 g MAR	50.11±18.23[a]	70.14±13.10[a]
	10 g MAR	50.11±17[a]	92.60±18.60[b]
Triglycerides (mg/dL)	Control	225.00±50.34[ab]	249.19±35[b]
	2.5 g MAR	184.04±38.48[a]	191.37±48[a]
	5 g MAR	230.99±59.40[ab]	208.60±31[ab]
	10 g MAR	244.25±47.24[b]	244.41±48[b]
Creatinine (mg/dL)	Control	0.45±0.210[a]	0.35±0.10[a]
	2.5 g MAR	0.44±0.19[a]	0.37±0.07[a]
	5 g MAR	0.39±0.12[a]	0.38±0.10[a]
	10 g MAR	0.51±0.21[a]	0.33±0.08[a]

Effects of different concentrations of *Althaea officinalis* extract as supplement (0, 0.25, 0.5 and 1 % per 1 kg food) on some blood biochemical parameters determined in common carp after 30 and 60 days. Effects of different concentrations of *Althaea officinalis* extract on some blood biochemical parameters were analyzed using a one-way ANOVA. Significant differences between treatment and control groups were represented by alphabets ($p<0.05$). Values represent mean ± S.D.

Plasma total protein and albumin as shown in table 5 significantly increased in fishes treated with *A. officinalis* at doses of 10 g/kg ($P < 0.05$) compared to the control group which received only normal diet on day 60. The significant increase in the level of these parameters is an induction that the *A. officinalis* extract stimulated their synthesis in the liver. The result indicates that *A. officinalis* extract administration caused a significant increase in globulin levels in fishes in the 2.5 g/kg dose on day 60 ($P < 0.05$).

Plasma cholesterol in the treated group was also significantly decreased at the 5 and 10 g/kg dose levels of *A. officinalis* extract. Plasma triglyceride levels were affected by the *A. officinalis* extract (at 2.5 g/kg) administration for 30 days as shown in table 5. Diminishing effect of *A. officinalis* extract on plasma cholesterol and triglyceride in this study is an indication of the involvement of the flower extract in mechanisms involved in elimination of the lipids from the body, thus confirming its potential hypolipidaemic effects.

The levels of creatinine in the treated fishes did not show any significant difference with respect to the control levels, an induction that flower extract of *A. officinalis* is not nephrotoxic at the dose levels used in this study.

4. Conclusion

Measuring blood biochemical changes and hematological indices in carp treated with different concentration of marshmallow extract proves the safety of this drug at concentrations of 2.5 and 5 g in preclinical stages, although the concentration of 10 g may lead to cytotoxicity.

5. References

Abbaszadeh, S., Sharifzadeh, A., Shokri, H., Khosravi, A.R., Abbaszadeh, A. 2014. Antifungal efficacy of thymol, carvacol, eugenol and menthol as alternative agents to control the growth of food-relevant fungi. *Journal of Medical Mycology*. 24(2): 51-56.

Abdelwahab, A.M., El-Bahr, S.M. 2012. Influence of black Cumin seeds (*Nigella sativa*) and Turmeric (*Curcuma longa* Linn.) mixture on performance and serum biochemistry of Asian Sea Bass, *Lates calcarifer. World Journal of Fish and Marine Sciences*. 4(5): 496-503.

Ahmadi, K., Banaee, M., Vosoghei, A.R., Mirvaghefei, A.R., Ataeimehr, B. 2012. Evaluation of the immunomodulatory effects of silymarin extract (*Silybum marianum*) on some immune parameters of rainbow trout, *Oncorhynchus mykiss* (Actinopterygii,Salmoniformes, Salmonidae). *ActaIchthyol. Piscat*. 42(2): 113–120.

Al-Salahy, M.B. 2002. Some physiological studies on the effect of onion and garlic juices on the fish, *Clarias lazera. Fish Physiology and Biochemistry*. 27: 129–142.

Ardó, L., Yin, G., Xu, P., Váradi, L., Szigeti, G., Jeney, Z., Jeney, G. 2008. Chinese herbs (*Astragalus membranaceus* and *Lonicera japonica*) and boron enhance the non-specific immune response of Nile tilapia (*Oreochromis niloticus*) and resistance against *Aeromonas hydrophila. Aquaculture*. 275 (1–4): 26–33.

Asadi, M.S., Mirvaghefei, A.R., Nematollahi, M.A., Banaee, M., Ahmadi, K. 2012. Effects of Watercress (*Nasturtium nasturtium*) extract on some immunological parameters of rainbow trout (*Oncorhynchus mykiss*). *Open Veterinary Journal*. 2(1): 32-39.

Astani, A., Reichling, J., Schnitzler, P. 2010. Comparative study on the antiviral activity of selected monoterpenes derived from essential oils. *Phytotherapy Research*. 24(5): 673-679.

Banaee, M. 2010. *Influence of silymarin in decline of sublethal diazinon-induced oxidative stress in rainbow trout (Oncorhynchus mykiss)*. Ph.D. Thesis, Aquaculture and Environmental Department, Natural Resource Faculty, Natural Resource and Agriculture Collage, Tehran University, Iran, 149 pp.

Banaee, M., Mirvagefei, A.R., Rafei, G.R., Majazi Amiri, B. 2008. Effect of sub-lethal Diazinon Concentrations on Blood Plasma Biochemistry. *International Journal of Environmental Research*. 2(2): 189-198.

Banaee, M., Sureda, A., Mirvaghefi, A.R., Rafei, G.R. 2011. Effects of long-term silymarin oral supplementation on the blood biochemical profile of rainbow trout (*Oncorhynchusmykiss*). *Fish Physiology and Biochemistry*. 37: 887-896.

Bilia, A.B., Santomauro, F., Sacco, C., Bergonzi, M.C., Donata, R. 2014. *Essential oil of Artemisia annua L, An extraordinary component with numerous antimicrobial properties*. Hindawi Publishing Coporation. Evidence-Based Complemetary and Alternative Medicine ID: 159819. 7 pp. Doi:10.115/2014/159819.

Burt, S.A., Vlielander, R., Haagsman, H.P., Veldhuizen, E.J.A. 2005. Increase in activity of essential oil components carvacrol and thymol against *Escherichia coli* O157:H7 by addition of food stabilizers. *Journal of Food Protection*. 68(5): 919-926.

Divyagnaneswari, M., Christybapita, D., Dinakaran, M.R. 2007. Enhancement of nonspecific immunity and disease resistance in *Oreochromismossambicus* by *Solanumtrilobatum* leaf fractions. *Fish & Shellfish Immunology*. 23: 249-259.

Ebrahimi, A. 2005. *Clinical Explanation of Laboratory Testes*. Tehran, Iran: Teimorzadeh, Tabib Publisher. 628 pp.

Elmastas, M., Ozturk, L., Gokce, I., Erenler, R., Aboul-Enein, H.Y. 2004. Determination of antioxidant activity of marshmallow flower (Althaea officinalis L.). *Bioanalytical.* 37(9): 1859-1869.

Foster-Swanson, A., Swartzentruber, M. and Roberts, P. 1994. Refrence interval studies of the rate-blancked creatinine, Jaffe method on BM /Hitachi Systems in Six U.S. Laboratories (Abstract). *Clinical Chemistry.* No. 361.

Gannam AL, Schrock RM. 1999. Immunostimulants in fish diets. *J. Appl. Aqua.* 9: 53- 89.

Garcia, F., Pilarski, F., Makoto, E., Moraes, F., Martins M.L. 2007. Hematology of *Piaractus mesopotamicus* fed diets supplemented with vitamins C and E, challenged by *Aeromonas hydrophila. Aquaculture.* 271: 39–46.

Ji, S.C., Jronh, G.S., Gwang-Soon, I.M., Lee, S.W., Yoo, J.H., Takii, K. 2007. Dietary medicinal herbs improve growth performance, fatty acid utilization, and stress recovery of Japanese flounder. *Fisheries Science.* 73(1): 70-76

Johnson, A.M., Rohlfs, E.M., Silverman, L.M. Proteins. In: Burtis CA, Ashwood ER, editors. Tietz Textbook of Clinical Chemistry. 3rd ed. Philadelphia, W.B. Saunders Company 1999. p. 477-540.

Jun, H.J., Lee, J.H., Kim, J., Jia, Y., Kim, K.H., Hwang, K.Y., Yun, E.J., Do, K.R., Lee, S.L. 2014. Linalool is a PPARα ligand that reduces plasma TG levels and rewires the hepatic transcriptome and plasma metabolome. *Journal of Lipid Resaerch.* 55: 1098-1110.

Kubiça, T.F., Alves, S.H., Weiblen, R., Lovato, L.T. 2014. In vitro inhibition of the bovine viral diarrhea virus by the essential oil of *Ocimum basilicum* (basil) and monoterpenes. *Brazilian Journal of Microbiology.* 45(1): 209-214.

Martins, M.L., Moraes, F.R., Miyazaki, D.M., Brum, C.D., Onak, E.M., Fenerick, J.J., Bozzo, F.R. 2002. Alternative treatment for *Anacanthorus penilabiatus* (*Monogenea*: Dactylogyridae) infection in cultivated pacu, *Piaractus mesopotamicus* (*Osteichthyes*: *Characidae*) in Brazil and its haematological effects. *Parasite.* 9: 175-180.

Moss, D.V., Henderson, A.R. 1999. Clinical enzymology. In: Burtis CA, Ashwood ER, editors. Tietz Textbook of Clinical Chemistry. 3rd ed. Philadelphia, W.B. Saunders Company. p. 617-721.

Murray, R., Bender, D., Botham, K.M. Kennelly, P.J., Rodwell, V., Weil, P.A. 2012. Harpers Illustrated Biochemistry 29th Edition. University of Toronto, Ontario, Canada: Mc Graw Hill Education. 818 pp.

Nafisi Bahabadi, M., Banaee, M., Taghiyan, M., Nematdoust Haghi, B. 2014. Effects of dietary administration of yarrow extract on growth performance and blood biochemical parameters of rainbow trout (*Oncorhynchus mykiss*). *International Journal of Aquatic Biology.* 2(5): 275-285.

Ndong, D., Fall, J. 2007. The effect of garlic (*Allium sativum*) on growth and immune responses of hybrid tilapia (*Oreochromis niloticus* x *Oreochromis aureus*), Document Scientifique du CRODT, 1–22.

Nya, E., Austin, B. 2009b. Use of dietary ginger, *Zingiber officinale* Roscoe, as an immunostimulant to control *Aeromonas hydrophila* infections in rainbow trout, *Oncorhynchus mykiss* (Walbaum) *Journal of Fish Disease.* 32: 971-977.

Nya, E.J., Austin, B. 2009a. Use of garlic, *Allium sativum*, to control *Aeromonas hydrophila* infections in rainbow trout, *Oncorhynchus mykiss* (Walbaum). *Journal of Fish Disease.* 32: 963-970.

Puri, A., Srivastava, P., Pandey, P., Yadav, R.S., Bhatt, P.C. 2014. Scopolamine induced behavioral and biochemical modifications and protective effect of *Celastrus paniculatous* and *Angelica glauca* in rats. *International Journal of Nutrition, Pharmacology, Neurological Diseases.* 4(3): 158-169.

Ramos, M., Beltrán, A., Peltzer, M., Valente, A.J.M, del Carmen Garrigós, M. 2014. Release and antioxidant activity of carvacrol and thymol from polypropylene active packaging films. *LWT-Food Science and Technology.* 58(2): 470-477.

Rifai, N., Bachorik, P.S. and Albers, J.J. 1999. Lipids, lipoproteins and apolipoproteins. In: Burtis CA, Ashwood ER, eds. *Tietz Textbook of Clinical Chemistry. 3rd ed. W.B. Saunders Company, Philadelphia. pp.* 809-861.

Sacks, D.B. 1999. Carbohydrates. In: Burtis CA, Ashwood ER, eds. *Tietz Textbook of Clinical Chemistry. 3rd ed. W.B. Saunders Company, Philadelphia. pp.* 766-85.

Sadighara, P., Gharibi, S., Moghadam Jafari, A., Jahed Khaniki, G.R., Salari, S. 2012. The antioxdant and flavonoids contents of *Althaea officinalis* L. flowers based on their color. *Avicenna Journal of Phytomedicine.* 2(3), 113-117.

Sahu, S., Das, B.K., Mishra, B.K., Pradhan, J., Sarangi, N. 2007a. Effect of *Magnifera indica* kernel as a feed additive on immunity and resistance to *Aeromonas hydrophila* in *Labeo rohita* fingerlings. *Fish & Shellfish Immunology*. 23: 109-118.

Sahu, S., Das, B.K., Mishra, B.K., Pradhan, J., Sarangi, N. 2007b. Effect of *Allium* sativum on the immunity and survival of *Labeo rohita* infected with *Aeromonas hydrophila. Journal of Applied Ichthyology*. 23: 80-86.

Sartoratto, A., Machado, A.L.M., Delarmelina, C., Figueira, G.M., Duarte, M.C.T., Rehder, V.L.G. 2004. Composition and antimicrobial activity of essential oils from aromatic plants used in Brazil. *Brazilian Journal of Microbiology*. 35: 275-280.

Secombes, C.J., Bird, S., Zou, J. 2005. Adaptive immunity in teleosts: cellular immunity. *Dev. Biol.* 121: 25-32.

Shalaby, A.M., Khattab, Y.A., Abdel Rahman, A.M. 2006. Effects of garlic (*Allium sativum*) and chloramphenicol on growth performance, physiological parameters and survival of Nile tilapia (*Oreochromis niloticus*). *J. Venom. Anim. Toxin Trop. Dis*. 12: 172-201.

Soltan, M.A., Hanafy, M.A, Wafa, M.I.A. 2008. An Evaluation of fermented silage made form fish by products as a feed ingredient for African catfish (*Clarius gariepinus*). *Global veterinaria*. 2: 80-86.

Suresh Kumar, S.V., Mishra, S.H. 2005. Hepatoprotective activity of rhizomes of *Cyperus rotundus* Linn. aganist carbon tetrachloride induced hepatotoxicty, *Indian Journal of Pharmaceutical sciences*. 67(1): 84-88.

Tešević, V., Vajs, V., Lekić, S., Dordević, I., Novaković, M., Vujisić, L., Todosijević, M. 2012. Lipid composition and antioxidant activities of the seed oil from three Malvaceae Species. *Arch. Biol. Science. Belgrade*. 64(1): 221-227.

Vázquez, G.R., Guerrero, G.A. 2007. Characterization of blood cells and hematological parameters in *Cichlasoma dimerus* (Teleostei, Perciformes). *Tissue and Cell.* 39: 151-160.

Veličković, D., Milenković, S., Stojanović, D. 2011. Enzymochemical and biochemical changes in the liver of rats induced by furfural. *Acta Medica Mediance*. 50(2): 34-38.

Wynn, S.G., Fougère, B.J. 2007. Veterinary herbal medicine. USA: Mosby Elsevier St. Louis. 736pp.

Yin, G., Ardó, L., Thompson, K.D., Adams, A., Jeney, Z., Jeney, G. 2009. Chinese herbs (*Astragalus radix* and *Ganoderma lucidum*) enhance immune response of carp, *Cyprinus carpio*, and protection against *Aeromonas hydrophila. Fish and Shellfish Immunology.* 26 (1): 140–145.

Yin, G., Jeney, G., Racz, T., Xu, P., Jun, X., Jeney, Z. 2006. Effect of two Chinese herbs (*Astragalus radix* and *Scutellaria radix*) on non-specific immune response of tilapia, *Oreochromis niloticus*. *Aquaculture*. 253 (1–4): 39–47.

Essential oil composition of *Elaeagnus angustifolia* and *Elaeagnus orientalis* from Sistan and Baluchestan, Iran

Malek Taher Maghsoodlou[1]*, Nasrin Kazemipoor[2], Rohallah Jafarazad[3], Nahid Rahneshan[4]

[1]*Professor, Department of Chemistry, University of Sistan and Baluchestan, Zahedan, Iran;*

***Email:** *mt_maghsoodlou@yahoo.com*

[2]*Associate Professor, Department of Agriculture, Shiraz University, Shiraz, Iran;*

[3,4]*Master of Science, Department of Chemistry, University of Sistan and Baluchestan, Zahedan, Iran;*

ARTICLE INFO

Topic: *Phytochemistry*

Key words:

- ✓ *Volatile constituents*
- ✓ *Elaeagnus angustifolia*
- ✓ *Elaeagnus orientalis*
- ✓ *hydro-distillation*
- ✓ *GC/MS*

ABSTRACT

Background & Aim: *Elaeagnus angustifolia* and *Elaeagnus orientalis* have a lot of medical utilization. In folk medicine, the fruit and flower of these plants are used as a tonic and antipyretic agent. The aim of the present study was to chemical analysis of volatile constituents of *E. angustifolia* and *E. orientalis* flowers.

Experimental: The essential oils of *E. angustifolia* and *E. orientalis* flowers collected from Zahedan in Sistan and Baluchestan province were obtained by hydro-distillation. Chemical composition of oils were determined by GC/MS.

Results & Discussion: 12 compounds representing 100% were identified in the essential oil of *E. angustifolia* flowers in which Ethyl cinnamate (73.24%), Cyclohexanecarboxylic acid, ethenyl ester (6.94%), Isobutyl cinnamate (4.74%), Palmitic acid (4.39%), Buthyl cinnamate (2.38%), Ethanol (2.24%) and Methyl 9,9- Dideutero- Octadecanoate (2.05%) were the major constituents. In the essential oil of *E. orientalis* flowers twelve constituents representing 100% were identified in which Ethyl cinnamate (84.80 %), Ethanol (7.86%), Tetra hydrogeranyl acetone (2.18%) and Phenantrenol (1.26%) were the major ones. The results showed that there are some differences and similarities between the oil compositions of *Elaeagnus* species growing in the same weather conditions. Although the main component of the essential oils of *Elaeagnus* species was Ethyl cinnamate, but its relative content was higher in the oil of *E. orientalis.* The percentage of Ethanol in the oil of *Elaeagnus* species also was less than 10%. Moreover, although the Isobutyl cinnamate, Buthyl cinnamate and Methyl 9, 9- Dideutero- Octadecanoate compounds were the main component of the essential oil of *E. angustifolia* flowers, but these compounds were not identified in the essential oil of *E. orientalis.*

Industrial and practical recommendations: The results of the present study showed that the *E. angustifolia* and *E. orientalis* flower oils can be utilized as cheap commercially sources to isolation Ethyl cinnamate. In addition, extraction of the identified components can be useful for medicinal uses.

1. Introduction

E. angustifolia (Russian olive, oleaster) belongs *to Elaeagnus* genus and *Elaeagnaceae* family. *E. angustifolia* is a shrub or tree with a height of up to 7 m and a capacity to grow under a wide range of environmental conditions (Klich, 2000). This species shows a broad geographical range, occurring widely in Asia and Europe, particularly in Turkey and Central Asia (Aksoy and Sahin, 1999). It is used as an ornamental tree in many European cities (Sastre *et al.*, 2004). Its fruits are used as diuretic, tonic, antipyretic, antidiarrheal and as a medication against kidney disorders in traditional Turkish medicine (Lev and Amar, 2002; Ahmadiani *et al,* 2000). Decoction and infusion of its fruits are considered to be a good remedy for fever, jaundice, asthma, tetanus and rheumatoid arthritis. Its flowers also are used in flavoring some liqueurs (Zargari, 1990).

E. orientalis belongs *to Elaeagnus* genus. It is a diffused shrub with small pale green leaves and a woody stem growing to 6-12 m. In Iran, this plant is in Mazandaran, Sistan and Baluchestan and Gilan province (Ghahraman, 1986). *E. orientalis* is used by local physicians for the treatment of tumours, certain type of cancer and viral diseases (Matthews, 1994).

For this reason, the importance of *E. angustifolia* and *E. orientalis* plants as an herbal medicine, the aim of the present study was to elucidate the chemical composition of the essential oil of *E. angustifolia* and *E. orientalis* flowers in Sistan and Baluchestan province. In order to study the complex chemical composition of volatile compound from plants, advanced analytical GC-MS techniques must be used, these allowing the identification of compounds even in minute quantities (Rădulescu and Oprea, 2008; Pavel *et al.*, 2009).

2. Materials and methods

E. angustifolia and *E. orientalis* flowers were collected from Zahedan in Sistan and Baluchestan province. In first step, the flower samples were dried away from sunlight and then powdered. Hydrodistillation using a Clevenger- type apparatus was used for essential oil extraction. For the extraction, 100 g of the *E. angustifolia* flower powder was hydrodistilled with 300 mL water in a Clevenger-type apparatus for 5h. Moreover, 40 g of the *E. orientalis* flower samples were hydrodistilled with 200 mL water in a Clevenger-type apparatus for 5h. The essential oils were dried over anhydrous Na_2SO_4 (Merk), stored in a dark glass bottle and kept at 4°C until analysis.

The essential oils were analyzed by GC-MS electron impact ionization (EI) method on GC-17A gas chromatograph (Shimadzu) coupled to a GC/MS QP 5050A Mass Spectrometer (Shimadzu). Compounds were separated on a 50m × 0.25mm fused-silica capillary column coated with a 0.32μm film tickness of DB-1 (Shimadzu). The data were acquired under the following conditions: the initial temperature and final temperature were 50 °C and 225 °C, respectively. The carrier gas was helium and the split ratio was 30 ml/min. For GC–MS detection, an electron ionization system with ionization energy of 70 eV was used. The components of the oils were identified by comparison of their mass spectra with those of a computer library (Wiley-v.7 database) or with authentic compounds.

3. Results and discussion

The oils from flowers of *E. angustifolia* and *E. orientalis* were examined by GC-MS. The chemical composition of the essential oils and their amount were shown in Table 1. In the essential oil of *E. angustifolia,* 12 constituents representing %100, were identified in which Ethyl cinnamate (73.24 %), Cyclohexanecarboxylic acid, ethenyl ester (6.94 %), Isobutyl cinnamate (4.74%), Palmitic acid (4.39%), Buthyl cinnamate (2.38%), Ethanol (2.24%) and Methyl 9, 9- Dideutero- Octadecanoate (2.05 %) were the major constituents (Table 1).

In total, 12 constituents in the *E. orientalis* flower oils representing %100, were identified in which Ethyl cinnamate (84.80 %), Ethanol (7.86%), Tetra hydrogeranyl acetone (2.18%) and Phenantrenol (1.26%) were the major ones (Table 1). The results showed that there are some differences and similarities between the oil compositions of *Elaeagnus* species growing in the same weather conditions.

There are no adequate literature data concerning chemical composition of the volatile oil of *E. orientalis* and *E. angustifolia* flower. Twenty six compounds were identified in the essential oil of *E. angustifolia* flower and ethyl cinnamate was the most dominant followed by

(E)-9-octadecenoic acid ethyl ester and n-hexadecanoic acid. In addition, relatively high amounts of n-propyl acetate, 2-pentadecyn-1-ol and 9-octadecenal (Z) were also found in the extract. Apart from ethyl cinnamate, aromatic alcohols and ketones appeared to contribute to the aroma of the essential oil (Hu and Guo-qiang, 2013). The presence of 4-hydroxybenzoic acid, phenolic acid, and acid caffeic also was reported in the *E. angustifolia* fruit (Ayaz *et al.,* 1999) and the significant amounts of flavonoid, terpenoid, and cytosterol compounds were derived from the *E. angustifolia* leaves (Dembinska-Migas and Gill, 1973). Total phenolic and flavonoid content of leaves and flowers were also determined in two *E. angustifolia* variants and reported that the amount of phenolic and flavonoids compounds in leaves were higher than flowers (Saboonchian *et al.,* 2014). Flavonoids have been considered one of the most important constituents in *E. angustifolia*. Antinociceptive and anti-inflammatory activities of some flavonoids have been reported previously (Ramezani *et al.*, 2001; Ahmadiani, 2000; Küpeli and Yesilada, 2007; Erdemoglu *et al.*, 2008). In another study Elaeagnoside, a new steroidal glucoside, has been isolated from the chloroform fraction of *E. orientalis*. The identified components showed significant inhibitory activity against the enzyme chymotrypsin (Ayaz *et al.*, 2009). The type and amount of the components are different in *Elaeagnus* species. These variations may be attributed mainly to variation in their agroclimatic and geographical conditions.

Table 1. Composition of the volatile oil of the *E. angustifolia* and *E. orientalis* flowers.

Compounds of *E. angustifolia*	%	Compounds of *E. orientalis*	%
Ethanol	2.24	Ethanol	7.86
2-propenoic,3-phenyl, ethyl ester	0.81	Cinnamic acid, isopropyl ester	0.35
Ethyl cinnamate	**73.24**	Ethyl cinnamate	**84.80**
Cyclohexanecarboxylic acid, ethenyl ester	6.94	Cyclohexanecarboxylic acid, ethenyl ester	0.94
Buthyl cinnamate (Cis or Trans)	0.66	1- Phenanthrenol	1.26
Pheylethyl tiglate 2	0.97	Megastigmatrinone 4	0.21
Isobuthyl cinnamate	4.74	Cycloheptan,1,3,5-tris(methylene)	0.51
Buthyl cinnamate (Cis or Trans)	2.38	Palmitic acid	0.94
2- phenylnitroethane	0.74	2-methyl-5-phenylpent-4-en-3-one	0.42
2-Phentadecanone	0.84	Hexahydropseudoionone (Tetra hydrogeranyl acetone)	2.18
Palmitic acid	4.39	Di-N-buthyl phthalate	0.32
Methyl 9,9-Dideutero-Octadecanoate	2.05	Octadecane	0.21

4. Conclusions

Here in, we reported the essential oil composition of *E. angustifolia* and *E. orientalis* flowers. The results of the present study showed that the *E. angustifolia* and *E. orientalis* flower oils can be utilized as cheap sources for the commercial isolation of Ethyl cinnamate. In addition, extraction of the identified components can be useful for medicinal uses. This study is a preliminary research for investigating the nutritional values and potential use of *E. angustifolia* and *E. orientalis*. Hopefully, it paves the way for further research projects.

5. Acknowledgement

We appreciate the university of Sistan and Baluchestan Research Council for its partial support.

6. References

Ahmadiani, A., Hosseiny, J., Semnanian, S., Javan, M., Saeedi, F., Kamalinejad, M. and Saremi, S. 2000. Antinociceptive and anti- inflammatory effects of *Elaeagnus angustifolia* fruit extract. *Journal of Ethnopharmacology,* 72: 287-92.

Aksoy, A. and Sahin, U. 1999. *Elaeagnus angustifolia* L. as a biomonitor of heavy metal pollution. *Turkish Journal of Botany,* 23: 83-87.

Ayaz, F. A., Kadioğlu, A. and Doğru A. 1999. Soluble sugar composition of *Elaeagnus angostiholio* L. var.

orientalis (L.) Kuntze (Russian olive) fruits. *Botany*, 23: 349-354.

Ayaz, M., Riaz, A., Malik, A., Ahmad, E., Fatima, I., Arif Lodhi, M. and Iqbal Chaudhary, M. 2009. Elaeagnoside, chymotrypsin inhibiting steroidal glucoside from *Elaeagnus orientalis*. *Natural Product Research,* 23: 409-414.

Dembinska-Migas, W. and Gill, S. 1973. Flavonoids in leaves of *Elaeagnus angustifolia* L. *Polish Journal of Pharmacology and Pharmacy*, 25: 599-606.

Erdemoglu, N., Akkol, E.K., Yesilada, E. and Calls, I. 2008. Bioassay-guided isolation of anti-inflammatory and antinociceptive principles from a folk remedy, *Rhododendron ponticum* L. leaves. *Journal of Ethnopharmacology,* 119:172-78.

Ghahraman, A. 1986. *Flora of Iran.* Vol. 5. The Research Institute of Forests and Rangelands press.

Hu, Y. and Guo-qiang, G. 2013. Gas Chromatographic-Mass Spectrometric Analysis of Essential Oil Extracted by Supercritical CO2 from Flowers of *Elaeagnus angustifolia* L. *Food Science*, 34: 152-156.

Klich, M.G. 2000. Leaf variations in Elaeagnus *angustifolia* related to environmental heterogeneity. *Enviromental and Experimental Botany*, 44:171-183.

Küpeli, E. and Yesilada, E. 2007. Flavonoids with anti-inflammatory and antinociceptive activity from *Cistus laurifolius* L. leaves through bioassay-guided procedures. *Journal of Ethnopharmacology,* 112:524-30.

Lev, E. and Amar, Z. 2002. Ethnopharmacologicl survey of traditional drugs sold in the Kingdom of Jordan. *Journal of Ethnopharmacology*, 82:131-145.

Matthews, V. 1994. *The new plantsman*. Vol. 1. Royal Horticultural Society.

Pavel, M., Rădulescu, V., Ilieş, D.C. 2009. GC-MS analysis of essential oil obtained from the species *Thymus comosus* Heuff.ex Griseb (Lamiaceae). *Farmacia*, 57: 479-484.

Rădulescu, V. and Oprea, E. 2008. Analysis of volatile compounds of officinal *Tiliae flos* by gas chromatography coupled with mass spectrometry. *Farmacia*, 4: 129-138.

Ramezani, M., Hosseinzadeh, H. and Daneshmand, N. 2001. Antinociceptive effect of *Elaeagnus angustifolia* fruit seeds in mice. Fitoter, 72:255-62.

Saboonchian, F., Jamei, R. and Hosseini Sarghein, S. 2014. Phenolic and flavonoid content of *Elaeagnus angustifolia L.* (leaf and flower). *Avicenna journal of phytomedicine*, 4: 231-238.

Sastre, J., Lluch-Bernal, M., Bustillo, A.M.G., Carnes, J., Maranon, F., Casanovas M. and Fernandez-Caldas, E. 2004. Allergenicity and cross- reactivity of Russian olive pollen (*Elaeagnus angustifolia*), *Allergy*, 59: 1181-1186.

Zargari, A. 1990. *Medicinal plants,* vol.4. Tehran, Tehran Univercity Press, pp. 275-277.

Ethnobotanical study of medicinal plants of Sardasht, Western Azerbaijan, northwestern Iran

Hejraneh Azizi*[1], **Maryam Keshavarzi**[2]

[1]*Faculty of Biological sciences, Shahid Beheshti University, Tehran, Iran;*

[2]*Faculty of Biological sciences, Alzahra University, Tehran, Iran;*
***Email:** hejraneh.azizi@yahoo.com*

ARTICLE INFO

Topic: *Ethnobotany*

Key words:
- ✓ *Medicinal plants*
- ✓ *Ethnobotany*
- ✓ *Traditional medicine*
- ✓ *Sardasht*
- ✓ *Iran*

ABSTRACT

Background & Aim: The traditional knowledge about medicinal plants is the basic step in many drug productions. Traditional medicine and herbal drug have absorbed attraction of many world authorities. Using medicinal plants has developed in many countries even those with a vast use of chemical drugs. Ethno-botanical studies result in documentation of many useful plants. In these studies the main aim is to identify such plants and introduce their active and biologic ingredients. Iran is a proper case of ethno-botanical studies due to its different habitats and rich plant vegetation types. Nowadays using new medicinal plants components and optimized usage of rich natural resources is a necessity.
Experimental: In present project medicinal plants of Sardasht with local importance have been collected and identified during 2011 & 2012 growth seasons. Careful uses of medicinal herbs were determined by interview with native people. Scientific names and local medicinal uses are mentioned.
Results & Discussion: There were totally recognized 70 medicinal species of 29 families. Results of present study showed that local people mainly used Asteraceae and Apiaceae then Lamiaceae, Rosaceae and Fabaceae medicinal taxa. Medical plants in this region are mainly used to treat circulatory system problems such as Diabetics and blood lipid.
Industrial and practical recommendations: According to results of this study, the preservation and conservation of some herbs species is essential. This document can play a role in preserving the indigenous knowledge of using these plants.

1. Introduction

From the early days of human history he tried to recognize the plants in order to use them as food, shelter and medicine or avoid from toxic ones. Plants are always considered as an eternal source of human needs. Science development provides a new insight to use natural products as food and medicine. World plant vegetation comprises more than tens of thousands of species but only a minority of these has been considered by researchers in biological pharmacological and phyto-chemical studies (Qureshi *et al.*, 2006). One of the most effective and proper methods to select plants for such studies is the use of people traditional knowledge in different parts of the world. Such kind of native knowledge and experience is inherited generation by generation and nowadays is used to improve scientific and practical researches. Ethnobotany as a practical field of study is trying to link human culture and ecosystem (Jorjani, 2001). With the findings of these studies, plant usage in different societies are gathered and studied in order to conserve the thousand years of human experience about plants properties and their implications in treatments and to improve botany in the other hand (Goleniowski *et al.*, 2006). Medicinal extracts as taxol, Curcomine, Cochysine, Aspirine, Digoxcine, ephedrine, quinine, quinidine etc. are some of these approaches. The more ancient the history and culture of a nation the more it reaches the aims of such studies. Iran community with a history of several thousand years of cultural and ethnic diversity, climate and weather diversity and a richness of more than 8000 species is a proper case of ethonobotanical study. Phytotrapy is initiated from early medieval in Western countries although it was not tangible progress at first but after appearance of Salerne doctrine it was improved rapidly. They used not only their native plants but also plants of Persian and Arabic celebrity doctors (Omid beige, 2000; Safizadeh, 1982; Razi, 1990). Chemical drugs are used extensively nowadays but medicinal plants are used increasingly and its production and composed a significant value. Prolonged use of chemical substances may have side effects, sometimes as severe as disease itself, while using medicinal plants component has not such side effects. Thalidomide in Europe is best sample for this bad effects (Daryaie, 2006).

Sardasht is a borderline city of West Azerbaijan province, Iran with a vast Kurdish settlement. This city is situated between 36°9′ latitude and 45° 32′ longitude. Sardasht is located at the southwest of the Orumiyeh Lake, 1500 meters above sea level. Sardasht area is about 1411 km^2 which is about 7% of the province area (Fig. 1). People language of Sardasht is Kurdish (Soorani, mikeriani accent). Neighboring cities are Piranshahr and Mahabad (at N and NE), Bookan (at E) and Baneh (at SE). The studied area is near Rania and Dize at west (Arbil, Iraqi Kurdistan) and soleymaniyeh (at south) and Gir and out (at east). The population of the Sardasht is about 111590 based on 2010 Census. Its geographical position and the annual rainfall prepare the proper situation to have plant vegetation richness. There is an important forest region of the province in Sardasht over than 80000 hectares. One third of these forest zone is very dense, one third is sparse and remaining part is of disturbed and destroyed forests. The main forest type of this region is Oak, quince, peer and wild grapes. The economic importance of these forests is based on oak and its accessories as gall nut, manna, turpentine and medicinal materials. Due to the ancient culture of this region, and the historical interest of Kurdish people to use medicinal plants, the aim of present study is to collect and identify the medicinal plant of the Sardasht region.

2. Materials and methods

Samples were collected from the entire studied region during two growth seasons of 2011 & 2012 from April to September. For each plant complete parts were gathered and dried to make herbarium specimens. Studied and sampled specimens are deposited at Herbarium of Alzahra University. Plants were identified by use of local and other floras (Rechinger, 1988; Mozaffarian, 2009; Parsa, 1948-1960; Ghahreman, 1975-2000). Traditional medicinal and local implications of plants were achieved by interviews with old local people.

3. Results and discussion

Totally 70 species were identified in studied region. Details of samples and their scientific name are indicated in Tab. 1. In order to study the ethnobotany of a region one should live with them to know the perfect implication of herbal materials. Ethnobotanist not only deals with medicinal but also with edible, coloring agent, toxical and ornamental plants. Based on field study in Sardasht region with all its villages, there were totally recognized 70 medicinal species of 29 families. Results of present study showed that local people mainly used Asteraceae and Apiaceae then Lamiaceae, Rosaceae and Fabaceae medicinal taxa (Fig. 2). According to the conducted studies on the medicinal plants in other provinces of Iran, these families were also in the first or second rank in terms of medicinal plants (Akbarinia *et al.*, 2006; Mirdavodi & Babakhanlo, 2007). Due to the diversity and spread of this family in the flora of Iran, this is not unexpected (Asadi *et al.*, 1998-2008).

These plants are mainly used to treat circulatory system problems such as Diabetics and blood lipid with frequency of 22.85 percent and the reason can be considered and investigated. At the next step studied plants are used in medical treatment of digestive problems and as analgesic with frequency of 20 percent. The frequency application of medicinal plants for treating Soothing was 17%, as Skin and hair was about 11%, Anti infection, Respiratory system, Menstruation and fertility was 10%, as an Kidney and urinary tract was 8%, for Teeth and Gums was 5.75%, for was Vision 4%, for anti-Cancer was 1%. (Fig. 3).

Due to the vegetation richness of Sardasht region in Iran, and the presence of medicinal plants special attention should be paid on collection, identification and cultivation of local medicinal plants to prepare the proper and standard form of drugs. Plants provide a great comfort and shelter for human being with a vast genetic diversity and medicinal properties. Only 5000 plants out of 250 – 300 thousands specie have been studied as medicinal ones.

Table. 1. List of medicinal plant species and their uses

Scientific name	Family	Local name	Used parts	Medicinal application
Achillea eriophora DC.	Asteraceae	Bozhana	Leaves	Anti-diarrheal
Allium sativum L.	Aliaceae	Sire	Shoots	Anti-hypertensive
Allium affine Ledeb.	Aliaceae	Pivaz	Shoots	Strengthen the teeth and gums
Allium Akaka Gmel.	Aliaceae	Losha	Shoots	Anti-infection and kidney stones
Althaea officinalis L.	Malvaceae	Hero	Flowers, roots and leaves	Regulate menstruation, , anti-migraine headache and Diabetes
Amygdalus scoparia L	Rosaceae	Bayam	Fruit & leaves	Strengthen hair
Anethum graveolens L.(dill)	Apiaceae	Toragh	Leaves	Treatment of Diabetes
Arctium lappa L.	Asteraceae	Chaghl	Root	Strengthen hair and Blood Purifier
Artemisia aucheri Boiss.	Asteraceae	Dermana kevi	Leaves	Anti-Cough
Bunium spp.	Apiaceae	Zirah	Shoots	Strengthen the stomach
Berberis spp.	Berberidaceae	Zrishk	Fruit	Blood thinners
Beta vulgaris L.	Chenopodiaceae	Chavandar	Leaves	Anti-hemorrhoids and constipation
Brassica Napus L.	Brasicaceae	Kolza	Leaves	Anti-Cough, Diabetes and night blindness
Cardaria draba(L.) Desv.	Brassicaceae	Tef ba sar	Leaves	Diuretic
Caryophillium aromaticus	Caryophylaceae	Mikhak	Fruit	Toothache pain and strengthen the vision
Cerasus vulgaris Mill.	Rosaceae	Belalok	Fruit	Blood purification
Chamaemelum nobile(L.) All.	Asteraceae	Gola hajiana	Flower	Menstrual pain
Cirsium arvense (L.)Scop.	Asteraceae	Kengeri vahshi	Root	Strengthen the stomach
Coriandrum sativum L.	Apiaceae	Geshniz	Fruit	Avar rule and Painkiller
Corylus avellana L.	Betulaceae	Fandogh	Leaves	Strengthen hair
Cratagus monogyna Jacq.	Rosaceae	Goizh	Fruit	Anti-Blood lipid
Cydonia vulgaris L.	Rosaceae		Fruit	Antihypertensive

Cynara scolymus L.	Asteraceae	Kenger	Leaves	Strengthen the digestive system
Daucus carota L.	Apiaceae	Gezar	Root	Vision amplifiers
Descurainia Sophia L.	Brassicaceae	Khak shir	Fruit sand seed	Laxatives and strengthen the stomach
Dianthus spp.	Caryophylaceae	Mikhak	Seed	Tooth Pain Relief
Echium amenum Fisch. & Mey	Boraginaceae	Gozervan	Leaves	Burning pain relief
Euphorbia helioscopia L.	Euphorbiaceae	Gia kala	Shoots	Anti-arthritic and rheumatic
Vicia faba L.	Fabaceae	Baghla	Fruit and seed	Tooth Pain Relief
Ficus carica L.	Moraceae	Hanjir	leaves	Agglutination
Foeniculum vulgare Mill.	Apiaceae	Razianah	Leaves, Fruit	Relieve abdominal pain in children and increase breast milk
Fumaria officinalis L.	Fumariaceae	Shatarah	Shoots	Anti-parasite and fever
Fumaria parvifora Lam.	Fumariaceae	Shatarah	Shoots	Anti-Acne
Glycyrrhiza glabra L.	Fabaceae	Giah balak	Root	Treatment of Ulcer
Heliotropium ramosissimum (Lehm.) DC.	Boraginaceae	Tav parast	Leaves	Treatment of snake bites
Hordeum vulgare L.	Poaceae	Jou	Fruit	Anti-Diabetes
Juglans regia L.	Juglandaceae	Gveze	Leaves and fruit	Anti-headaches, high blood pressure, anti-worm
Lamium album L.	Lamiaceae	Gaz gaz spi	Leaves	Anti-Diabetes
Lawsonia inermis L.	Lathyraceae	Khana	Leaves	Anti-headaches, migraines and strengthening hair follicles
Lepidium sativum L.	Apiaceae	Taratizah	Leaves	Arthritis pain reliever
Lens culinaris L.	Fabaceae	Nisk	Fruit	Increasing breast and colon strengthen
Malva sylvestris L.	Malvaceae	Tolaka	Leaves	Anti-abdominal pain in infants
Medicago sativa L.	Fabaceae	Venja	Leaves	Vision amplifiers
Mentha longifolia (L.) Huds.	Lamiaceae	Naana	Leaves	Asthma and respiratory tract
Morus alba L.	Moraceae	Tou	Fruit	Refrigerant
Morus nigra L.	Moraceae	Toua gaya	Fruit	Hematopoietic
Nymphaea alba L.	Nymphaceae	Nilufar	Leaves	Anti-Cough
Ocimum basilicum L.	Lamiaceae	Rehana	Leaves	Anticonvulsant and to increase breast milk
Ornithogalum sintenisii L.	Liliaceae	Shir morgh	Leaves	Soothing
Phasaeolous vulgaris L.	Fabaceae	Lubia	Fruit	Strengthening the heart
Pirus communis L.	Rosaceae	Harmeh	Fruit	Anti-kidney stones and fever
Pistacia atlantica Desf.	Anacardiaceae	Ghazvan	Fruit	Stomach ulcers and stomach pain
Pistacia khinjuk L.	Anacardiaceae	Khinjuk	Leaves	Hemorrhoid Treatment
Plantago major L.	Plantaginaceae	Baza rishi	Leaves and roots	Wound healing and anti-infection
Plantago lanceolata L.	Plantaginaceae	Baza risha barik	Leaves	Anti-diarrheal
Portulaca oleracea L.	Portulaceae	Perperah	Shoots	Blood purification and cleansing the skin
Prangos ferulacea Lindl.	Apiaceae	Marzah	Shoots	Anti-parasitic and anti-cancer
Ricinuscommunis L.	Euphorbiaceae	Karchak	Seed	Skin Booster
Rosa canina L.	Rosaceae	Shilan	Flower	Anti-Infections and kidney stones

Rumex thyrsiflorus Fingerth.	Polygonaceae	Tershoka	Leaves	Strengthen the digestive system
Salvia spp.	Lamiaceae	Maryam goli	Flower	Anti-infection
Sclia sibirica Haw.	Liliaceae	Najm abi	Leaves	Soothing
Scrophularia spp.	Scropholariaceae	Gol mimoni	Flower	Anti-asthma
Tanacetum spp.	Asteraceae	Babone gavi	Flowers and leaves	Strengthen the digestive system
Thymus vulgaris L.	Lamiaceae	Jatrah	Leaves	Anti-itch and anti-abdominal pain
Trifolium pretense L.	Fabaceae	Shavar	Leaves	Increase Fertility
Urtica dioica L.	Urticaceae	Gaz gaz	Leaves	Soothing Foot Pain and anti-Kidney Stones
Vicia sativa L.	Fabaceae	Mash	Seed	Refrigerant
Vitis vinifera L.	Vitaceae	Meve	Shoots	Kidney infection treatment and prevention of hair loss
Ziziphora spp	Lmiaceae	Kakoti	Flower	Anti-Cough

Unfortunately many plant species are endangered or become extinct before even a preliminary study. It seems that valuable nature resource is devastating rapidly (Fransworth and Morris, 1976; Fransworth *et al.*, 1985). Two type of medicinal plants are used in Iran: first a well identified group with a definite common name and a second group composed of unrecognized plants with empirical usage in different parts. So it seems necessary to study the medicinal plants more seriously (Poyan, 1989).

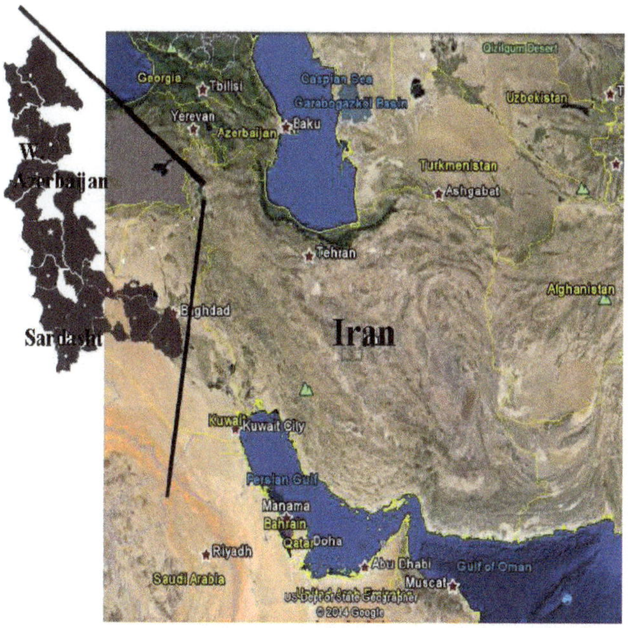

Fig. 1. Map of Iran, Western Azerbaijan province (gray color), Sardasht.

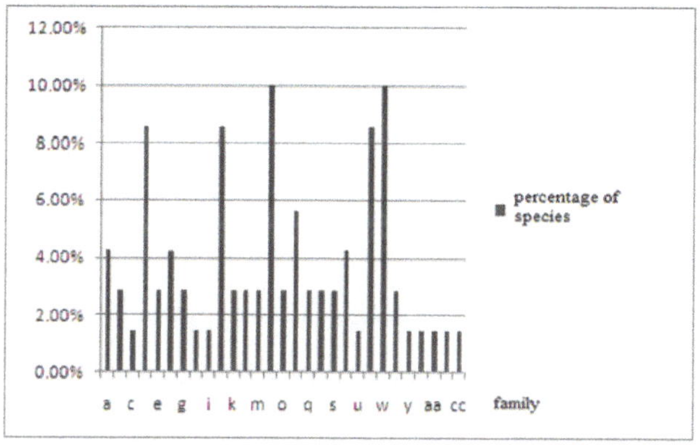

Fig. 2. Families with their medicinal importance (as percentage) in studied area. a. Aliaceae, b. Malvaceae, c. Chenopodiaceae, d. Rosaceae, e. Ephurbiaceae, f. Moraceae, g.Fumariaceae, h. Juglandaceae, i. Lathyraceae, j. Lamiaceae, k. Liliaceae, l. Anacardiaceae, m. Plantaginaceae, n. Apiaceae, o. Punicaceae, p. Polygonaceae,q. Urticaceae, r. Vitaceae, s. Boraginaceae, t. Brasicaseae, u. Nymphaceae,v. Fabaceae, w. Asteraceae, x. Caryohyllaceae, y. Betulaceae, z. Portulaceae, aa. Berberidaceae, bb. Poaceae, cc. Schropholariaceae.

In present study, we have compared our ethnobotanical data with the data present in Iranian Medicinal plant literatures (Afshar, 1990; Amin, 1991; Ayiineh Chii, 1989; Ghahreman1987-198918; Ghasemi Pirbalouti, 2009 a,b; Ghasemi *et al.*, 2013; Ghorbani, 2005; Hovayzeh *et al.*, 2001; Miraldi *et al.*, 2001; Mir-Heidari, 1993; Rojhan, 1991; Salehi Surmaghi *et al.*, 1992; Zargari, 1989–1992 28). Most of the plants indicated by the interviewees are reported in Iranian literature, but not in every occasion were the actions attributed to a plant the same. Traditional knowledge should therefore feature more often in the agendas of nature reserves besides biological richness as a value to preserve for the future. In general, the people of the study area still have a strong belief in the efficiency and success of medicinal plants.

The results of our study reveal that some of the plant species do play an important role in the primary healthcare system of this tribal community.

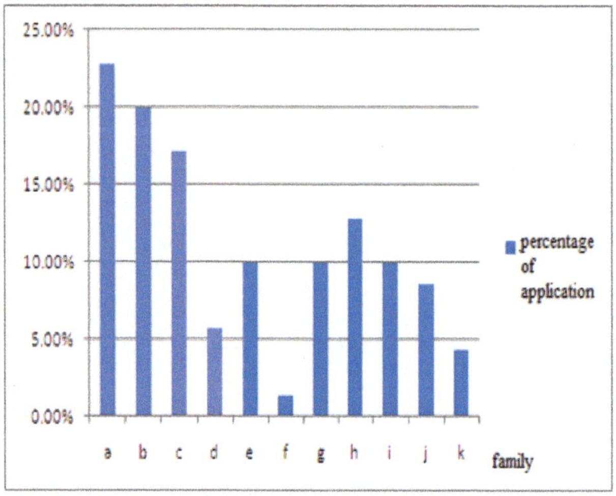

Fig. 3. Medicinal plants application in different human disease treatments (in percentage).

A: Circulatory system,b: Digestive System, c: Soothing, d: Teeth and Gums, e: Anti infection, f: anti-Cancer, g: Respiratory system, h: Skin and hair, i: Menstruation and fertility, j: Kidney and urinary tract, k: Vision.

4. Conclusion

Most of the plants mentioned in Table 1 have been used as medicinal herbs in folkloric medicine in present and past. The dialectical relationship between indigenous knowledge and practices shapes the ecosystem and affects the constituent plant population. By incorporating indigenous knowledge and use in the process of scientific research, new hypotheses for the sustainable conservation of resources can be developed. Indigenous knowledge and use have to be analyzed to develop appropriate management measures that build on both scientific and local knowledge. Due to lack of interest among the younger generation as well as their tendency to migrate to cities for lucrative jobs, there is a possibility of losing the wealth of knowledge in the near future. It thus becomes necessary to acquire and preserve the traditional system of medicine by proper documents and identification of specimens. This first report can play a role in identification and preserving of specimens the indigenous knowledge of using these plants.

5. References

Afshar, I. 1990. The Iranians Traditional Medicine. Homa Press.

Akbarinia, A., Babakhanlo, P. and Mozafarian, V. 2006. Evaluation of floristic and biological characteristics of medicinal plants Qazvin. *Journal of Pajouhesh va Sazandegi.*, 72: 70-76.

Amin, G. 1991. Popular Medicinal Plants of Iran. Iranian Research Institute of Medicinal Plants press.

Asadi, M., Masomi, A., Khatam saz, M. and Mozafarian, M. 1998-2008. *Flora of Iran. Research Institute of forests and pastures press.* 1-59 (in Persian).

Ayiineh Chii, Y. 1989. *Medicinal Plants and Materia Medica.* University press.

Daryaie, M. 2006. *Miracles of healing herbs in Iranian Medicine.* Creative Visualization press. pp: 31-186.

Fransworth, N., Morris, R.1976. Higher plants the sleeping gaint of drug development, *American J ournal of Pharmacy.*, 148: 46-52.

Fransworth, N.R., Akerel, O., Beingel, A.S., Soejarto, D.D., Guo, Z. 1985. Medicinal plants in thrapy. *Bulletin of the World Health Organization.*, 63: 965-81.

Ghahreman, A. 1987-1989. *Flora of Iran. Department of Botany.* Institute of Forest Sciences press.

Ghahreman, A. 1975-2000. *Colored Flora of Iran*, Vol. 1-20. Research institute of forests and rangelands press.

Ghasemi Pirbalouti, A. 2009a. Medicinal plants used in Chaharmahal and Bakhtyari districts Iran. *Herba Polonica.*, 55: 69-75.

Ghasemi Pirbalouti, A. 2009b. *Iranian Medicinal and Aromatic Plants.* Islamic Azad University Press.

Ghorbani, A. 2005. Studies on pharmaceutical ethnobotany in the region of Turkmen Sahra, north of Iran. *Journal of Ethnopharmacology.*, 102: 58-68.

Goleniowski, M.E., Bongiovanni, G.A., Palacio, L., Nunez, C.O., Cantero, J.J. 2006. Medicinal plants from the (sierra de comechingones). *Argentina. Journal of Ethnopharmacol.*, 107: 324- 41.

Hovayzeh, H., Dinarvand, M. and Sahlehi, J. 2001. Ethnobotany of medicinal plants in Khuzestan province. *Pajouhesh va Sazandegi.*, 53: 12-16.

Jorjani, E. 2001. *Save the kharazmshahi.* Academy of Medical Sciences press. Iran. pp: 10-150.

Miraldi, E., Ferri, S. and Mostaghimi, V. 2001. Botanical drugs and preparations in the traditional medicine of west Azerbaijan (Iran). *Journal of Ethnopharmacology.*, 75: 77-87.

Mirdavodi, H. and Babakhanlo, P. 2007. Identification of medicinal plants of central province. *Iranian Journal of Medical and Aromatic Plants*., 23(4): 554-559.

Mir-Heidari, H. 1993. *Encyclopedia of Medicinal Plants of Iran*. Islamic Culture Press.

Mozaffarian, V. 1996. *Encyclopedia of Iranian Plants.* Farhang Moaser Publication, Tehran, Iran.

Mozaffarian, V. 2008. *Flora of Ilam*. Farhang Moaser Publication, Tehran, Iran.

Mozaffarian, V. 2009. *Culture names of Iranian plants.* Farhang Moaser press.

Omid beigi, R. 2000. *Approaches to the production and processing of medicinal plants*. Designers press. pp: 56.

Parsa , A. 1948-1960. *Flora de L Iran*. Ministre de L educatioation press.

Poyan, M. 1989. *Medicinal Plants of South Khorasan.* nashre danesh press. pp. 78.

Qureshi, R., Waheed, A., Arshad, M., Umbreen, T. 2006. Medico- ethnobotanical inventory of tehsil chakwal. *Pakistan Journal of botany*., 41: 529-53.

Razi, A. 1990. Alhavi, Vol.10. *Pharmaceutical Institute Alhavi press*. pp: 15.

Rechinger, KH. 1988. Flore iranica, Vol. 1. Graz – Austeria: Akademische Druck- und verlagsanstalt.

Rojhan, M. S. 1991. *Herbal Drugs and Treatment with Medicinal Plants.* Marshal Press.

Safizadeh, S. 1982. *Traditional medicine among the Kurds*. attai press. pp: 6.

Salehi Surmaghi, M. H., Aynehchi, Y., Amin, G. and Mahmoodi, Z. 1992. *Survey of Iranian plants for saponins.* alkaloids.

Zargari, A. 1982-1992. *Plants*, Vol. 1-6. University press. Iran.

Study of qualitative characteristics of saffron cultivated in different regions of Iran

Nasibeh Sharifi, Mohammad Hojjatoleslamy*, Maryam Jafari

Department of food Science and Technology, Islami Azad University, Shahrekord branch, Shahrekord, Iran;
*Email: *mohojjat@gmail.com*

ARTICLE INFO

Topic: *Medicinal Plants*

Key words:

- ✓ *Gallic acid*
- ✓ *Crocin*
- ✓ *Picrocrocin*
- ✓ *Safranal*

ABSTRACT

Background & Aim: Saffron is one of the expensive spices known since antiquity for its color, flavor and medicinal properties. Saffron is the dried stigma of *crocus sativus* plant. The three basic components of the stigma on which the qualitative characteristics of saffron depend are crocin (color), picrocrocin (taste), and safranal (aroma). The quality of saffron is a function of climatic conditions, soil type, as well as method of drying, packaging, and storage.

Experimental: In this research, the saffron growing in different regions of Iran including Kerman, Shiraz, Arak, Natanz, Ghaen, Shahrekord, and Dolatabad has been studied with regard to its humidity, ash, phenolic compounds, crocin, safranal, and picrocrocin for its classification.

Results & Discussion: The saffron of Shiraz and that of Kerman showed the maximum and minimum amount for ash with a value of 8.02% and 5.38%, respectively. With a view to moisture content, Natanz and Shahrekord saffron showed the highest and the lowest moisture content with a value of 11.97% and 9.7%, respectively. The phenolic compounds were determined by spectrophotometry and ranged from 17.43 mg gallic acid/g dry weight of saffron in Kerman sample to 8.87mg gallic acid/g dry weight in Dolatabad saffron. The highest level of safranal, crocin, and picrocrocin belonged to Shahrekord, Dolatabad, and Shahrekord saffron with a rate of 84.43, 234.4 and 38.4 (strength/ g dry matter) based on the most absorption over three wavelengths of 257, 440, and 330nm, respectively.

Industrial and practical recommendations: With regard to variable applications of saffron as flavoring and coloring in food industry, the results of this study can be used for appropriate usage of saffron cultivated in different regions according to their specifications.

1. Introduction

Saffron is one of the most expensive seasonings all over the world. It is obtained by drying the stigma of saffron plant, scientifically named *Crocus sativus* (Shahidi & Bolandi, 2008). Saffron is a perennial plant of Iridacea family flowering in fall season (Caballero-Ortega *et al*, 2007). This plant often has 1 to 3 violet-colored flowers and its stalk is very short hiding beneath soil (Shahidi & Bolandi, 2008). Saffron grows in Mediterranean climate with mild cold winters and dry and hot summers; the suitable soil for its growth is clay (Khoddami *et al*., 2013). There are two different types of saffron, i.e. strand and cut strand saffron. Strand saffron consists of stigma along with a section of style, while the style is separated from the stigma in the cut strand saffron (Nazari & Keifi, 2011). The origin of saffron whose reputation dates back to about 2500 years ago is the Alvand and Zagross mountainsides (Caballero, 2007). Iran is one of the greatest producers of saffron in the world, and other countries such as Turkey, Greece, Italy, Spain, France, Egypt, Israel, Iraq, and Pakistan also cultivate saffron (Nazari & Keifi, 2011). Saffron contains carbohydrate, vitamins, carotenoid, protein, fat, flavonoids, and one triterpene aromatic named Safranal (Shahidi & Bolandi, 2008). The phenolic compounds that contain one aromatic ring with one or several more hydroxyl groups in plants are generated as a response to physiological pressures such as pathogens, attack of insects, and ultraviolet light (Hadizadeh *et al.*, 2010). Flavonoids are one of the most important phenolic compounds and mostly play a role along with carotenoids in the formation of orange, yellow, and red colors (Caballero- Ortega *et al.*, 2007). Stigma contains flavones, flavanols, iso-flavanols, anthocyanins and catechin (Mohamad *et al.*, 2015).

The most important compounds present in saffron stigma are crocin, picrocrocin and safranal (Mozzafar *et al.*, 2014). Crocin is a 20-carbon carotenoid of the glycoside derivatives of crocetin producing a red-orange color when dissolved in water forming about 6 to 16 percent of the dry weight of saffron; it is the effective material responsible for the saffron color (Nazari & Keifi, 2011). Crocin is used for the production of color in beverage industry and flour products (Khodadadi, 2014). The bitter taste of saffron is derived from glycoside picrocrocin, which is a colorless monoterpene aldehyde (Caballero-Ortega *et al.*, 2004). Due to the binding of one molecule of glucose to hydroxy trimethyl cyclohexene carboxaldehyde, picrocrocin is produced and over the process of saffron drying stages, picrocrocin is hydrolyzed and changed into volatile Safranal, which is the factor for the aroma of saffron and consisting of about 30 to 72% of the aroma compounds of the stigma (Emadi & Saiedirad, 2011). The saffron stigma contains the carotenoids of hydrophile and lipophile. Due to the presence of antioxidants in its stigma, saffron has anti-cancer properties and reduces heart attacks and depression (Karimi *et al.*, 2010). The quality of saffron is a function of different factors such as climate conditions, harvesting conditions, storing conditions, method of drying, and packaging (Caballero-Ortega *et al*, 2004). Saffron usually tolerates high temperatures, but it is sensitive to light and oxygen. Therefore, it is necessary to place it in suitable packages like polyethylene with cellophane covering (Hadizadeh *et al.*, 2010). The quality of saffron is decided by the rate of its color, and compounds of aroma and taste which are affected by different factors such as climate conditions, harvesting conditions, storing conditions, method of drying, and packaging (Caballero-Ortega *et al.*, 2004; Hadizadeh *et al.*, 2010). Zarrinkamar *et al.* (2011) showed that the great altitude and the average low temperature of a region had positive effects on the qualitative specifications of Ghaen and Tabas saffron. The phenolic contents of Natanz Karcass saffron was measured on the basis of gallic acid by Goli *et al.* (2012) who showed that the methanol extract of saffron had the most phenol compounds. Joki *et al.* (2012) studied the rate of Picrocrocin and Safranal of different regions in Khorasan Province and showed that the most crocin and Picrocrocin belonged to Torbateheidarieh. In another research, Tajik (2011) specified that the qualitative specifications of regions with 3 years of saffron cultivation were better than those of regions with 6 years of saffron cultivation (Sariri *et al.*, 2011). Atefi (2012) showed that different methods of drying affected the qualitative specifications of saffron. With regard to the importance of Iranian saffron in the world trade and the spread of this product in different regions of Iran, no comprehensive research has yet been conducted to study the qualitative specifications of saffron in different regions of Iran. The goal of this research is to compare the saffron of different regions of Iran in terms of color, aroma, taste, phenolic compounds, moisture, and ash.

2. Materials and Methods

2.1. Sampling

Saffron samples were taken from each of the provinces of Isfahan (Natanz and Dolatabad), Fars (Estahban), Kerman (Baft), Yazd (Beniz), Markazi (Arak), Khorasan (Ghaen), and Chaharmahal and Bakhtiari (Farrokhshahr).

2.2. Chemicals

All solvents and chemicals used were of analytical grade and obtained from Sigma Chemical Co. (St Louis, MO).

2.3. Determination of moisture and ash contents

259-2 National Standard was employed for determination of moisture and ash. The moisture content was measured by drying the sample in an oven at 100–105°C to constant weight and ash by incinerating in a furnace at 550°C.

2.4. Determination of qualitative specifications with spectrophotometer

Extract preparation: About 500 g of saffron was mixed with 900 ml distilled water and placed on a magnetic stirrer at 1000 rpm for one hour. Then, 20 ml of the solution brought to volume of 200 ml with distilled water. The solution was filtered with filer paper and the absorption of the solution was read with spectrophotometer (Shimadezo, 2100). The results of the solution absorption reading of the three wavelengths of 257, 330, and 440 nm were calculated according to the following formula for safranal, picrocrocin and crocin, respectively.

$$E^{1\%}\,(\lambda_{max}) = \frac{D \cdot 10000}{m(100-w)} \qquad (1)$$

Where D is the absorbance of the sample, m and w are the mass and moisture content of saffron samples. The results were expressed as strength/ g dry matter.

2.5. Determination of total phenolics (Folin-Ciocalteu)

Extract preparation: About 50 mg of the saffron sample were mixed with 5 ml distilled water and 5ml of 98% methanol and placed in a refrigerated incubator (German Aqualytic) equipped with a shaker for 24 hours in a dark space. The supernatant was then separated and placed in a centrifuge at 1500 rpm for 20 minutes. The solution was filtered with filter paper, its surrounding was covered with aluminum foil, and it was placed in a refrigerator.

To perform the test, first, 0.5 ml of the extract was diluted with 20 ml of distilled water; then, 2.5 ml of folinciocalteu (10% by volume) and 0.5 ml of 7.5% sodium carbonate solution were added to it and kept for 30 minutes at ambient temperature until the light blue color appeared. Then, the absorption of the solution was measured along the wavelength of 765nm. Total polyphenol content was expressed as mg of gallic acid per g of dry matter. A calibration curve of gallic acid in methanol was performed in a concentration range of 25–100 mg/l.

2.6. Statistical analysis

Results were shown as the mean ±SD of three separate determinations. The data were statistically analyzed by ANOVA program in SPSS software, version 22. The means evaluation was done using Duncan test at 5% probability level.

3. Results and discussion

3.1. Moisture and ash contents

The results for the moisture and ash contents of saffron samples are presented in Table 1. As seen, no significant difference was observed between the moisture content in the samples of Yazd and Natanz saffron at the probability level of 5%. There was also no significant difference ($p<0.05$) among the samples taken from Arak, Shahrekord, Dolatabad, Ghaen, and Kerman. Among samples, Natanz saffron showed significantly ($p<0.05$) higher moisture content with a value of 11.97% and Shahrekord saffron showed the lowest value with a rate of 9.7%. The most important factors affecting the moisture content are the method of drying, duration of drying, and storage conditions. There are different methods of drying such as drying in the shade, toasting, freeze drying, microwave, and solar drying. These values were higher than those obtained by Atefi (2012) in which the saffron moisture was measured through three methods of drying, i.e. roasting, oven, and shade (5.26%, 6.4%, and 5.5%). Since the saffron drying method is traditionally done in the shade in the two mentioned regions, we may conclude that the duration of drying process was probably different and unsuitable packing cause to an increase in moisture of saffron during storage and transportation.

In terms of ash, no significant difference ($p<0.05$) was observed among the saffron samples of Shahrekord, Arak, Natanz, and Dolatabad. Ash content of the samples ranged from 5.3% to 8.02% showing that ash level of Shiraz saffron was significantly($p<0.05$) higher than that of the other samples which implies higher amount of minerals in this saffron. Ash is indicative of the presence of minerals in saffron depending on the type of soil and climatic conditions as well as the rate of the pollutants existing in air. Values found in this study were similar to the range reported by some researchers (Atefi *et al.,* 2012).

Table 1. Moisture and ash contents of saffron samples

Region	Moisture (%)	Ash (%)
Shiraz	10.96±0.15^{b}	8.02±0.15^{a}
Shahrekord	9.70±0.26^{d}	5.90±0.08^{d}
Kerman	10.13±0.23^{c}	5.38±0.07^{e}
Yazd	11.86±0.11^{a}	6.39±0.06^{c}
Arak	9.90±0.10^{cd}	5.95±0.16^{d}
Natanz	11.97±0.05^{a}	5.77±0.01^{d}
Dolatabad	10.03±0.05^{cd}	5.81±0.06^{d}
Ghaen	9.83±0.28^{cd}	7.10±0.07^{b}

Lowercase letters in the same column represent significant difference (p<0.05).

Table 2. Crocin, picrocrocin and safranal level (strength/ g of dry matter) of saffron samples.

Region	Crocin	Picrocrocin	Safranal
Shiraz	185.5±0.50^{g}	79.66±0.57^{d}	30.83±0.76^{e}
Shahrekord	234.36±1.70^{b}	84.43±0.40^{a}	38.40±0.52^{a}
Kerman	218.73±0.46^{e}	83.03±0.25^{b}	36.86±0.23^{b}
Yazd	140.96±0.15^{h}	72.06±1.00^{e}	21.16±0.20^{f}
Arak	229.26±0.66^{c}	84.40±0.52^{a}	37.53±0.50^{b}
Natanz	211.76±0.76^{f}	70.60±0.52^{f}	30.33±0.57^{e}
Dolatabad	236.40±0.52^{a}	81.93±0.90^{c}	35.70±0.26^{c}
Ghaen	225.80±0.80^{d}	83.83±0.28^{ab}	33.73±0.46^{d}

Lowercase letters in the same column represent significant difference (p<0.05).

3.2. Safranal, crocin and picrocrocin contents in saffron samples

According to Table 2, there is a significant difference (p<0.05) among all the saffron samples in terms of crocin content. The highest level of crocin was found in Dolatabad saffron (234.4 based on the strength/g of dry matter) and Yazd saffron showed the lowest level (140.96 strength/g of dry matter). On Our results were less than that found by Salari *et al.* (2012) who measured the crocin of saffron as 250.26 (strength/g of dry matter). There was no significant difference (p<0.05) in safranal concentration between the saffron samples of Arak and Kerman. Furthermore, no significant difference was found between Natanz and Shiraz samples. The highest value for safranal was found in Shahrekord saffron (38.4, based on strength/ g of dry matter) and the lowest amount was found in Yazd saffron (21.16 based on strength/ g of dry matter). In terms of the picrocrocin content, no significant difference (p<0.05) was observed among the saffron samples of Shahrekord, Arak, and Ghaen and also among Ghaen and Kerman saffron samples. The highest level of picrocrocin was found in Shahrekord saffron sample (84.43 strength/g of dry matter) and the lowest level was found in Natanz saffron (70.6, strength/g of dry matter). The level of these three compounds in saffron is a function of different factors such as method of drying, climatic conditions, altitude, plant age, time of harvest, storage ambient temperature, type of packaging, and plant species. The amount of picrocrocin and safranal in Shahrekord saffron was more than that presented by Atefi *et al.* (2012) who reported it 81.25 and 17.62 (strength/ g of dry matter) for picrocrocin and safranal, respectively. In addition, Salari *et al.* (2012) also measured the picrocrocin and safranal content of Southern Khorasan saffron and reported them as 112.9 and 27.24 (strength/ g of dry matter), respectively. Regarding the effect of altitude, Zarrinkamar *et al.* (2011) studied two regions of Ghaen with an altitude of 1400 meters and Tabas with an altitude of 700 meters. The results showed that the amount of the three factors was more in Ghaen with a higher altitude than that in Tabas. According to Zarrinkamar *et al.* (2011) it is expected that Shahrekord shows the most rate of crocin while having the highest altitude, but only the two factors of safranal and picrocrocin of Shahrekord saffron are higher than those of Dolatabad. Therefore, it can be concluded that since the drying method for all the saffron is traditional (in shade); therefore, other factors such as average temperature of the region, plant age, type of soil, type of saffron bulb, rate of rainfall, climate, and the time of saffron flower harvest could affect the range of these three factors of color, aroma, and taste.

3.3. Total phenolic compounds

The results of phenolic compounds of saffron samples are presented in Table 3. Total phenol content ranged from 17.43 mg gallic acid/g of dry weight (Kerman saffron) to 8.87 mg/g of dry weight (Dolatabad saffron). No significant difference (p<0.05) was observed between the saffron samples of Shiraz and Dolatabad and also between Shiraz and Arak. Phenolic compounds produced in plants as a response to physiological pressures such as pathogens, insect attacks, and ultraviolet irradiation. According to the results obtained by Karimi *et al.* (2010) the highest amount of phenolic compounds based on gallic acid was found in Kerman saffron with a value of 17.43 mg/g and the lowest amount was found in Dolatabad saffron with a value of 8.89 mg/g which were similar to our results. They also reported that phenolic compounds of methanol and ethanol extracts of Kashmar saffron were 6.5 and 6.3mg gallic acid/g of dry weight of saffron, respectively. phenolic compound based on caffeic acid of saffron reported by Gismondi *et al.* (2012) was 53.52 µg/mg. Asymopolo *et al.* (2005) concluded that the saffron with higher crocin and safranal had higher antioxidant property since the methanol solution of crocin had 65% antioxidant activity (DPPH free radical scavenging) and safranal had 36% antioxidant activity.

Table 3. Total phenolic content of saffron samples.

Region	TPC(mg gallic acid/g of dry matter)
Shiraz	9.24±0.24[fg]
Shahrekord	9.89±0.20[e]
Kerman	17.43±0.18[a]
Yazd	10.78±0.11[d]
Arak	9.32±0.10[f]
Natanz	15.88±0.20[b]
Dolatabad	8.89±0.11[g]
Ghaen	13.90±0.47[c]

Lowercase letters in the same column represent significant difference ($p<0.05$).

4. Conclusion

With regard to the importance of Iranian saffron and the spread of the planting of this valuable plant in different regions of the country, it is necessary to classify and compare the saffron of different regions with regard to their qualitative specifications. The results of this research showed that the qualitative specifications of saffron of different regions of Iran are influenced by different factors such as the quality of saffron bulb, type of soil, altitude of the region, average temperature of the region, age of saffron plant, climatic conditions, storage conditions, packaging, and method of drying.

5. References

Atefi, M. 2012. Effect of drying on chemical properties of saffron. *Journal of Food Science*, 3: 201-208.

Assimopoulou, A., Sinakos, Z., Papageorqiou, V. P. 2005. Radical scavenging activity of crocus sativus extract and its bioactive constituents. *Phytotherapy Research*, 19(11): 997-1000.

Caballero- Ortega, H., Pereda-Miranda,R., Abdullaev, F. I. 2007. HPLC quantification of major active components from11 different saffron source. *Food Chemistry,* 100(3): 1126-1131.

Caballero-Ortega, H. Pereda-Miranda, R., Riverón-Negrete, L., Hernández, J. M., Medécigo-Ríos, M., Castillo-Villanueva, A., Abdullaev, F. I. 2004. Chemical composition of saffron (*crocus sativus* L.) from four countries . *Journal of Food Science, 20*: 322-328.

Emadi, B., Saiedirad, M. H. 2011. Moisture dependent physical properties of saffron flowe. *Journal of Agriculture and ScienceTechnology, 13*: 387-393.

Gismondi, A., Serio, M., Canuti, L., Canini, A. 2012. Biochemical,antioxidant and antineoplastic properties of Italian saffron . *American Journal of Plant* Sciences, 3: 1573-1580.

Goli, A. Mokhtari, F., Rahimmalek, M. 2012. Phenolic Compounds and Antioxidant Activity from Saffron petal. *Journal of Agricaltural Science,4*: 175-184.

Hadizadeh, F., Mohajeri, S. A., Seifi, M. 2010. Extraction and purification of crocin from saffron stigmas employing asimple and efficient crystallization method. *Journal of Biological Science,* 13(14): 691-698.

Joki, M., Khazaei, N., Tavakolipoor, H., Rajabifar, S., Motamedisedeh, F., Kalbasi, A. 2012. Determination of chemical characteristics of saffron in different area of Iran. *Current Research Journal of Biological Science,* 4(1): 71:74.

Karimi, E., Oskoueian, E., Hendra, R., Jaafar, H. Z. 2010. Evaluation of crocus sativus L. stigma phenolic and flavonoid compounds and its antioxidant activity. *Molecules,* 15(9): 6244-6256.

Khodadadi, M. 2014. Heavy metals concentration (copper,chromium, cadmium and zinc) in saffron of south Khorasan. *Environmental Biology*, 12: 628-631.

Khoddami, A., Wilkes, M. A., Roberts, T. H. 2013. Techniques for analysis of plant phenolic compounds. *Molecules,* 18(2): 2328-2375.

Mohamad, I., Shukla, S. K., Shakeel, W. 2015. Rapid detection of adulteration in indigenous saffron of Kashmir ValleyIndia ".*Research Journal of Forensic Sciences,* 3(3): 7-11.

Mozzafar, S., Zaman Khan, K., Javid, S., Ahmed, A. 2014. Effect of drying methods on the colour of Kashmir saffron (*Crocus sativus* L.) and simultaneous method validation. *Chemical Science Review,* 3(12): 995-997.

Nazari, S., Keifi, N. 2011. Saffron and various fraud manners in its production and trade. *ISHS Acta Horticulturae*, 1-7.

Salari, R. 2012. Effect of storage time on physiochemical and microbial properties of saffron. *Journal of Food Chemistry,* 2: 61-68.

Sariri, R., Sabbaghzadeh, R., Poumohamad, F. 2011. *In-vitro* antioxidant and anti-tyrosinase activity of methanol extracts from crocus sativus flowers. *Pharmacologyonline*, 2: 1205-1215.

Shahidi, F., Bolandi, M. 2008. Shelf-life Determination of Saffron Stigma:water activity and temperature studies . *World Applied Science Journal*, 5: 132-136.

Sobolev, A. P., Carradori, S., Capitani, D., Vista, S., Trella, A., Marini, F., Mannina, L. 2014. Saffron samples of different origin: an NMR study of microwave-assisted extracts. *Journal of Food Technology,* 3: 201-208.

Tajik, C. 2011. Determination of crocin, picrocrocin and safranal in Ghaen saffron. *Journal of Food Science*. 3: 1-7.

Zarrinkamar, F., Tajik, S., Soleimanpour, S. 2011 . Effects of altitude on anatomy and concentration of crocin, Picrocrocin and Safranal in saffron. *Journal of Crop Science,* 5(7): 831-838.

Ethnomedicinal plants of Farouj district, North Khorasan province, Iran

Atena Eslami Farouji, Hamed Khodayari*

Department of Biology, Faculty of Science, Lorestan University, 5Km Khorramabad toward Tehran, Khorramabad, Iran;

Email: *hamedkhodayari75@yahoo.com

ARTICLE INFO

Topic: *Medicinal Plants*

Key words:
✓ *Ethnobotany*
✓ *Farouj*
✓ *Iran*
✓ *North Khorasan*
✓ *Medicinal plants*

ABSTRACT

Background & Aim: Medicinal plants are one of the most valuable resources in Iran, having a scientific knowledge and proper use; they can play an important role in community health. Some of the significant aims of ethnobotany project are to indicate the most common medicinal species, finding out the exact application of the plant species from various population of the area, and proving the knowledge of ethnobotany among human beings.

Experimental: To achieve these goals, the project has been conducted in Farouj, North Khorasan province, Iran in 2014-2015. To acquire ethnobotanical data of the studied area, several steps were taken such as the accumulation of plants, interviews with native people, and distribution of the questionnaires. Some important indices such as the relative frequency of citation (RFC), informant agreement ratio (IAR), and cultural important index (CI) were estimated. Furthermore, a traditional null hypothesis testing was adopted.

Results & Discussion: A total of 91 taxa belonging to 29 families were identified, 73 of which are grown naturally in the studied area. Asteraceae and Brassicaceae were the most detected families with 16 and 9 genera, respectively. Other diseases and digestive ones are the most curable ailments in Farouj County. Most of the parts of the plants that were collected consist of leaves (22%), whole plants (18%) and seeds (14%), orderly. *Vitis vinifera* L. has the maximum relative frequency of citation and cultural importance indices. Farouj area has a great potential in the growing of pharmaceutical plants. This research has been done for the first time in this area.

Industrial and practical recommendations: Plant extracts can be used as cure for many diseases and some extracts might have new beneficial effects on illness.

1. Introduction

Human indigenous knowledge about medicinal herbs is dynamic and complex (Reyes-Garcia *et al.*, 2013). Contemporary and historical documents allow the use of medicinal plants in different times (Ameri *et al.*, 2015; Hamedi *et al.*, 2013). Gathering medical information lead to recall many experiences and combining it with the past, present and future knowledge (Breitbach *et al.*, 2013; Giorgetti *et al.*, 2011; Medeiros & Albuquerque, 2014). Due to increasing industrialization and human need to find a suitable replacement for treating diseases safely and without any side effects, many researchers have an especial tendency on medical plants (Turner *et al.*, 2011). However, such enthusiasm have been more seen in Asian countries (Kim & Song, 2013; Song *et al.*, 2013).

According to World Health Organization (WHO), around 80% of the population in developing countries rely on traditional healing herbs to treat diseases, maintaining and improving the lives of their generation (Calixto, 2005; WHO, 2002). Based on several studies, around 442000 flowering plants were identified, of which just 50000 of them are applied for medicinal purposes and only 5000 of these plants have been scrutinized in terms of phytochemistry (Mahmood & Tabassum, 2011).

Since the beginning of human civilization, plants were used as medicinal resources for many body disorders (Chung *et al.*, 2013). Increasing the price of synthetic drugs not only multiplied the interests of people to utilize these plants, but also the number of researchers who are following them are intensified (Ahmad *et al.*, 2014; Bibi *et al.*, 2014; Mann *et al.*, 2008; Shrivastava & Kanungo, 2013; Sulaiman *et al.*, 2011).

On the basis of broad sense, ethnobotany means the study of complex relationships between people and plants (Hurrell & Albuquerque, 2012). This science is deal with the past and current knowledge of medicinal herbs (Pochettino & Lema, 2008), and for the first time; it was used by the American botanist (Harsh Berger) in 1896. Ethnobotany is composed of two words including ethno (people) and botany (plant). Rate of infectious diseases have been increased with growing technology in the world (Carballo *et al.*, 2002). Interestingly, using herbal medicines for treatment of various diseases have considerable economic benefits. About 74% of herbal medicines have been detected by botanists in field studies (Azaizh, 2003). It can be considered that the traditional knowledge plays an important role in defining the use of plants in large human communities.

Identifying and analyzing the characteristics of the natural environment and plants of each area is one of the fundamental steps in investigation of health of indigenous people and traditional customs. However, ethnobotany attracts the attention of many scientists through time, for instance; Abel & Busia (2005) had an exploratory ethnobotanical study of the practice of herbal medicine by the Akan people of Ghana. Manjula & Mamidala (2013) concerned about an ethnobotanical survey of medical plants used by traditional healers of Thadvai, Warangal district, Andhra Pradesh, India. Safa *et al.*, (2012) have studied Hormozgan Province in Iran, Abbasi *et al.*, (2012) concerned about the ethnobotanical study of medicinal plants in Natanz region (Kashan), Iran.

North Khorasan Province with an area of 28179 square kilometers comprise seven cities is located in North East of Iran including Farouj, Shirvan, Esfarayen, Jajarm, Garmeh, Maneh and Semelghan. Farouj city is the gate of North Khorasan province from holy Mashhad and terminated to some other cities such as Bajgiran (North), Esfarayen (South), Shirvan (from West) and Quchan (East). This city with an area of 1736 square kilometers has 2 cities, 2 districts, 5 subdistricts and 77 villages by latitude: 37 °13'N and longitude: 58 ° 13'E, 1182 meter above sea level (Fig. 1). Moreover, it has a pleasant climate, fertile soil and appropriate position because of Atrak River, Shah-e jahan (South) and Hezar masjed (North) Mountains. Because of water resources, including Atrak River, Agriculture has flourished and become an important center of oilseeds and nuts. Some meteorological data of the studied region (from 1977 to 2015) are as follow: average maximum and minimum temperature are 6.9 and 19.8 ℃; Average maximum and minimum humidity are 80 and 40 in percent, respectively.

The main aims of this study are as follow: 1. To dedicate most common medicinal species in Farouj (Faruj or Faroj) district (North Khorasan, Iran); 2. Find out the exact application of the species from local population of the area; 3. How the people use these plants and where are the most important part of these species to cure diseases; 4. Maintain the correct usage of wild, cultivated plants, and 5. Prove the knowledge of ethnobotany among human beings.

2. Material and Methods

To acquire ethnobotanical data of studied area, several steps have done such as accumulation of plants, interviews with native people (experienced people like herbal therapists; local people, especially elderly ones), and distribution a questionnaire. This project was lasted from April 2014 to November 2015.

The questions which utilized are as follow: what is your name, how old are you, do you know any medicinal plants in Farouj, what is the local name of these plants, which part of the plant, how and what diseases can be used for treatment. The participants have selected randomly (amateurs) and intentionally (professionals) in various locations such as villages, farmlands, streets, homes and spicy stores. Totally, 53 informants were participated with an approximate average of 61 years old (28-95 years), among which 37 were women and 16 men. Of these, 53 are belonging to elderly people or a medical traditional therapist whom has enough knowledge about herb healings.

Personally, during the interviews, several places (gardens, orchards, agriculture fields) were cautiously checked out. Careful observation and collection of samples were taken place using different methods (random-stratified, transect tape, and etc) through determined time. The size of plots was 1.5 × 1.5 m^2. Normally, a transect line set up across the studied area where there were transparent environmental gradients. Each species which touch the line or occurred in plots were accumulated. After gathering information from amateur and professional people of Farouj, a field walk was done along some transects; in order to distinguish environmental properties of collected samples. Unknown species were transported to Lorestan University Herbarium for more detailed studies using authoritative floras including Flora Iranica (Rechinger, 1963-2013).

2.1. Data analysis

The final information was obtained from questionnaires and other collected data. In addition some indices (relative frequency of citation (RFC), index of informant agreement ratio (IAR), Cultural importance index (CI) were measured using some variables like i, u and s. s is a species which the informant (i) put it in an especial category like u.

RFC is estimated with separating frequency of citation (FC) (the number of informants who mention the use of the species) to total number of informants in the research (N). This value alters from zero (nobody refers to the plants as useful) to one when all informants prove the beneficial of species (Tardio & Pardo-de Santayana, 2008).

$$1.\quad RFC = \frac{FC}{N}$$

Following formula is considered to measure the index of informant agreement ratio (IAR). It dedicate the range of agreement about usefulness of medicinal plants among informants (Trotter & Logan, 1986). IAR transparent the relationship between n_t (number of taxa) and n_{ur} (number of citation in each use category) (Collins *et al.*, 2006). More IAR shows higher agreements among participants.

$$2.\quad IAR = \frac{n_{ur} - n_t}{n_{ur} - 1}$$

The last index is cultural importance index (CI) (Tardio & Pardo-de Santayana 2008) which calculated the proportion of informants. Vividly, it sums the number of informants that noticed the use of each species divided by total number of informants (N). This index concerned about the number of participants whom use medicinal plants.

$$3.\quad CI = \sum_{u=u_1}^{u_{NC}} \sum_{i=i_1}^{i_N} \frac{URui}{N}$$

To investigate the relationship between medical usage and participant recovery from ailment, a traditional null hypothesis test was prepared using IBM SPSS Statistics 22 x86/x64. In null hypothesis (H_0) the researcher tries to accept or reject a concept. As a result, the hypothesis of this project was determined as follow:

H_0: People who use medical plants for disease therapy do not show serious symptoms of it than people who do not.

3. Results and discussion

A total of 91 species belonging to 80 genera and 29 families were identified, 73 of which grow naturally in the studied area and classified as wild edible plants (*Artemisia siberi* Bessr, *Carthamustinctorius* L., *Centaurea solstitialis* L., *Echinopsritrodes* Bunge, *Gundelia tournefortii* L., etc), but other species are cultivated (*Ficus carica* L., *Juglansregia* L., *Helianthustuberosus* L., *Vitisvinifera* L., etc). The scientific names, plant families, local names, medical applications, part uses, frequency of citation (FC), number of use reports (UR), number of uses (NU) are available in Table 1. Based on Figure 2 Asteraceae family with 15 species (20%), Brassicaceae and Lamiaceae each with 9 species (12%) were the most described families. The preference of these two families is mainly due to some especial properties such as secondary metabolites.

Table 1. Ethnopharmacology of plants in Farouj area. FC, frequency of citation; UR, use reports and NU, number of use.

Family name	Scientific name	Local name	Parts used	medicinal uses	FC	UR	NU
Amaranthaceae	*Amaranthus caudatus* L.	Tajkhorous domgorbeie, baroutak	whole plant	Treatment of hemorrhoids, Blood purification, Painful and slow urination	2	1	1
Apiaceae	*Ferula latisecta* Rech. f. Aell.	Anghouzeh	whole plant	Analgesic, Anti-tumor, Cure digestive diseases, Carminative, Fungicides, Reduction of blood pressure	9	10	7
Aspleniaceae	*Asplenium Ruta-muraria* L.	Sarakhs panjeie	whole plant	Pain relief, Astringent, Treatment of lung infection, Bactericidal, Antipyretic, Anti-inflammatory, Urinary tract antiseptic, Pain relief, Insecticide, Lowering fat and sugar, Cold treatment	1	-	-
Asteraceae	*Anthemis cotula* L.	Babouneh bahari	flowers, leaves	Antiepileptic, Headaches treatment, Diarrhea, Dysentery, Increased sleeping, Shortness of breath	8	9	5
Asteraceae	*Artemisia siberi* Bessr	Dermaneh	whole plant	Treatment of burns, Earache	4	2	2
Asteraceae	*Calendula officinalis* L.	Hamisheh bahar	flowers, leaves	Blood purification, Anticancer, Wound treatment, Analgesic, Vermifuge, Antibacterial, Anti-retroviral, Heart tonic,	1	1	1
Asteraceae	*Carthamus tinctorius* L.	kajireh	flowers, leaves	Analgesic, Anti-plot adhesion, Antipyretic, Anti-tumor, Heart tonic, Eye problems, Sedative, Rheumatism treatment	5	4	2
Asteraceae	*Centaurea behen* L.	Gol gandome talaei	flowers, roots	Strengthening, Jaundice treatment, Heart diseases, Antidote, Relief impotence, Palpitations, Increase sperm volume, Heart strengthen, Refreshing, Jaundice, improve memory loss	2	2	2
Asteraceae	*Centaurea depressa* M. B.	Gole gandom	whole plant	Neurasthenia treatment	3	1	1
Asteraceae	*Centaurea solstitialis* L.	Gole gandome zard	flower, roots	Refrigerant, Stomach tonic	9	6	4
Asteraceae	*Cichorium intybus* L.	Kasni	leaves, roots	Anti-bacterial, Carminative, Heart tonic, Liver protection, Nerves reinforcing, Lowering blood sugar, Anti-anemia, Skin disorders, Digestive, Jaundice treatment, Stomach ache	3	1	1
Asteraceae	*Echinops ritrodes* Bunge	Shekar tighal	whole plant	Treatment of skin diseases, Prevention of cough	2	2	2
Asteraceae	*Gundelia tournefortii* L.	Kangar	leaves	Sedative, Eaten with rice	8	7	7
Asteraceae	*Helianthus annus* L.	Aftabgardan	flower, seeds, leaves, roots	Refrigerant, Disposal of lung diseases, Diuretic and mucosa creative, Hypoglycemia, Stomach pain	6	5	5
Asteraceae	*Helianthus tuberosus* L.	Sibzamini torshi	glands	Lowering blood sugar and blood urea	5	5	3
Asteraceae	*Lactuca sativa* L.	Kahoo	stems, leaves, seeds	Cool agent, Blood purifier, Analgesic, Appetizer, Hypnotic, Anti-cough, Hypoglycemic, Liver cleaning, Treatment of neuritis, Mental weakness, Iron deficiency, Treatment of whooping	1	1	1

				cough, Nervous cough treatment, Asthma, Diabetes, Hyperemia, Gout, Constipation			
Asteraceae	*Onopordon acanthium* L.	Khar panbeh	flowers, stems, roots	Cancer treatment, Skin wounds, Stomach tonic, Appetizer, treat baldness	1	1	1
Asteraceae	*Silybum marianum* (L.) Gaertn	Khar maryam	seeds	Hypoallergenic, Anti-cancer, Anti-depressant, Anti-oxidants, Resistant prostate diseases, Anti-virus, Laxative, Expellant, Digesting food, Fat blockers, Treatment of chronic hepatitis	1	2	1
Brassicaceae	*Brassica rapa* L.	Shalgham	fruits, roots, leaves	Rheumatic muscle treatment, Bronchitis treatment, Inhibition the growth of bacteria and fungi, Anti-cancer, Anti-microbial, Anti-virus, Diuretic, Treatment of kidney stones, Uric acid reduction, Gout treating, Soothing breathing problems	2	1	1
Brassicaceae	*Brassica oleracea* L.	Kalame mamouli	leaves, seeds	Laxative, Stomach tonic, Appetizer, Vermifuge, Gout treating, Rheumatism, Pus draining, Contusion, Adolescent pimples, Vascular disorders, Eyelid inflammation, Heart disease	1	1	1
Brassicaeae	*Eruca sativa* Miller	Mandab	whole plant	Stimulant and tonic for the digestive system, Sexual motivation	1	1	1
Brassicaceae	*Erysimum repandum* L.	Khakshir	seeds	Fever reduction, Relieve abdominal pain	1	-	-
Brassicaceae	*Lepidium sativum* L.	Tartizak, Shahi	roots, seeds, leaves	Treatment of Asthma, Anti-cough and stomach ache, Carminative, Decreasing the stimulation of intestinal mucous layer, Back pain and rheumatism, Fix hiccups, Appetizer, Eaten with rice.	3	2	2
Brassicaceae	*Raphanus raphanistrum* L.	Torob vahshi	whole plant	Eliminating redness of the skin, Stimulant, Appetizer	4	4	3
Brassicaceae	*Raphanus sativus* L.	Torobche noghli	roots, leaves, seeds	treatment of Urinary and gastrointestinal pain, Laxative, Digestion stimulating, Strengthen the digestive system, Curing headaches and insomnia	4	3	3
Brassicaceae	*Sinapis arvensis* L.	Khardal biabani	seeds	Gastric mucosa stimulation, Anti-rheumatism, Hypnotic, Analgesic, Antibacterial, Carminative, Digestive, Fungicides, Anti-cancer	1	-	-
Brassicaceae	*Sisymbrium altissimum* L.	Khakshir laghzan	flowers, leaves	Mucosa, Nourishing, Antipyretic, Relieving cough and asthma	5	1	1
Chenopodiaceae	*Spinacia oleracea* L.	Esfanaj	whole plant	Decrease blood sugar, Treatment of anemia, Vermifuge, Expellant, Antipyretic	2	4	4
Convolvulaceae	*Convolvulus arvensis* L.	Pichake sahraei	whole plant	Very toxic and causing gastro-intestinal sensitivity, Expellant	1	2	2
Cucurbitaceae	*Benincasa hispida* (Thunb. Ex Murray) Cogn.	Kadouye moumi	fruits, seeds,	Vermifuge, Treatment of wound, Anti-cough, dermatology diseases, Anti-wrinkle, Prevent sunburn	1	1	1
Cucurbitaceae	*Citrullus lanatus* (Thunb.) Matsum. & Nakai	Hendevaneh	fruits	Cool agent, Sedative, Fortifying, Vermifuge	2	1	1
Cucurbitaceae	*Cucumis melo* L.	Kharbozeh	fruits, roots, seeds	Expellant, Nutritious, Remove freckles, Sedative, Relieve indigestion, Fix eczema, Cool agent, Urinary tract	1	2	2

				infection and painful urination, Treatment of gastro-intestinal disorders, Anti-fungal, Treatment of urinary disorders			
Cucurbitaceae	*Cucumis melo* L. var. flexuosus	Khiar chanbar	fruits	Cooling and cleaning the skin, Treatment of burns and scratches, Fortifying, Refrigerant, Anti-cough, Strong digestive, Vermifuge, Expellant	4	4	3
Cucurbitaceae	*Cucumis melo* L. var. reticulatus	Talebi	fruits	Strong digestive, Treatment of burns and scratches, Fortifying, Cooling and cleaning the skin, Refrigerant, Stomach tonic, Anti-cough, Vermifuge, Expellant, Sedative, Remove freckles, Relieve indigestion, Fix eczema, Cool agent, Treat urinary tract infection, Anti-fungal, Treatment of biliary disorders	1	1	1
Cucurbitaceae	*Cucurbita moschata* Duchesne	Kadou halvaei	Seeds, fruits	Vermifuge, Relieve abdominal cramps, Improving inflation	1	1	1
Elaeagnaceae	*Elaeagnus angustifolia* L.	Senjed	leaves, fruits	Stomach disorders, Diarrhea, Asthma, Anti-fever, Anti-cancer	1	2	2
Euphorbiaceae	*Ricinus communis* L.	Bid anjir	leaves, roots, seeds	Expellant, Antibacterial, Analgesic, Fungicides, Treatment of constipation Anti-tumor, Anti-cough, Lowering blood sugar, Jaundice treatment, Stomach pain, Blister treatment, Joint pain relief	1	-	-
Fumariaceae	*Fumaria officinalis* L.	Shahtareh	whole plant	Fortifying, Blood purification, Liver regularity, Treatment of vascular disorders, Anti-hyperemia, Vermifuge, Jaundice, Anti-histamines, Disinfectants, Appetizer, Fortifying	1	-	-
Geraniaceae	*Erodium moschatum* L' Her. ex Aiton	Noklaklaki	whole plant	Stop internal bleeding, Wound healing, Diarrhea, Astringent	2	3	3
Juglandaceae	*Juglans regia* L.	Gerdou	flowers, leaves, barks	Pancreas stimulation, Blood purification, Anemia, Diabetes, Gout, Vermifuge, Anti-cancer, Anti-tumor, Antifungal, Anti-virus, Appetizer	1	1	1
Lamiaceae	*Lavandula angustifolia* Miller subsp. *angustifolia*	Ostokhoddo us	whole plant	Analgesic, Nerve and Heart paregoric, Blood pressure decreasing	1	1	1
Lamiaceae	*Mentha longifolia* (L.) Hudson	Pouneh	leaves, flowers	Anti-asthma, Carminative, Stimulant, Refrigerant, Headache, Treatment of digestive disorders	1	2	1
Lamiaceae	*Ocimum basilicum* L.	Reihan	flowers	Fortifying, Anti-spasm, Asthma, Pertussis, Paralysis, Migraine, Gout, Epilepsy, Treatment of neurasthenia, Treatment of anorexia, Alzheimer's prevention, Fortifying, Anti-arthritis, Anti-cancer, Anti-fungal	1	1	1
Lamiaceae	*Rosmarinus officinalis* L.	Rozmari	leaves	Stimulating the adrenal glands, Blood pressure increasing, Anti-cough, Anti-diarrhea, Heart fortifying, Anti-rheumatism pains, Pertussis, Common cold, Prevention from obstruction of the bile ducts, Stomach disorders, Epilepsy, Paralysis, Healing of wounds and scalds	1	1	1
Lamiaceae	*Calamintha officinalis* Moench	Nana ziba	whole plant	Carminative, Causing hiccups, Fever lowering, Cough improvement, Common cold	1	1	1

Lamiaceae	*Dracocephalum moldavica* L.	Badranjbouyeh	seeds, leaves, stem	Fever lowering, Food digestion, Wound healing, Paregoric Sedative	2	2	2
Lamiaceae	*Satureja laxiflora* C. Koch	Marzeh	leaves	Analgesic, Anti-arthritis, Anti-herpes virus, Disinfectant, Food digestion, Carminative, Vermifuge, Anti-cancer, Expellant, Anti-diarrhea	1	1	1
Lamiaceae	*Thymus serpyllum* L.	Avishane vagheei	whole plant	Improving visual impairment, Curing toothache, Carminative, Nervous headache treatment, Pertussis, Angina treating	1	1	1
Lamiaceae	*Ziziphora persica* Bunge	Kakouti Irani	stems,leaves	Decreasing fever, Mucosa creative, Carminative, Improving digestive system, Heart fortifying, Bloody diarrhea	8	8	6
Liliaceae	*Allium cepa* L.	Piaze khoraki	bulbs	Arthritis, Disinfectant, Common cold, Indigestion, Decrease fat, Prevention of premature aging, Analgesic, Lowering blood sugar, Rheumatism	7	9	5
Liliaceae	*Allium hirtifolium* Boiss.	Mousir	bulbs	Lowering blood pressure	5	5	5
Liliaceae	*Allium sativum* L.	Seer	bulbs	Lowering blood pressure and heart beat, Appetizer, Common cold, Lowering blood fat, Anti-gout, Pertussis, Disinfection, Prevention of premature aging, Asthma, Anti-cough, Rheumatism, Antipyretic, Anti-amoeba, Sudoriferous	7	6	4
Malvaceae	*Alcea fasciculiflora* Zohary	Khatmi	flowers,	Anti-cough, Common cold	1	1	1
Malvaceae	*Malva sylvestris* L.	Panirake ghermez	leaves, flowers	Laxative, Mucosa creative, Constipation treatment, Common cold, Improve tongue inflammation, Paregoric	1	1	1
Moraceae	*Morus alba* L.	Toote sefid	Leaves, barks, roots, fruits	Sudoriferous, Expellant, diarrhea, Many stings, Stimulant, Stomach fortifying, Mucosa creative, Laxative, Vermifuge, Sore throat treatment, Relief thirst and fever, Reduce depression, Headache, Dizziness, Indigestion	2	2	1
Moraceae	*Morus nigra* L.	Shahtoot	leaves, fruits, barks, roots	Refrigerant, Diuretic, Mucosa creative, Blood pressure reduction, Tapeworm, Pest and Sore throat treatment, Anti-depressant, Vermifuge, Decrease blood pressure, Lowering blood sugar, Analgesic, Inflammation of oral mucosa, Antipyretic	1	1	2
Moraceae	*Ficus carica* L.	Anjir	fruits, roots, barks	Sedative, Anemia treatment, Vermifuge, Constipation, Wart removing, Laxative, Expellant	1	1	1
Nyctaginaceae	*Mirabilis jalapa* L.	Laleh abbasi	roots, leaves, glands	Laxative, Mucosa creative, Jaundice, Refrigerant, Treatment of anemia, Blain disinflation, Sputum reduction, Asthma, Vermifuge, Diarrhea, Stomach fortifying	1	1	1
Papaveraceae	*Papaver bracteatum* Lindl.	Khashkhashe kabir	flowers, leaves, seeds	Anti-addiction, Strong hypnotic, Paregoric, Lung infections, Bronchitis, Pneumonia, Treatment of sore throat, Food digestion, Eyelid inflammation, Anti-cough, Sedative, Rheumatism pains, Paregoric, Analgesic, Anti-spasm, Asthma	1	1	1
Papilionaceae	*Alhagi*	Kharshotor	whole	Sudoriferous, Laxative, Mucosa creative	1	1	1

	mannifera Desf.		plant				
Papilionaceae	*Cicer arietinum* L.	Nokhode abgoushti	seeds, leaves	Vermifuge, Renal colic, Opening and healing the festering wounds, Treatment of sprained joints, Thirst resolving, Burns treatment	1	1	1
Papilionaceae	*Coronilla varia* L.	Yonjeh baghi	whole plant	Expellant	1	1	1
Papilionaceae	*Glycyrrhiza glabra* L.	Shirin bayan, Choub shirin	roots	Antihistamines, Mucosa creative, Anti-inflammatory, Nervous cough treatment, Anti-ulcer, Anti-depressant, Expellant, Anti-tumor	1	1	1
Papilionaceae	*Medicago sativa* L.	Yonjeh	whole plant	Antimicrobial, Carminative, Cholesterol lowering, Arthritis therapy, Anti-anemia	6	3	3
Papilionaceae	*Pisum sativum* L.	Nokhod farangi, Nokhod sabz	fruits	Lowing blood sugar, Meningitis treatment, Nervous system problems, Cramp, Tremor, Walking problems, Paralysis	5	4	2
Papilionaceae	*Psoralea drupacea* Bunge	Loubiaye Khorasani	whole plant	Antimicrobial, Antibacterial	1	1	1
Papilionaceae	*Trigonella foenum-graecum* L.	Shanbelileh	whole plant	Treatment of small-pox, Heart fortifying, Disinfectant, Carminative, Rheumatism Lowering blood pressure, Small pox treatment	1	1	1
Poaceae	*Cynodon dactylon* (L.) Pers.	Margh	whole plant	Epilepsy treatment, Skin disorders, Cool agent, Nosebleed prevention, Improvement of fresh wounds, Treatment of inflamed glands and Sedative, Stop bleeding, Appetizer, Inflammation, Gout, Liver diseases, Delusion, Rheumatism, Reduce burn feeling, Vomiting	1	1	2
Poaceae	*Panicum miliaceum* L.	Arzan	whole plant	Recover wounds	1	1	1
Poaceae	*Hordeum vulgar* L.	Jo		Antipyretic, Digestive, Diuretic, Stomach fortifying, Mucosa creative, Stimulate blood circulation	1	1	1
Poaceae	*Triticum aestivum* L.	Gandom	seeds	Appetizer, Disinfectant, Anti-jaundice, Anti effects of alcohol, Lowering blood fat, Intestine stimulating, Expellant, Remove thirst, Antipyretic	1	1	1
Poaceae	*Zea mays* L.	Zorrat, Balal	whole plant	Rheumatism, Losing weight, Analgesic, Burn treatment, Sedative, Inflation and Wound, Fortifying, Expellant	1	1	1
Polygonaceae	*Polygonum aviculare* L.	Alafe haftband	roots	Vermifuge, Astringent, Reduce intestinal secretion, Anti-diabetic, Blood purification, Treatment of gallstones and urinary	6	6	4
Polygonaceae	*Rheum ribes* L.	Rivas	stems	Joyful and Cooling	6	4	4
Polygonaceae	*Rumex crispus* L.	Torshake mavvaj	roots	Fortifying, Anti-anemia, Diabetes treatment, Tuberculosis and liver diseases, Disinfectant, Sore throat treatment, Anti-tumor, Blister and Scorch, Vermifuge, Laxative, Anti-cancer	5	3	1
portulacaceae	*Portulaca oleraceae* L.	Khorfeh	leaves	Diarrhea, Appetizer, Headache, toothache, Anti-spasm, Asthma, Vermifuge, Recover rash, Snake bite, Jaundice	1	1	1
Rosaceae	*Amygdalus conmmuis* L.	Badame talkh	leaves, flowers, barks	Paregoric, Vermifuge, Pain relief, Gum revival	1	1	1

Rosaceae	*Armeniaca vulgaris* Lam.	Zardalou	fruits	Anti-cough, Mucosa creative, Anti-cramp, Asthma therapy, Analgesic, Liver diseases, Earache	1	1	1
Rosaceae	*Cerasus avium* (L.) Moench	Gilas	stems, fruits	Treatment of cystitis, Arthritis, Laxative	1	1	1
Rosaceae	*Cerasus vulgaris* Miller	Albalou	flowers	Liver diseases, Kidney swelling, Chronic inflammation of the digestive system	3	3	3
Rosaceae	*Cotoneaster nummularioides* Pojark.	Shirkheshte sekkehei	whole plant	Expellant, Refrigerant, Mucosa creative, Recover chest and throat discomfort, Laxative, Anti-cough	1	1	1
Rosaceae	*Cydonia oblonga* Miller	Beh, Shal beh	fruits, seeds	Stomach tonic, Anti-cough, Refrigerant, Mucosa creative, Inflammation reduction, Heart Fortifying	1	1	1
Solanaceae	*Capsicum annuum* L.	Felfel dolmeei	fruits	Stomach tonic, Indigestion, Nausea, Paralysis, Analgesic, Anti-platelet adhesion, Insecticide, Enhancing capillaries diarrhea, Rheumatism	1	1	1
Solanaceae	*Datura innoxia* Miller	Datoureh	leaves, seeds	Highly toxic, Anti-spasm, Analgesic, Hypnotic, Anti-anxiety, Anti-Asthma, Pupil dilation, Blister and Ulcer treatment, Earache Sedative	1	1	1
Solanaceae	*Ipomoea purpurea* (L.) Roth.	Niloufar	roots	Expellant	1	1	1
Solanaceae	*Nicotiana tabacum* L.	Tanbakou	leaves	Laxative, Narcotic, Vermifuge, Carminative, Bronchitis treatment, Fortifying, Relief muscle pain, Skin disorders, Healing wound, Pain treatment, Asthma, Anti-cancer, Paregoric, Nerves strengthen	1	1	1
Solanaceae	*Solanum melongena* L.	Bademjan	roots, leaves, fruits, seeds	Asthma, Anti-spasm, Stimulant, Therapy, Nasal ulcer treatment, Narcotic, Cholesterol-lowering	1	1	1
Solanaceae	*Solanum tuberesum* L.	Sibzamini	leaves, glands	Analgesic, Antibacterial, Heart strengthen, Blood pressure, Scorch healing, Appetizer, decreasing, Treatment of gingivitis	1	1	1
Urticaceae	*Urtica dioica* L.	Gazaneh	leaves	Rheumatism, Joints improvement, Blood pressure decreasing, Anti-dandruff, Asthma, Anti-histamines, Antiepileptic, Disinflation, Blood pressure decreasing, Analgesic, Anti-cancer	1	1	1
Vitaceae	*Vitis vinifera* L.	Angour	fruits, leaves, stem	Sedative, Laxative, Heart diseases, Anti-fever, Relieve sore throat, Jaundice, Thirst removing, Skin disorders, Constipation, Cold treatment, Slimming.	9	9	8
Violaceae	*viola tricolor* L.	Banafsheh sehrang	whole plant	Laxative, Mucosa creative, Treatment of kidney inflammation, Rheumatism, Skin disorders, Muscle relaxants, Detoxification, Diarrhea	1	-	-

Table 2. Comparison of significant medicinal plants utilizing indices and species ranking according to each index in Farouj area.

Family	Scientific name	CI	RFC	CI ranking	RFC ranking
Vitaceae	*Vitis vinifera*	0.5112	0.3953	1	1
Apiaceae	*Ferula latisecta*	0.5112	0.3523	1	2
Lamiaceae	*Ziziphora persica*	0.4832	0.2932	2	3
Asteraceae	*Gundelia tournefortii*	0.4612	0.2932	3	3

Liliaceae	*Allium cepa*	0.4476	0.2932	4	3
Liliaceae	*Allium sativum*	0.4332	0.2429	5	4
Asteraceae	*Centaurea solstitialis*	0.3712	0.2340	6	5
Asteraceae	*Anthemis cotula*	0.3732	0.2340	6	5
Asteraceae	*Helianthus annus*	0.3511	0.1834	7	6
Brassicaceae	*Sisymbrium altissimum*	0.3382	0.1713	8	7
Cucurbitaceae	*Cucumis melo*	0.2919	0.1713	9	7
Asteraceae	*Helianthus tuberosus*	0.2637	0.1552	10	8
Asteraceae	*Carthamus tinctorius*	0.2110	0.1101	11	9

RFC: relative frequency of citation CI: index of cultural importance.

Table 3. Informant's agreement factor for different use categories in Farouj area.

IAR	n_t	n_{ur}	Use category
0.562	15	33	Other diseases
0.518	14	28	Digestive diseases
0.409	14	23	Sugar and Fat reduction
0.375	11	17	Respiratory disease
0.285	6	8	Urinary tract
0.2	5	6	Skin disease
0.0	4	4	Eye disease
0.0	2	2	Oral disease

n_t: number of taxa; n_{ur}: number of citation in each use category. IAR: informant agreement ratio.

Other pharmaceutical dominant families are Papilionaceae, Cucurbitaceae, Rosaceae, and Solanaceae (Table 1). Asteraceae was the most abundant families in many previous projects like Ghasemi Pirbalouti *et al*., (2012).

In Figures 3 and 4, the usages of medicinal plants are described. According to Figure 3, other diseases (23%), digestive diseases (22%), sugar and fat reduction (17%), respiratory disease (15%), skin diseases (11%) are the most ailments which treated with healing herbs. Moreover, as illustrated in Figure 4 the most collected plant parts belonging to leaves (22%), whole plants (18%) and seeds (14%), orderly. As mentioned leaves are allocated the most part for drugs consumption, that probably due to the ease of access and being fresher than the other parts of plants (Bonet & Valles, 2002). The highest and the lowest part of the plant used as medicinal purposes are the leaves and bulbs. Obviously, many diseases can be cured (from common to complicated sickness) using these medicinal plants and most of these plants can treat a variety of current diseases (Figures 3 and 4). Leaves is one of the most usable parts in medical purposes as Mosaddegh *et al*., (2012) research. Nevertheless, roots are the most abundant applicable medical part in Traditional Chinese Medicine (Weckerle *et al*., 2009).

3.1. Medicinal and non-medicinal uses

Of 91 species discovered in Farouj district, some species have two properties (medicinal and non-medicinal). *Ferula latisecta* Rech. f. Aell., is using for making kind of broth. *Gundelia tournefortii* L. and *Allium cepa* L. have been eaten with rice. *Brassica* species using in salads. Some species use as vegetables such as *Lepidium sativum* L, *Cucumis melo* L., *Mentha longifolia* (L.) Hudson, *Satureja laxiflora* C. Koch, and *Spinacia oleracea* L., *Ziziphora persica* Bunge have been drink with tea. *Morus alba* L., *Morus nigra* L., *Ficus carica* L., *Cerasus avium* (L.) Moench, *Cerasus vulgaris* Miller, *Cydonia oblonga* Miller, *Vitis vinifera* L. applied as fruits. Additionally, animals are feeding with *Medicago sativa* L. and *Amygdalus conmmuis* L. utilize for making baskets.

3.2. Compare estimated indices

Ferula latisecta has the highest number of informants. It shows that it is the most distinguished species in the studied area. *Vitis vinifera* and *Carthamus tinctorius* have the maximum and minimum number of use-reports with 10 and 4 use-reports, orderly. The position of *Ferula latisecta* and *Vitis vinifera*are changed in Figures 6 and 7 due to the independence of CI index to the number of informants, in contrast with RFC.

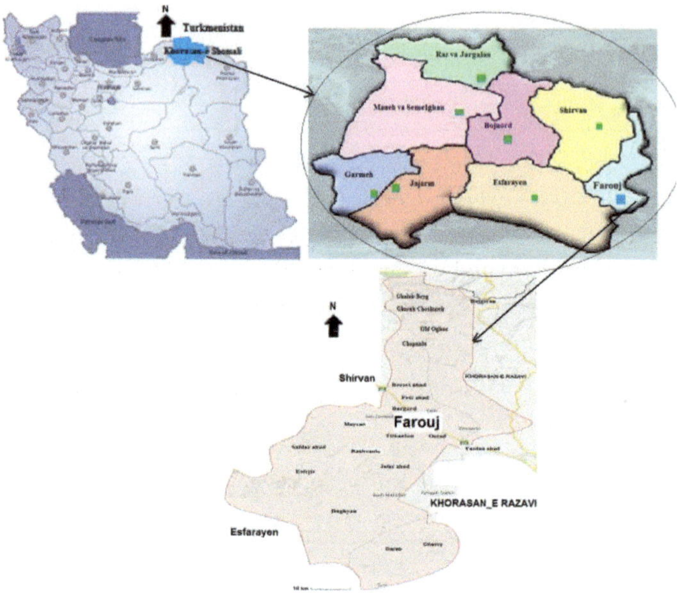

Fig. 1. The position of the studied area (Farouj district), in North Khorasan province, Iran.

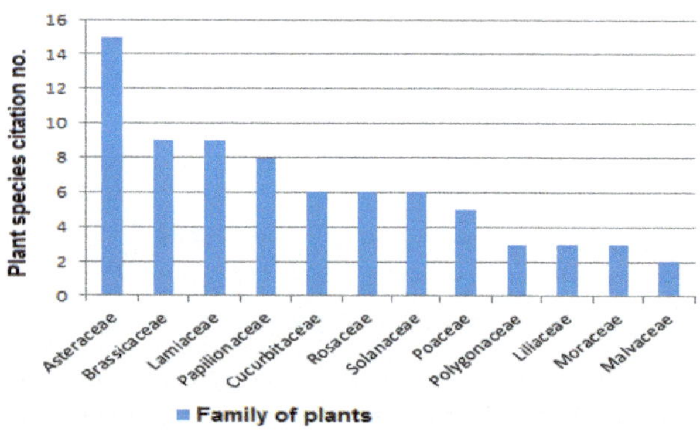

Fig. 2. Plants families with the highest number of cited species in Farouj area.

Based on Table 2, the ranking indices are different among species. Obviously, informant agreement factor (IAR) have displayed in Table 3. IAR (informant agreement ratio) estimated using n_t (number of taxa) and n_{ur} (number of citation in each use category). IAR is zero for two categories (eye and oral diseases) because of the same number of plants and citation for each species. It shows lack of agreement among informants on species usage. The disagreement is probably due to the long history of mankind and lack of attention on using medical plants. Similar results with present research have reported in Kohghiluyeh and Boyer Ahmad, (Mosaddegh *et al.*, 2012) and china (Ghorbani *et al.*, 2011).

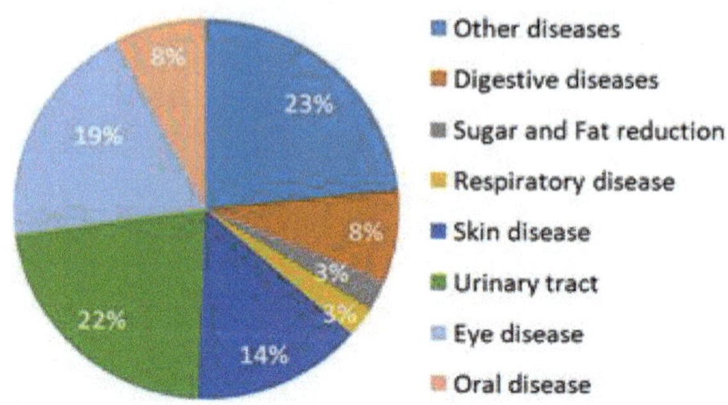

Fig. 3. Chart abundance of medicinal plants in treatment of various diseases in Farouj area.

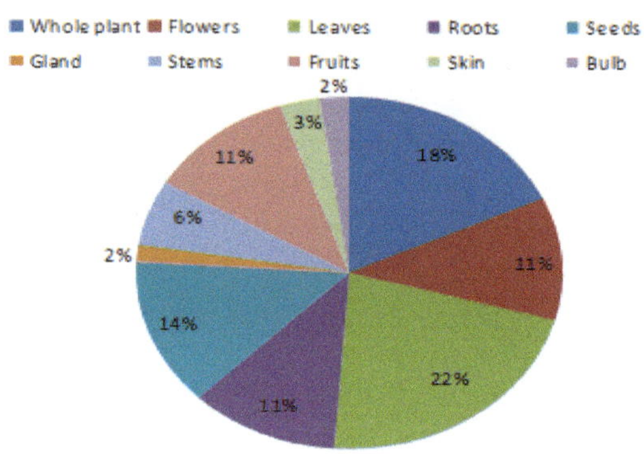

Fig. 4. The most frequently used part of the plants in the studied area, Farouj area.

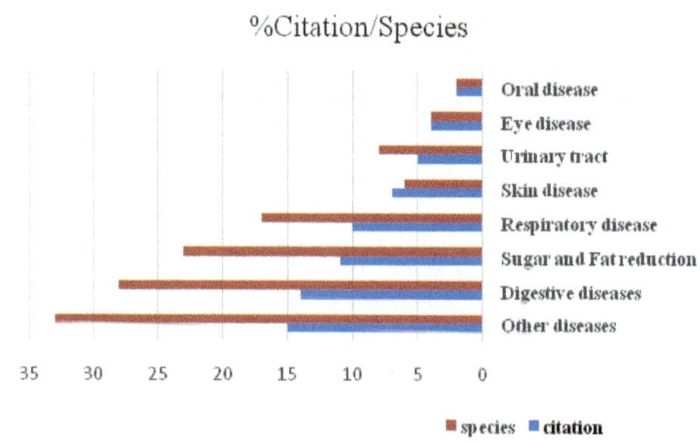

Fig. 5. Percentage of species and citation in each use category in Farouj area.

The maximum IAR indices are mainly pertain to other diseases and digestive disorders, respectively. More IAR value is mostly because of high rate of these ailments over successive generations and as a result more frequent applications of these medicinal plants. High IAR values are also reported from Indian Mexicans (Heinrich *et al.*, 1998), Thailand and China (Inta *et al.*, 2008), SW of Iran (Mosaddegh *et al.*, 2012).

Statistic results fit the null hypothesis because the significance tests generate 95% or 99% likelihood, then the hypothesis is accepted. It means that people who use medical plants for disease therapy will soon recover their health than people who do not.

3.3. Most cited plants and some pictures of the studied area, farouj area

Vitis vinifera L., *Ferula latisecta* Rech. f. Aell., and *Ziziphora persica* Bunge are the most prevalent plants which introduced by people. Some important properties are as follow sedative, laxative, heart diseases, anti-fever; relieve sore throat, jaundice, thirst removing, skin disorders, constipation, cold treatment, slimming.

3.4. Importance of medicinal plants usage in urban and rural regions

Many researchers interested in ethnobotany field. The results of some researchers are accordance with many prior projects. For instance; leaves were the most frequent plant part for curing diseases in some parts of Colombia (Cadena-Gonzalez *et al.*, 2013).

Choudhary and his counterparts (2008) studied medicinal plants in India. They noted "that 2500 plant species have medicinal value". Other scientists like Mesfin *et al.*, (2013) had a research on Northern Ethiopia. They concluded "that a total of 31 medicinal species are grown there (less species than present study)". Moreover, Jeruto *et al.*, (2008) dedicated that around 40 medicinal plants are present in Nandi Forests in Kenya. Some other scientists like Lagos (2005) and Neves with his colleagues studied Imbituba, Santa Catarina, Brazil Zank, and Hanazaki. They agreed that digestive disorders such as stomach pains are one of the most illnesses which can be treated in the studied areas (Zank & Hanazaki 2011). Rajaei & Mohammadi (2012) were look over SE of Iran (Hezar Mountain). Similar to present research, they have recorded "about 92 species; the most common remedy was related to digestive disorders". Amiri & Joharchi (2013) investigate traditional medicinal plants in Mashhad. Approximately, 269 species were discovered. In this research, plants are mostly used for curing digestive disorders that is in accordance with our research.

In contrast with existent experiment, Bahmani *et al.*, (2014) evaluate 30 medicinal plants in Uremia which Lamiaceae family was the most abundant family (in accordance with Amiri & Joharchi). Similarly, leaves were the most part used in disease remedy. They also considered that many of mentioned species have active potential to improve diabetes. Abbasi *et al.*, (2012) examined Natanz region (Kashan). In total, 65 medicinal plants were identified. They mentioned "that because of livestock grazing and inappropriate climate, most species are supposed to be endangered".

Compare with the present research, a total of 122 genera was investigated in Dehloran and Abdanan districts, Ilam Province. Asteraceae was the most abundant family correspondingly to present project. Digestive pains and leaves are the main disease and plant part, respectively (Ghasemi Pirbalouti *et al.*, 2012). In contrast with our study the fruits of these species are used most often and the region is ample with Lamiaceae family (Khajoei Nasab & Khosravi, 2014). In another research a notable amount of medical plants (around 45 species) have conducted. Asteraceae and Fabaceae were dominant families in Hamedan. The most treated disorders (similar to our results) were digestive pains (Naghibi *et al.*, 2014). Additionally, Khodayari *et al.*, (2014) investigated the medical plants of South East of Khuzestan Province. They detected about 174 species owing to 65 families. Asteraceae family had the most value in medicinal treatments especially digestive disorders which are correspond positively with our results.

Some more researches from Iranian projects which involved in ethnobotany are as follow: Ghelichnia (2005) studied the East of Khuzestan province. He considered "more than 86 medical species in that area that is less than the detected species in Farouj". Lamiaceae, Rosaceae, and Asteraceae were the most abundant families there. Traditionally, Kohkilouyeh and Boyerahmad had 138 used plants. Similar to our research Asteraceae was dominant (Mosaddegh *et al.*, 2012), Ghasemi Pirbalouti (2009) discloses 61 species in Chaharmahale Bakhtiari. Lamiaceae, Asteraceae, and Fabaceae were the most common families, in another research, 91 species were investigated in Kazeroun. Lamiaceae and Asteraceae were commonly used in this region (Dolatkhahi *et al.*, 2014), in Boushehr city, 63 species belonging to 55 genera and 36 families have recognized. Asteraceae family was the largest taxon with nine species (Dolatkhahi & Nabipour 2013), 227 medical plant were found out in Markazi Province. Asteraceae, Lamiaceae and Brassicaceae conclude more usable taxa (Mirdavoodi, 2008), some other ethnobotanists studied Kordestan, and discovers 144 medical plant species (Hooshidari 2009). Ilam has about 122 plants that can be used as ailment therapy. Asteraceae and Lamiaceae were claimed to be the most taxa which contain these plants (Ghasemi Pirbalouti *et al.*, 2012), 394 species of medicinal plants is also grown in Hamedan Province among which the most common family is Asteraceae (Kalvandi, 2007).

It should be noticed that, based upon excessive use of some medicinal plants, they might be unprotected and vulnerable in near future. These species can be conserved by domestication and revival techniques. Obviously, there are some more phenomena that abrogate medicinal plants such as fire, browsing, grazing, grass cutting, lopping, climatic factors, wild animals and insects, agriculture, and etc. Generally, depend on the type of diseases that people meet, different plants might be exposed to danger, for example Njoroge *et al.*, (2010) reported that "*Crassia edulis* is threatened by overuse to cure many disorders such as stomach problems in Ethiopia" (CRAF-PROSEA network). As a result, overutilization of plants can be a parameter to detect threatened species.

4. Conclusion

Farouj district has a great potential in the growing of pharmaceutical plants. This research has been done for the first time in this area. Some striking knowledge has been accumulated about traditional medical plants which will be in use in near future.

Entirely, more plants belonging to angiosperms (except Aspleniaceae). Two families (Liliaceae and Poaceae) fit to monocotyledons, the rest belong to dicotyledonous.

Transparently, women (69%) have more knowledge about medicinal herbs than men (31%), and a more number of questionnaires were completed by them, which is probably due to the fundamental role of women in maintaining family health. Most people in the studied area claimed that they had used these medicinal plants a long time ago, when they were very young, and the plants which are now used only for food consumption not pharmaceutical ones.

Iran with great experience in traditional medical plants is one of the most appropriate countries in this field and has a growing potential in preparation, production, and export of pharmaceutical plants. On the other hand, collecting medicinal plants in their natural habitat need enough knowledge and experience. Great efforts made in this paper have highlighted the drug habits of Farouj city from past to present.

5. References

Abbasi, S., Afsharzadeh, S. Mohajeri, A. 2012. Ethnobotanical study of medicinal plants in Natanz region (Kashan), Iran. *Journal of Herbal Drugs*, 3 (3): 147-156.

Abel, C. and Busia, K. 2005. An exploratory ethnobotanical study of the practice of herbal medicine by the Akan people of Ghana.*Alternative Medicine Review*, 10 (2): 112-122.

Ahmad, M., Sultana, S., Fazl-i-Hadi, S., Hadda, T. B., Rashid, S., Zafar, M. Yaseen, G. 2014. An ethnobotanical study of medicinal plants in high mountainous region of Chail valley (District Swat-Pakistan).*Journal of Ethnobiology and Ethnomedicine*, 10 (1): 36.

Ameri, A., Heydarirad, G., Mahdavi, J. J.,Ghobadi, A., Rezaeizadeh, H. Choopani, R. 2015. Medicinal Plants Contain Mucilage Used in Traditional Persian Medicine (TPM). *Pharmaceutical Biology,* 53 (4): 615-623.

Amiri, M. S. Joharchi, M. R. 2013. Ethnobotanical investigation of traditional medicinal plants commercialized in the markets of Mashhad, Iran. *Avicenna Journal of Phytomedicine*, 3 (3): 254-271.

Azaizh, H. 2003. Ethnobotanical knowledge of local Array practioners in the Middle Eastern region. *Fitoterapia*, 74: 98- 108.

Bahmani, M., Zargaran, A., Rafieian-Kopaei, M. Saki, K. 2014. Ethnobotanical study of medicinal plants used in the management of diabetes mellitus in the Urmia, Northwest Iran. *Asian Pacific Journal of Tropical Medicine,* 7(1): 348-354.

Bibi, T., Ahmad, M., Tareen, R. B., Tareen, N. M., Jabeen, R., Rehman, S. U., Sultana, S., Zafar, M. Yaseen, G. 2014. Ethnobotany of medicinal plants in district Mastung of Balochistan province-Pakistan. *Journal of Ethnopharmacology,*157: 79–89.

Bonet, M. A. Valles, J. 2002. Use of non-crop food vascular plants in Montseny biosphere reserve (Catalonia, Iberian Peninsula). *International Journal of Food Science Nutrition,* 53: 225–248.

Breitbach, U. B., Niehues, M., Lopes, N. P., Faria, J. E. Brandão, M. G. L. Q. 2013. Amazonian Brazilian Medicinal Plants Described by C.F.P. von Martius in the 19th Century. *Journal of Ethnopharmacology*, 147 (1): 180-189.

Cadena-González, A. L., Sørensen, M. Theilade, I. 2013. Use and valuation of native and introduced medicinal plant species in Campo Hermosoand Zetaquira, Boyacá, Colombia. *Journal of Ethnobiology and Ethnomedicine,* 9: 23.

Calixto, J. B. 2005. Twenty five years of research on medicinal plants in Latin America: a personal review. *Journal of Ethnopharmacology*, 100: 131-134.

Carballo, L. J., Hernandez-inda, L. Z., Perzer, P. Gravalos, M. D. 2002. A comparison between two brine shrimp assays to detect *in vitro* cytotoxicity in marine natural products. *Biology Medicine Central,* 2 (1): 17.

Choudhary, K., Singh, M. Pillai, U. 2008. Ethnobotanical Survey of Rajasthan - An Update. *American-Eurasian Journal of Botany*, 1(2): 38-45.

Chung, J. M., Park, K. W., Jeong, H. R., Soo, S. K., Kim, H. J., Choi, K., Lee, C. H., Shin, C. H. Kim, S. S. 2013. Ethnobotany in Korea—the traditional knowledge and use of indigenous plants. *Korea National Arboretum*, Gyeonggi-Do (in Korean).

Collins, S., Martins, X., Mitchell, A., Teshome, A. Arnason, J. T. 2006. Quantitative ethnobotany of two East Timorese culture. *Economic Botany*, 60: 347–361.

CRAF-PROSEA network: World Agroforestry Centre, Agroforestry Tree Database. Available on Internet at:*http://www.worldagroforestry.org/treedb2/AFTPDFS/Carissa_edulis.pdf.*

Dolatkhahi, M. Nabipour, I. 2013. Systematically study of medicinal plants in Bushehr province, Southern Iran. *Journal of herbal drugs*, 3 (4): 209-222. (In Persian).

Dolatkhahi, M., Ghorbani, M., Mehrafarin, A. Amininejad, G. 2014. Ethnobotanical Study of Medicinal Plants in Kazeroon: identification, distribution and traditional uses. *Journal of medicinal plants,* 11(2): 163-178. (In Persian).

Ghasemi Pirbalouti, A. 2009. Medicinal plants used in Chaharmahal and Bakhtyari districts, Iran. *Herba Polonica*, 55: 69-75.

Ghasemi Pirbalouti, A., Momni, M. Bahmani, M. 2012. Ethnobotanical Study of Medicinal Plants Used by Kurd Tribe in Dehloran and Abdanan Districts, Ilam Province, Iran. *African Journal of Traditional, Complementary and Alternative Medicines* (AJTCAM), 10 (2): 368-385.

Ghelichnia, H. 2005. Traditional and public beliefs about medicinal plants province. National conference on stable development of medicinal plants, Mashhad 565-566. (In Persion).

Ghorbani, A., Langenberger, G., Feng, L. Sauerborn, J. 2011. Ethnobotanical study ofmedicinal plants utilised by Hani ethnicity in Naban River Watershed National Nature Reserve, Yunnan, China. *Journal of Ethnopharmacology*, 134: 651–667.

Giorgetti, M., Rossi, L. Rodrigues, E. 2011. Brazilian Plants with Possible Action on the Central Nervous System: A Study of Historical Sources from the 16th to 19th Century. *Revista Brasileira de Farmacognosia*, 109 (2): 338-347.

Hamedi, A., Zarshenas, M. M., Sohrabpour, M. Zargaran, A. 2013. An Herbal medicinal oils in traditional Persian medicine. *Pharmaceutical Biology,* 51 (9): 1208-1218.

Heinrich, M., Ankli, A., Frei, B., Weimann, C. Sticher, O. 1998. Medicinal plantsin Mexico: Healers consensus and cultural importance. *Social Science and Medicine*, 47: 1859-1871.

Hooshidari, F. 2009. Medicinal plants of Kordestan Province. *Iranian Journal of Medicinal and Aromatic Plants*, 25 (1): 90-103 (In Persian).

Hurrell, J. A. Albuquerque, U. P. 2012. Is Ethnobotany an Ecological Science? Steps towards a complex

Ethnobotany. *Ethnobiology and Conservation*, 1, 4. Disponible: <http://ethnobioconservation.com> [Consulta: 8-IX-2013].

Inta, A., Shengji, P., Balslev, H., Wangpakapattanawong, P. Trisonthi, C. 2008. A comparative study on medicinal plants used in Akha's traditional medicine in China and Thailand, cultural coherence or ecological divergence? *Journal of Ethnopharmacology*, 116: 508–517.

Jeruto, A., Lukhoba, C., Oumaa, G., Otieno. A. Charles, M. 2008. An ethnobotanical study of medicinal plants used by the Nandi people in Kenya.*Journal of ethno-pharmacology*, *Elsevier,* 116: 370-376.

Kalvandi, R. 2007. Identification of Medicinal plants of Hamedan Province. *Iranian journal of Medicinal and Aromatic Plants,* 23 (3): 350-374. (In Persian).

Khajoei Nasab, F. Khosravi, A. R. 2014. Ethnobotanical study of medicinal plants of Sirjan in Kerman Province, Iran. *Journal of Ethnopharmacology,* 154 (1): 190-197.

Khodayari, H., Amani, Sh. Amiri, H. 2014. Ethnobotanical study of medicinal plants in the Northeast of Khuzestan province: identification and traditional uses. *Journal of Echophytochemical of medical plants,*8 (4): 12-26. (In Persian).

Kim, H. Song, M. J. 2013. Ethnobotanical analysis for traditional Knowledge of wild edible plants in North Jeolla Province (Korea). *Genetic Resources Crop Evolution*, 60 (4): 1571–1585.

Lagos, L. M. 2005. Especies con propiedades medicinales encontradas en lascolecciones del herbario UPTC y su uso actual en Tunja y en losmunicipios de Chíquiza, Cómbita, Oicatá, Sora y Soracá (Boyacá). Revista De La Asociación Colombiana De Herbarios. *Universidad del*

Mahmood, A. Tabassum, A. 2011. Ethnomedicinal survey of plants from District Sialkot, Pakistan. *Journal of Applied Pharmacology*, 2: 212-220.

Manjula, S. Mamidala, E. 2013. An ethnobotanical survey of medical plants used by traditional healers of Thadvai, Warangal district, Andhra Pradesh, India. *International journal of medical research and health science*, 2 (1): 40-46.

Mann, A., Amupitan, J. O., Oyewale, A. O., Okogun, J. I., Ibrahim, K., Oladosu, P., Lawson, L., Olajideand, I. Nnamdi, A. 2008. Evaluation of invitro anti mycobacterial activity of Nigerian plants used for treatment of respiratory diseases. *African Journal of Biotechnology*, 7 (11): 1630–1636.

Medeiros, M. F. T. lbuquerque, U. P. 2014. Food Flora in 17th Century Northeast Region of Brazil in Historia Naturalis Brasiliae. *Journal of Ethnobiology and Ethnomedicine,* 10: 50.

Mesfin, K., Tekle, G. Tesfay, T. 2013. Ethnobotanical Study of Traditional Medicinal Plants Used by Indigenous People of Gemad District, Northern Ethiopia. *Journal of Medicinal Plants Studies,* 1 (4): 32-37.

Mirdavoodi, H. R. 2008. Identification of Medicinal plants of Markazi Province. *Iranian Journal of Medicinal and Aromatic Plants*, 23 (4): 544-559. (In Persian).

Mosaddegh, M., Naghibi, F., Moazzeni, H. Pirani, A. 2012. Ethnobotanical survey of herbal remedies traditionally used in Kohghiluyeh va Boyer Ahmad province of Iran. *Journal of Ethnopharmacology,*141: 80- 95.

Naghibi, F., Esmaeili, S., Malekmohammadi, M., Hassanpour, A. Mosaddegh, M. 2014. Ethnobotanical survey of medicinal plants used traditionally in two villages of Hamedan, Iran. *Research Journal of Pharmacognosy,*1 (3): 7-14.

Njoroge, G. N., Joroge, G. N., Kaibui, I. M., Njenga, P. K. Odhiambo, P. O. 2010. Utilization of priority traditional medicinal plants and local people's knowledge on their conservation status in arid lands of Kenya (Mwingi District).*Journal of Ethnobiology Ethnomedicine,* 6: 22.

Pochettino, M. L. Lema, V. 2008. La variable tiempo en la caracterización del conocimiento botánico tradicional. *Darwiniana*, 46: 227-239.

Rajaei, P. Mohamadi, N. 2012. Ethnobotanical Study of Medicinal Plants of Hezar Mountain Allocated in South East of Iran. *Iran Journal Pharmacy Restoration*, 11 (4): 1153-1167.

Rechinger, K. H. 1963-2013. *Flora Iranica*. nos: 1-178. Akademische Drucku. Varlasanstalt, Graz. *Austria,*Vol. 1-174.

Reyes-García, V., Luz, A. C., Gueze, M., Paneque-Gálvez, J., Macía, M. J.,Orta-Martínez, M. Pino, J. 2013. Secular Trends on Traditional Ecological Knowledge: An Analysis of Changes in Different Domains of Knowledge among Tsimane' Men. *Learning and Individual Differences*, 27: 206-212.

Safa, O., Soltanipoor, M. A., Rastegar, S., Kazemi, M., Nourbakhsh Dehkordi, K. Ghannadi, A. 2012. An ethnobotany survey on Hormozgan Province in Iran. *Journal of phytomedicine*, 3 (1): 64-81.

Shrivastava, S. Kanungo,V. K. 2013. Ethnobotanical survey of Surguja District with special reference to plants used by uraon tribe in treatment of respiratory diseases. Int,*Journal of Herbal Medicine,*1(3): 131–134.

Song, M., Kim, H., Brian, H., Choi, K. H. Lee, B. 2013. Traditional Knowledge of wild edible plants on Jeju Island, Korea. *Indian Journal of Traditional Knowledge*, 12: 177–194.

Sulaiman, S. F., Zahariluddin, A. S. M. Noor, S. S. M. 2011. Anti-tuberculosis potential of some ethnobotanically selected Malaysian plants. *Journal of Ethnopharmacology,* 133: 1021–1026.

Tardio, J. Pardo-de Santayana, M. 2008. Cultural importance indices: a comparative analysis based on the useful wild plants of southern Cantabria (northern Spain). *Economic Botany,* 62: 24–39.

Trotter, R. T. Logan, M. H. 1986. Informant consensus: a new approach for identifying potentially effective medicinal plants. In: Etkin, N.L. (Ed.), Plants in Indigenous Medicine and Diet. Redgrave Publishing Company, Bedford Hill New York 91-112.

Turner, N. J., Łuczaj, Ł. J., Migliorini, P., Pieroni, A., Dreon, A. L., Sacchetti, L. E. Paoletti, M. G. 2011. Edible and tended wild plants, traditional ecological knowledge and agroecology. *Critical Reviews in Plant Sciences* 30 (1–2): 198–225. doi:10.1080/07352689.2011.554492.

Weckerle, C. S., Ineichen, R., Huber, F. K. Yang, Y. 2009. Mao's heritage: medicinal plant knowledge among the Bai in Shaxi, China, at crossroads between distinct local and common widespread practice. *Journal of Ethnopharmacology*, 123: 213–228.

WHO, 2002. Traditional Medicine: Growing Needs and Potentials, Geneva. Available on Internet at: *http://www.who.int/emc-documents/Growing needs and potentials /docs /EGlobalStrat. pdf.*

Zank, S. Hanazaki, N. 2011. Exploring the links between Ethnobotany, Local Therapeutic Practices, and Protected Areas in Santa Catarina Coastline. *Evidence Based Complement Alternative Medicine:* Brazil; doi:10.1155/2012/563570.

Effects of different sources of nitrogen fertilizer and applied rates on essential oil content and composition of peppermints

Adel Poshtdar[1*], Alireza Abdali Mashhadi[1], Foad Moradi[2], Seyed Ata Siadat[1], Abdolmehdi Bakhshandeh[1]

[1]*Department of Agronomy, Ramin Agriculture and Natural Resources University of Khouzestan, Khouzestan, Iran;*
***Email:** *adelposhtdar@gmail.com*
[2]*Agricultural Biotechnology Research Institute of Iran, Karaj, Iran;*

ARTICLE INFO

Topic: *Medicinal Plants*

Key words:
- ✓ *GC/MS*
- ✓ *Menthapiperita*
- ✓ *Menthol*
- ✓ *Phytochemical*
- ✓ *UAN*

ABSTRACT

Background & Aim: Peppermint known for its healing properties is a plant from the Labiatae family. Currently, different rates of nitrogenous fertilizers are used in production of peppermint while there is no precise information available about how much of nitrogen fertilizer is the optimum rate for this plant. The main purpose of this research was to evaluate the response of peppermint chemical composition to different nitrogen rates and type of nutrition strategy (with control and conventional chemical sources).
Experimental: Samples collected from different mint nutrition strategy [conventional: four nitrogen levels from three fertilizers source (UAN, urea and ammonium sulfate), and control (no added fertilizer) in the Khouzestan province at the southwest of Iran.
Results: Nitrogen supply led to increase of fresh and dry yield of peppermint. Maximum essential oil obtained from 210 kgN/ha of nitrogen fertilizer in UAN which showed the best results compared to urea, ammonium sulfate and control. The GC/MS data showed that the qualitative of the components appeared to be not constant in different nutrient strategy. Moreover, remarkable variations were found in the amounts of the major of essential oil constituents. A total thirty-five components, comprising 98.87, 97.62, 98.09 and 97.98% of the obtained total essential oils were characterized in control, UAN, urea and ammonium sulfate samples, respectively. Also Menthol (41.22, 33.7, 30.62 and 33.23%), menthone (16.32, 26.25, 27.33 and 26.7 %), menthofuran (4.09, 4.74, 5.81 and 5.14 %) and isomenthone (6.47, 7.48, 7.26 and 7.43%) were the main components of peppermint oil.
Recommended applications/industrie: Since, essential oil of peppermint, particularly menthol component, has many application in pharmaceutical and perfumery industry due to antiviral, antibacterial and antispasmodic activity, UAN fertilizers is recommended to be used in addition to control in view of the increasing in quality and quantity of essential oil.

1. Introduction

Consumer demand for organic foods has continuously increased because of the perception that they might contain greater amounts of beneficial components than their conventionally produced counterparts. Conflicting findings on the quality and nutritional values of organic foods compared to their conventional counterparts have been reported. For instance, a human crossover intervention study involving 16 subjects demonstrated that organic and conventional fruits and vegetables differed in their concentrations of five selected flavonoids and resulted in different urinary excretions of the major dietary flavonoids (Grinder-Pedersen *et al.*, 2003). In contrast, a systematic review concluded that there was no evidence indicating the nutrition quality difference between organic and conventional foods (Dangour *et al.*, 2009). Mints comprise a group of species of the genus *Mentha* belonging to the family Lamiaceae. The aerial parts of the herb on distillation yields essential oil containing a large number of aroma chemicals like menthol, menthone, isomenthone, menthofuran, carvone, linalool, linalyl acetate and piperitenone oxide which are used in pharmaceutical, food, flavour, cosmetics, beverages and allied industries (Verma *et al.*, 2010). Peppermint (*Mentha x piperita* L.) oil is one of the most popular and widely used essential oils, mostly because of its main components menthol and menthone. Peppermint oil is used for flavouring pharmaceuticals and oral preparations. The annual world production of *Menthaarvensis* L. and *M. piperita* L. oils are 22,000 and 7500 mt, while India is producing 16000 and 100 mt per year, respectively (Khanuja, 2007; Patra *et al.*, 2002). And it was found that the chemical composition is influenced by various factors, such as geographical location (Murray *et al.*, 1988), environmental conditions (Chalchat *et al.*, 1997) and agro-climatic requirements of the crops (Chand *et al.*, 2004).Cultivation techniques have a great influence on plant growth (biomass production) and the quality and quantity of secondary metabolites. There is an absolute N requirement for plant growth, and crop yields and quality depend upon substantial N inputs. Chemical N fertilizers were first used in agriculture in the 19th century, and subsequently to a much greater extent after the development of the Haber Bosch process at the beginning of the 20th century. At the present time, more than half of the chemically fixed N is used by agriculture, amounting to in excess of 80 Mt per year, worldwide (Hawkesford, 2014). Most authors report that significantly higher dry matter and essential oil yields for corn mint, peppermint and spearmint were obtained with higher nitrogen application but that the application of nitrogen did not affect the chemical composition of the essential oil (Saxena & Singh, 1995). Other authors have reported that a decrease in menthol and an increase in menthone and menthyl acetate in peppermint and corn mint has been found with increased application of N (Duhan *et al.*, 1977; Hornok, 1983). According to Kothari & Singh (1995), carvone and limonene concentrations in Scotch spearmint (*M. gracilis*) were affected by levels of N, and in general, an increase of N decreased carvone but increased limonene in oil. This is not quite in agreement with Singh & Singh (1986) who reported that the application of N increased carvone in spearmint oil. Marotti and co-authors (1994) used different levels of nitrogen and phosphorus in peppermint trials. They reported that mineral fertilization seemed to increase the menthol content of essential oil compared with untreated plants. Hornok (1983) reported that the most effective treatment on yield of peppermint regarding to fertilizers was achieved first by the level of nitrogen and second by the level of calcium. Phosphorus fertilization had no effect on yield. However, a high quality of peppermint oil in any region requires the optimum use of fertilizers and water to maintain herbage growth and delay maturity as long as possible so that the herbage may be harvested with a minimum of flowers (Murray *et al.*, 1988).

Nitrogen may be applied in various forms to fertilization strategies including organic manures and various inorganic fertilizers such as ammonium and nitrate salts, urea, and anhydrous ammonia. Critically the management practices for the type and time of fertilizer application should minimize volatile or leaching losses (Matson *et al.*, 1998). Nitrification is the conversion of ammonia into nitrate, the latter having a higher propensity for leaching from agricultural soils. Much of the N applied worldwide is in the form of ammonium and slowing the conversion to nitrate may facilitate more efficient capture (Hawkesford, 2014). Ammonium may be a better source of N for the plant as less energy is required for assimilation. Chemical nitrification inhibitors are available, but are costly. Some plant species produce exudates which are nitrification inhibitors and the transfer of this trait more widely has been proposed as a mean of improving NUE (Subbarao *et al.*, 2013). It has been shown that application of N fertilizers increases the productivity of peppermint.

There is a lack of information on the influence of nitrogen fertilizer sources on peppermint phytochemical and agronomic responses. Therefore, the purpose of this research was to evaluate the biochemical and agronomy response of peppermint to different rates of nitrogen fertilizer form applied, grown in semi-arid tropical climate (Ahvaz station).

2. Materials and Methods

2.1. Experimental site preparation

The field experiment was conducted during 2015, at the Research Station, Faculty of Agronomy, Ramin Agriculture & Natural Resource University of Khuzestan, Iran (31°35′ 7.67″ N, 48° 53′ 0.81″ E, elevation 25 m above sea levels) in a semi-arid tropical climate. Before conducting the experiment, soil samples were taken from the depth of 0–30 cm to determine the physicochemical characteristics of the experimental site. Soil information is presented in Table 1.

2.2. Experimental layout and treatments

The experiment was laid out in a factorial randomized block design with three replications. There were conventional fertilization strategy including four levels of nitrogen (70, 140, 210, 280 kg N/ha) of three nitrogen fertilizer sources (urea, ammonium sulfate, urea ammonium nitrate (UAN)) and control (no added fertilizer). The intent was to use a wide enough range of nitrogen to exceed that for maximum plant requirements. N was applied in four equal splits in 15 days interval in the form of urea, ammonium sulfate and nitrate liquid. P_2O_5, in the form of triple superphosphate at the rate of 200 kg/ha was applied in each plot of the experiment. Peppermint (*Menthapiperita*) was planted on 10th February 2015 in field plots at a spacing of 30 cm. Weekly irrigation was applied, depending upon the climatic conditions. Weeds were removed by hand and farms was kept weed free during the experiment.

2.3. Plant measurements

The crop was harvested 5 cm above the ground level during the budding -flowering stage and fresh yields was recorded from an area of 1 m^2. Plant material was dried at 65°C until dry mass remained constant and biomass determined. Then leaf dry yield and essential oil yield of peppermint were recorded. The oil concentration in the air-dried herbage was estimated using Clevenger's apparatus (Mitchell and Farris, 1996).

2.4. Essential oil and GC-MS analysis

Essential oil from *Menthapiperita* was analyzed using GC/MS. The GC/MS analysis was performed on an Agilent (MS 5875 C, GC7890) system. The capillary column used was a HP-5MS (30 m × 0.25 mm, film thickness 0.25 μm). The oven temperature program was initiated at 50°C, held for 5 min then raised up to 240°C at a rate of 3°C/min, then 240- 300°C at a rate of 15°C/min. Helium was used as the carrier gas at a flow rate 1 ml/min. The compounds of the oil were identified by comparison of their retention indices (RI), with data published in the literature (Adams, 2004).

2.5. Statistical analysis

The data were subjected to statistical analysis following analysis of variance (ANOVA) and regression technique as applied to factorial randomized block design (Snedecor and Cochran, 1989).

3. Results and discussion

3.1 Agronomic response of peppermint oil

Analysis of variance revealed significant differences between the nitrogen form and rates based on the fresh yield, dry yield and oil concentration of peppermint (Table 2). Maximum fresh and dry biomass yield obtained by 210 and 280 kgN/ha, while UAN exhibited better results than urea and ammonium sulfate. In control (no added fertilizer), fresh and dry yield biomass were 1150 and 379 g/m^2, respectively, but increased by adding 210 kg of nitrogen (4238, 4041, 3523 g/m^2fresh yield and 986, 982, 797g/m^2 dry yield for UAN, urea and ammonium sulfate, respectively). Result showed that all three forms of nitrogen fertilizer increased yield quantity (Figure 1a and b).Nitrogen is one of the most important modifiers of peppermint productivity and oil composition. Generally, higher N application rates were associated with high biomass yields.

Peppermint essential oil percentage in control (no added fertilizer) was 1.52 percent, while the use of 210 kgN/ha from UAN, urea and ammonium sulfate increased peppermint essential oil to 3.11, 2.65 and 2.19%, respectively. The use of more than 210 kg/ha nitrogen fertilizer led to leaf essential oil reduction (2.65, 2.36 and 1.74 by the source of UAN, urea and ammonium sulfate, respectively). The maximum percentage of essential oil obtained from 210 kg of UAN fertilizer (Figure 2).

Table 2. Analysis of variance (mean squares) of peppermint characteristics at different nitrogen rates and fertilizer form.

Source of variation	df	Fresh yield(g/m²)	Dry yield(g/m²)	Essential oil (%)
Block	2	3573652	210634	0.7115
N level	3	6672750**	285972**	0.7613**
N sources	2	214320^{ns}	7334^{ns}	1.164**
N level × N sources	6	302546*	30006*	0.124*
Error	22	98394	8196	0.03604
CV%	-	9.4	11.3	8.3

ns = not significant., * = P<0.05, ** = P<0.01.

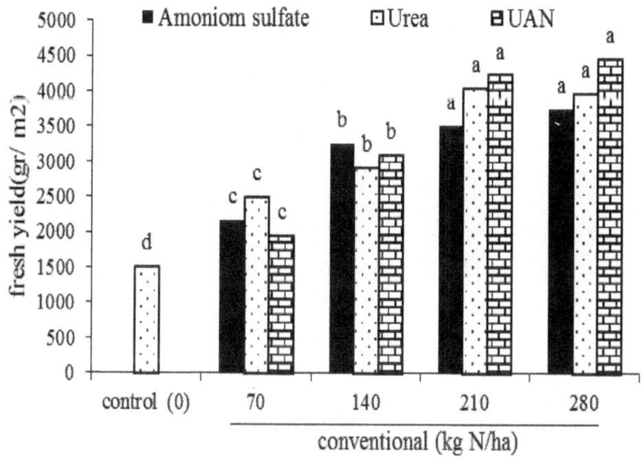

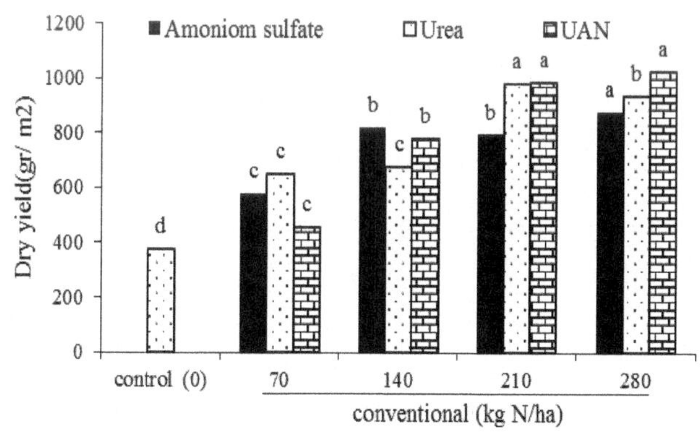

Fig. 1. Fresh (a) and dry (b) yield (g/m²) of peppermints in control and samples with conventional fertilization.

In literatures it was reported that the most effect on peppermint yield was achieved first by the level of nitrogen and second by the level of calcium (Hornok, 1983). Saxena *et al.* (1995) reported the higher essential oil yield for corn mint, peppermint and spearmint with higher nitrogen application.

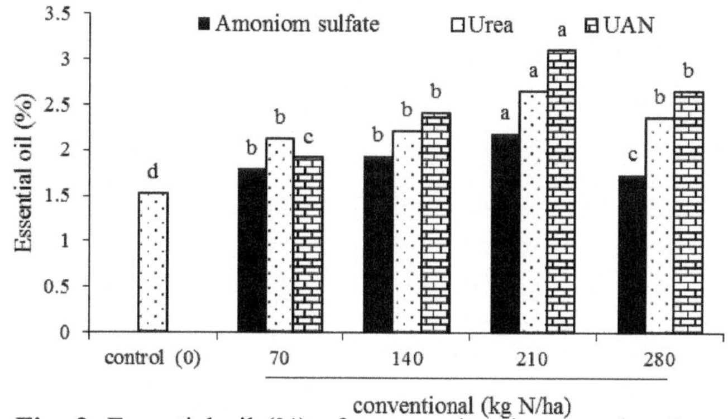

Fig. 2. Essential oil (%) of peppermints in control and samples with conventional fertilization.

3.2 Chemical composition of peppermint oil

Essential oil compounds in control and samples with 210 kg/ha of nitrogen intake was evaluated. Thirty five components were identified in peppermint oil accounting for 99% of total oil (Table 3). The essential oils from four samples (Control, 210 kg/ha UAN, urea and ammonium sulfate) were characterized according to what is listed below, respectively.

Menthol (41.22, 33.17, 30.62 and 33.23%), menthone (16.32, 26.25, 27.33 and 26.7 %), menthofuran (4.09, 4.74, 5.81 and 5.14%) and isomenthone (6.47, 7.48, 7.26 and 7.43%) were the main components of peppermint oil followed by ciscarvone oxide (8.99, 5.43, 5.74 and 5.57 %), pulegone (2.5, 2.76, 3.61 and 2.95 %), 1,8 cineole (2.71,5.79, 4.61 and 5.22%), and limonene (0.96, 1.47, 1.33 and 1.41%), trans piperitolacetatte (4.49, 3.03, 3.48 and 2.83%) and D-germacrene (3.64, 2.23, 2.5 and 2.17 %). Many studies reported the menthol as the main component of peppermint oil (Behnam *et al.*, 2006; Hawkesford, 2014; Hornok, 1983; Singh *et al.*, 1988), menthone and limonene as the second component of peppermint oil (Iscan *et al.*, 2002; Hussain *et al.*, 2010), but some others reported the β-terpinene and piperitone oxide as the main components of peppermint oil (Yadegarinia *et al.*, 2006).

Table 1. Soil physical and chemical properties of experimental area.

Treatments	Soil texture	Total N(%)	Organic Carbon(%)	E.C(dS/m)	pH	Available K (mg kgG¹)	Available P (mg kgG¹)
0-30	Silty clay	0.079	0.71	2.23	7.5	6.27	3.07

Table 3. Chemical composition (%) of the essential oils of *menthapiperita* samples

No.	Compound	KI	Control peppermint (No added fertilizer)	Conventional peppermint (Chemical fertilizers at 210 kg/ha nitrogen)		
				UAN	Urea	Ammonium sulfate
1.	α-pinene	939	0.08	0.51	0.45	0.5
2.	sabinene	975	0.23	0.44	0.4	0.41
3.	β-pinene	979	-	0.86	0.77	0.82
4.	myrcene	991	0.11	0.13	0.12	0.13
5.	octanol 3-	991	-	0.12	0.1	0.08
6.	limonene	1029	0.96	1.47	1.33	1.41
7.	1,8-Cineole	1031	2.71	5.79	4.61	5.22
8.	β-ocimene (z)	1037	0.11	0.16	0.15	0.13
9.	sabinene hydrate cis	1070	0.61	0.75	0.79	0.76
10.	trans-sabinene hydrate	1090	0.06	-	0.24	-
11.	linalool	1097	0.25	0.24	0.24	0.22
12.	isopulegole	1148	0.11	0.11	0.12	0.11
13.	menthone	1153	16.32	26.25	27.33	26.7
14.	menthofuran	1164	4.09	4.74	5.81	5.14
15.	menthoneiso	1163	6.47	7.48	7.26	7.43
16.	menthol	1172	41.22	33.7	30.62	33.23
17.	terpinen-4-ol	1177	0.35	-	0.68	0.63
18.	neo iso menthol	1187	0.73	0.42	0.36	0.42
19.	Iso- menthol	1183	0.15	0.1	0.08	0.1
20.	α-terpieol	1189	0.66	0.51	0.53	0.53
21.	pulegone	1237	2.5	2.76	3.61	2.95
22.	piperitone	1253	0.41	0.41	0.44	0.43
23.	Trans- piperiton epoxide	1254	0.45	0.29	0.3	0.31
24.	Cis- carvone oxide	1263	8.99	5.43	5.74	5.57
25.	Trans- carvone oxide	1276	0.33	0.15	0.15	0.16
26.	limonene 10 ol	1290	0.29	0.13	0.17	0.12
27.	Cis-piperitolacetatte	1335	0.31	0.14	0.19	0.13
28.	Trans- piperitolacetatte	1346	4.49	3.03	3.48	2.83
29.	α-humulene	1455	0.23	0.13	-	0.13
30.	β-farnesene	1457	0.51	0.33	0.39	0.32
31.	germacrene d	1485	3.64	2.23	2.5	2.17
32.	germacrene A	1509	0.49	0.24	0.28	0.26
33.	germacrene B	1561	0.38	0.2	0.23	0.18
34.	germacrene D 4 ol	1576	0.88	0.43	0.46	0.39
35.	β-elemenonecis	1590	0.17	-	-	-

Therefore, menthol is not always the primary component of peppermint oil. The chemical composition of peppermint oil from this study is comparable to Iscan *et al.* (2002). Menthol and menthone are the main components of the oil. Totally menthone, menthofuran, isomenthone, pulegone, 1,8 cineole and limonene increased with increasing in nitrogen fertilizer, but menthol, ciscarvone oxide and trans piperitol acetate and D-germacrene showed the reverse trend. Researchers have reported that a decrease in menthol and an increase in menthone and menthyl acetate in peppermint and corn mint has been found with increasing in nitrogen level (Duhan *et al.*, 1977; Hornok, 1983). According to Kothari & Singh (1995), carvone and limonene concentrations in Scotch spearmint (*M. gracilis*) were affected by levels of N, and in general, an increase of N caused a decrease in carvone content but an increase in limonene content in essential oil. This is not quite in agreement with Singh & Singh (1986) who reported that the application of N increased carvone in spearmint oil.

4. Conclusion

Quality of peppermint essential oil was close in samples treated by chemical sources of nitrogen fertilizer including UAN and urea while it was much higher in control (no added fertilizer) treatment. Quality and quantity of essential oil in plots which were fertilized by UAN was higher than urea and ammonium sulfate. The qualitative composition of the components appeared to be constant in the three different nitrogen sources and no remarkable variation was found in the amounts of the essential oil major constituents.

5. References

Adams, R.P. 2004. *Identification of Essential Oil Components by Gas-Chromatography/Mass Spectroscopy*. Allured Publishing, Carol Stream, USA, 456p.

Behnam, S., Farzaneh, M., Ahmadzadeh, M. and Tehrani, A.S. 2006. Composition and antifungal activity of essential oils of *Menthapiperita* and *Lavendulaangustifolia* on post-harvest phytopathogens. *Communications in Agricultural and Applied Biological Sciences*., 71(3): 1321-1326.

Chalchat, J.C., Garry, R.P., Michet, A. 1997. Variation of the chemical composition of essential oil of *Menthapiperita* L. during the growing time. *J. Essent. Res.,* 9: 463–465.

Chand, S., Patra, N.K., Anwar, M., Patra, D.D. 2004. Agronomy and uses of menthol mint (*Menthaarvensis*) Indian prospective. Proc. *Indian Nat. Sci. AcadB.,* 70 (3): 269–297.

Dangour, A. D., Dodhia, S. K., Hayter, A., Allen, E., Lock, K., Uauy, R. 2009.Nutritional quality of organic foods: a systematic review. *Am. J. Clin. Nutr.,* 90: 680–685.

Duhan, SPS., Bhattacharya, AK., and Husain A. 1977. Effect of N and its methods of application on the herb and quality of corn mint. *Indian Perfume*., 21: 135–138.

Grinder-Pedersen, L., Rasmussen, S. E., Gel, S. B., Jorgensen, L. V., Dragsted, L. O., Gundersen, V., Sandstrom, B. 2003. Effect of diets based on foods from conventional versus organic production on intake and excretion of flavonoids and markers of antioxidative defense in humans. *J. Agric. Food Chem*., 51: 5671−5676

Hawkesford. M. J. 2014. Reducing the reliance on nitrogen fertilizer for wheat production. *Journal of Cereal Science*., 59: 276e283

Hornok L. 1983. Influence of nutrition on the yield and content of active compounds in some essential oil plants. *Acta Horticulturae*., 132: 239–247.

Hussain, A.I., Anwar, F., Nigam, P.S., Ashraf, M. and Gilani, A.H. 2010. Seasonal variation in content, chemical composition and antimicrobial and cytotoxic activities of essential oils from four *Mentha* species. *Journal of the Science of Food and Agriculture*., 90: 1827-1836.

Iscan, G., Kirimer, N., kurkcouglo M., Baser K.H. and Demirci, F. 2002. Antimicrobial Screening of *Menthapiperita* Essential Oils. *Journal of Agricultural and Food Chemistry*., 50: 3943-3946.

Khanuja, S.P.S. 2007. Aroma vision 2020: Technology path of cultivating today for a fragrant tomorrow. National convention & seminar on business enabling of aromatic plants & products at Dehradun, India. November., 21-22.

Kothari SK & Singh UB. 1995. The effect of row spacing and nitrogen fertilization on scotch spearmint (*Menthagracilis* Sole). *Journal of Essential Oil Research*., 7: 287–297.

Marotti. M., R., Piccaglia. W., Crout. K., Craufutd. And S. Deans. 2004. Effect of planting time and mineral fertilization on peppermint (*Menthapiperita* L.) essential oil composition and its biological activity. *Flavor and Fragrance Journal*., 9(3): 125-129.

Matson, P.A., Naylor, R., Ortiz-Monasterio, I. 1998. Integration of environmental, agronomic, and economic aspects of fertilizer management. *Science.*, 280: 112-115.

Mitchell, A.R. and N.A. Farris. 1996. Peppermint response to nitrogen fertilizer in an arid climate. *J. Plant Nutr.*, 19: 955–967.

Murray, MJ., Marble, P., Lincoln, D & Hefendehl, FW. 1988. Peppermint oil quality differences and the reasons for them. Flavors and Fragrances: Proceeding of the 10th International Congress of Essential oils, Fragrances and Flavors, Washington, DC, U.S.A. p 189– 208.

Patra, N.K., Kumar, B., Shukla, K., Ram, P. and Srivastava, H.K. 2002. *Problems and issues of Agrotechnology transfer in menthol mint: A case study with variety Kosi.* Proceedings of First National Interactive Meet on Medicinal & Aromatic Plants CIMAP, Lucknow. pp: 440-443.

Saxena, A. and Singh, J.N. 1995. *Effect of irrigation, mulch and nitrogen on yield and composition of corn mint (Menthaarvensis L. subsp. Haplocalyx var. piperascens) oil.* Blackwell Wissenschafts-Verlag - Berlin ISSN. 0931-2250, 183–188.

Singh, A.K., Naqvi, A.A, Singh, K. and Thakur, R.S. 1988. Transformation of menthol, menthone and menthyl acetate in cornmint with relation to age of plant. *Current Science*., 57: 480-481.

Snedecor, G.W., Cochran, W.G. 1989. *Statistical Methods*, 8th ed. Iowa State University Press, Ames, Iowa.

Subbarao, G.V., Sahrawat, K.L., Nakahara, K., Rao, I.M., Ishitani, M., Hash, C.T., Kishii, M., Bonnett, D.G., Berry, W.L., Lata, J.C. 2013. A paradigm shift towards low-nitrifying production systems: the role of biological nitrification inhibition (BNI). Ann. Bot. 112, 297-316.

Verma, R.S., Rahman L., Verma, R.K., Chauhan, A., Yadav, A.K. and Singh, A. 2010. Essential Oil Composition of Menthol Mint (*Menthaarvensis*) and Peppermint (*Menthapiperita*) Cultivars at Different Stages of Plant Growth from Kumaon Region of Western Himalaya. Journal of Medicinal and Aromatic Plants. 1(1): 13-18

Yadegarinia, D., Gachkar, L., Rezaei, MB.,Taghizadeh, M., AlipoorAstaneh, S.H. and Rasooli, I. 2006. Biochemical activities of Iranian *Menthapiperita* L. and *Myrtuscommunis* L. essential oils. *Phytochemistry*., 67: 1249- 1255.

17

Screening of the profiles of the essential oils from the aerial parts of *Nepeta racemosa* using classical and microwave-based methods: Comparison with the volatiles using headspace solid-phase micro-extraction

Majid Mohammadhosseini*

Department of Chemistry, Shahrood Branch, Islamic Azad University, Shahrood, Iran;
Email:** ***m_mhosseini@iau-shahrood.ac.ir ; majidmohammadhosseini@yahoo.com

ARTICLE INFO

Topic: *Medicinal Plants*

Key words:
- ✓ *Nepeta racemose*
- ✓ *Hydrodistillation*
- ✓ *Solvent-free microwave extraction*
- ✓ *Microwave assisted hydrodistillation*
- ✓ *Headspace solid-phase micro extraction*

ABSTRACT

Background & Aim: *Nepeta racemosa* is an herbal and medicinal plant and this report aims to identify chemical compositions of the essential oils and volatiles of its aerial parts through classical and advanced methods.
Experimental: Chemical profiles of the essential oils and volatile compounds from the aerial parts of *Nepeta racemosa* obtained through hydrodistillation (HD), solvent-free microwave extraction (SFME), microwave assisted hydrodistillation (MAHD) and headspace solid-phase microextraction (HS-SPME) methods were subsequently investigated by means of GC and GC-MS instruments.
Results: Totally, 25, 26, 24, and 24 components were identified in the chemical profiles, representing 98.1%, 96.6%, 97.7% and 96.4% of the total compositions when using the HD, HS-SPME, SFME and MAHD methods, respectively. In all samples, oxygenated monoterpenes were the major fractions of the chemical profiles with the exception of chemical composition of the essential oil of *N. racemosa* obtained by using the MAHD approach in which monoterpene hydrocarbons were dominant constituting compounds. In final, 4aα,7α,7aα-nepetalactone was the most abundant compound in the chemical profiles of HD, HS-SPME and SFME approaches while 4aα,7α,7aβ-nepetalactone oxygenated monoterpene was the most frequent compound in the MAHD profile.
Recommended applications/industries: Using the advanced separation methods for isolation of the essential oils are economic, time saving and eminently suited compared with the classical and traditional separation methods. Moreover, the significance of this study relates to the fact that the essential oils, which are rich in monoterpene hydrocarbons and oxygenated monoterpenes could be regarded as powerful food preservatives and novel antioxidants.

1. Introduction

The Asteraceae or Compositae as a great family of plants involves a large number of flowering plants, which have been classified in about 1600 genera altogether covering 23,000 species (Bessada *et al.*, 2015). It is commonly referred to as the aster, daisy, composite or sunflower family, as well. In terms of numbers of species, the plants belonging to the Asteraceae family are only comparable with those of the Orchidaceae family. A broad spectrum of medicinal and herbal plants of the Asteraceae family has been utilized as vegetables and in folk medicine, edible oils and pesticides. As shown in the literature, diverse plants in the Asteraceae family have considerable amounts of sesquiterpenoids particularly eudesmane-type having ones (Sharma & Goyal, 2011; Wu *et al.*, 2006). The genus *Nepeta* with the local Persian name of 'Punesa' belonging to the Lamiaceae family, subfamily Nepetoideae and tribe Mentheae consists of about 300 herbaceous perennial plants mostly having beautiful flowers and a pleasant odor (Mozaffarian, 1996; Zargari, 1989). Different species of this genus are mainly found in two areas of the world, namely Southwestern Asia (Turkey and Iran) along with Western Himalayas (Hindu Kush).

According to Jamzad *et al.* (2003), about sixty-seven species of this genus could be found in different parts of the country. In the Iranian traditional and folk medicine, different species of the *Nepeta* genus are frequently used and prescribed as potent diaphoretic, antitussive, diuretic, antispasmodic, anti-asthmatic agents and proper alternatives for chemical drugs with harmful side effects. The other promising traditional uses of this genus relate to their high astringent, antiseptic, febrifuge as well as sedative characteristics. More specifically, in the cutaneous eruptions of the children and snake and scorpion bites, they have been recognized as novel tropical remedies (Formisano *et al.*, 2011). As found in the literature, nepetalactones, iridoids and respective glucosides, diterpenes, triterpenes and flavonoids have been reported as major constituents of diverse *Nepeta* species (Asgarpanah *et al.*, 2014). Approximately, most of the *Nepeta* species are good sources to produce essential oils and organic extracts having a broad spectrum of biological activities involving insecticidal (Calmasur *et al.*, 2006), acaricidal (Calmasur *et al.*, 2006), anticancer (Aloqail *et al.*, 2014), antibacterial (Sonboli *et al.*, 2009), antioxidant (Adiguzel *et al.*, 2009), antimicrobial (Sonboli *et al.*, 2004), antiviral (Abad *et al.*, 2000), anticandidal (Iscan *et al.*, 2011), antinociceptive (Ali *et al.*, 2012a, b), analgesic (Hussain *et al.*, 2015), anti-seizure (Bhat *et al.*, 2012), anti-inflammatory (Hussain *et al.*, 2015; Ali *et al.*, 2012a, b), antiprotozoal (Dua *et al.*, 2011), neuropharmacological (Galati *et al.*, 2004), antifungal (Sonboli *et al.*, 2004), antiglycation, antiplatelets aggregation, cytotoxic and phytotoxic (Hussain *et al.*, 2010) activities. In view of many promising medical, phytochemical and pharmacological properties of the plants in the *Nepeta* genus, characterization and identification of the corresponding profiles seem highly justifiable.

The presents report aims at profiling chemical composition of the essential oils and volatiles obtained from the aerial parts of *N. racemosa* (Figure 1). Furthermore, to the best of my knowledge, there has been no report concerning the essential oil composition and volatile constituents of *N. racemosa* determined by the SFME and HS-SPME techniques up to present.

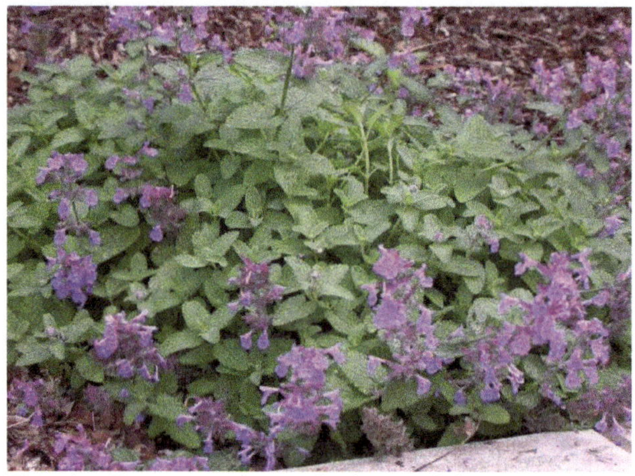

Fig 1. Representation of the aerial parts of *N. racemosa*.

2. Materials and Methods

2.1. Chemicals and supplies

The normal alkane mixtures were purchased from Fluka (Buchs, Switzerland). High purity helium and nitrogen carrier gases were used in the GC and GC-MS instrumentations.

2.2. Plant material and botanical identification

The plant material was collected while wearing polystyrene gloves during the flowering stage in April 2015, in the Afjeh, Lavasan, Tehran Province, at 51° 41' 28.00" E and 35° 51' 34.99" N. A voucher specimen was deposited at the Herbarium of the Research Institute of Forests and Rangelands, Tehran, Iran, for further authentication.

2.3. GC and GC-MS analyses

Gas chromatographic analyses were performed on a Shimadzu 15A gas chromatograph equipped with a split/splitless (ratio 1:30) injector and a flame ionization detector, both operating at 250 °C. In this separation process, high purity nitrogen with a flow-rate of 1 mL/min was utilized as the carrier gas across the capillary column which was of DB-5 type having dimensions of 50 m×0.2 mm and a film thickness of 0.32 µm. According to our temperature programming, the column temperature was first kept at 60°C for 3 min, then heated to 220 °C with a 5 °C/min rate and finally kept constant at 220 °C for 5 min. Relative percentage amounts were calculated from peak area using a CR5 Shimadzu CR pack without the use of correction factors.

GC/MS analysis was performed using a Hewlett-Packard 5973 instrument equipped with an HP-5MS column (30 m×0.25 mm, film thickness 0.25 µm). The effluent of the GC column was introduced directly into the source of MS. The column temperature programming was the same with the GC analysis. The flow-rate of helium carrier gas was set at 1 mL/min. Additionally, final temperature of the column was exactly 230 °C while detector temperature was set at 250 °C. All of the MS spectra were taken at 70 eV (E1) over the range 30-350 amu with an electron multiplier voltage of 1800 eV and scan times of 2 scans/ sec.

2.4. Hydrodistillation method

The collected plant material was dried in the dark room at ambient temperature in the absence of light. Then, 150-g portions of the air-dried aerial parts of *N. racemosa* were subjected to hydrodistillation in a Clevenger-type apparatus for 4 h. The obtained essential oils had pale yellowish colors and were subsequently dried using minimal amounts of anhydrous sodium sulphate and stored at 4 °C in the absence of daylight in brown vials until being analyzed (Mohammadhosseini & Beiranvand, 2013).

2.5. Solvent-free microwave extraction (SFME) method

The basic principles of the SFME approach have been extensively discussed in our previous reports (Mohammadhosseini, 2016; Mohammadhosseini, 2015a; Mohammadhosseini *et al.*, 2015; Mohammadhosseini & Nekoei, 2014; Nekoei & Mohammadhosseini, 2016a; Nekoei & Mohammadhosseini, 2016b). Accordingly, a Milestone SRL microwave oven was used for isolation of the oils operating at 2450 MHz. For performance of the SFME-extraction in the absence of any solvent, the aerial parts of *N. racemosa* were placed in the microwave oven interior cavity having dimensions of 29 cm × 37 cm × 40 cm. However, prior to the extraction, 80-g portions of the dried and ground aerial parts of *N. racemosa* were soaked in appropriate amounts of distilled water in our laboratory at 25 °C for 1 h., and immediately after the excess water was drained off. The main reason of this step was to hydrate the external layers of the plant material and to condition them for better extraction of the essential oils from the respective secretory glands.

In our used set up, a full glass made Clevenger system in the outside of the extraction vessel served as the distillate condenser during the extraction process. Moreover, to maintain the same conditions of temperature and humidity within the process and to restore the *in situ* water to the plant material, the condensed water was repeatedly returned to the isolation medium. To conduct the SFME technique, the aerial parts of *N. racemosa* were heated in the microwave oven using an optimized fixed power of 800 W for an optimized time of 30 min. The chemical compositions of the isolated essential oils were then determined by the GC-MS apparatus.

2.6. Microwave assisted hydrodistillation (MAHD)

The operational characteristics of the MAHD technique were described in some of our recent papers (Hashemi-Moghaddam *et al.*, 2015; Hashemi-Moghaddam *et al.*, 2014; Mohammadhosseini *et al.*, 2016a; Mohammadhosseini *et al.*, 2013; Mohammadhosseini *et al.*, 2016c). In our suggested methodology, we used a microwave oven (Samsung, South Korea) regulated at a frequency of 2450 MHz capable of maintaining a maximum power of 1000 W. To initiate the separation step, a proper power (800 W) was directly applied to the hydrodistillation apparatus. The MAHD assembly consisted of a modified microwave oven housing a 1000-mL flat bottom which was directly connected to the Clevenger apparatus via a hole located above the oven. In our proposed MAHD procedure, 75-g portions of the dried and ground aerial parts of the plant sample (*N. racemosa*) were placed in a distinct volume of distilled water (500 mL) and the extraction carried out at a power of 800 W for 30 min using the introduced system. A glass condenser in the outside of the microwave cavity continuously condensed the vapor flow within the apparatus. The MAHD process was performed several times and was repeated until the volume of the extracted essential oil became constant. In the next step, the obtained essential oil was collected in amber brown vials. It was then dehydrated with anhydrous sodium sulfate, capped under nitrogen and kept at 4 °C until the analysis time.

2.7. Headspace solid-phase microextraction method

The foundations of the SPME-based procedures have been given in the literature in detail (Arthur & Pawliszyn, 1990). This method which was first introduced by Pawliszyn has considerably developed in the recent decades (Pawliszyn, 1999; Pawliszyn, 2003; Setkova *et al.*, 2007; Vuckovic *et al.*, 2010). The sequential steps by which the volatile fraction is separated from the plant materials are similar in a variety of scientific reports (Mohammadhosseini, 2015b; Mohammadhosseini *et al.*, 2016b; Nekoei & Mohammadhosseini, 2014; Nekoei & Mohammadhosseini, 2016b). In our investigation, we employed a commercially available manual SPME (Supelco, Bellefonte, USA) apparatus having 75-µm diameter fibers and a modified syringe containing stainless steel microtubing within its syringe needle. The microtubing has an about 1-cm fused-silica fiber tip on which an organic polymer has been deposited involving polydimethylsiloxane combined with craboxene (binder) namely, PDMS-CAR. The positions of the coated silica fiber are variable in different situations inside and outside the needle through a plunger similar to a routine syringe. However, the mean diameter of the syringe needle housing the microtubing and coated silica fiber is highly restricted and miniaturized. The first experimental step corresponds to the conditioning step in which the fiber is placed in the GC injector at 250 °C for 30 min. The next step is heating step in which one gram portions of powdered plant sample are placed in a 20-mL sample vial sealed with septum-type caps (Supelco), and then heated at 70 °C for 15 min. In the third step (adsorption), the SPME needle pierces the septum immediately after the PDMS fiber is extended through the needle and exposed to the headspace above the sample for 15 min to trap the volatile compounds in the upper space of the vials. In the final step (desorption), the fiber is drawn into the needle, and then the needle is removed from the septum and directly inserted onto the injection port of the GC in the splitless mode (250 °C) for about five minutes. Penetration from the septum of the GC injection port is possible when the fiber is withdrawn into the syringe needle. Finally, the volatile parts are desorbed and transferred to the capillary columns after again moving the fiber to the position outside the syringe.

2.8. Characterization of the chemical profiles

In this investigation, identification and determination of the constituents of each profile were tentatively made through comparison of their mass spectral fragmentation patterns and retention indices (RI) relative to C_9-C_{25} *n*-alkanes both with those given in the literature (Adams, 2007) as well as those stored in the MS spectral literature data (Wiley 275). In addition, complementary identification was confirmed through the comparison of the mass spectral fragmentation patterns of the constituents in the profiles with those stored in the MS database (National Institute of Standards and Technology and Wiley libraries). In some cases, when possible, we used the conformity pattern of some spectral patterns as well as consistency of Kovatz indices regarding previous findings of our research group (Akhlaghi *et al.*, 2009; Mohammadhosseini *et al.*, 2008; Mohammadhosseini *et al.*, 2011; Akhlaghi *et al.*, 2012; Mohammadhosseini *et al.*, 2010). Relative percentages of the components were calculated from peak areas using a Shimadzu C-R4A chromatopac on the DB-5 column, without the use of a correction factor.

3. Results and discussion

3.1. Chemical profiles by the HD, SFME, MAHD and HS-SPME approaches

Although the chemical profiles of the hydrodistilled oils of *N. racemosa* have been reported previously, this study produced rather new profiles. Moreover, quantitative and qualitative analyses of the essential oils and volatile fractions from the aerial parts of *N. racemosa*, using the described methods, have resulted in recognition of several monoterpene hydrocarbons (MH), oxygenated monoterpenes (OM), sesquiterpene hydrocarbons (SH), oxygenated sesquiterpenes (OM) and non-terpene hydrocarbons (NH).

Table 1. Chemical composition of the essential oils from the aerial parts of *N. racemosa* obtained by using HD, SFME and MAHD approaches as well as the volatile constituents by HS-SPME method [a]

NO.	Compound	Class	RI [b]	HD (%)	HS-SPME (%)	SFME (%)	MAHD (%)
1	2-Hexenal	NH [c]	855	0.2	0.5	1.2	0.8
2	α-Thujene	MH [d]	930	0.1	-	1.7	1.5
3	α-Pinene	MH	939	**10.2**	**7.4**	**6.0**	**18.9**
4	Camphene	MH	954	2.0	0.7	1.1	**12.3**
5	β-Pinene	MH	979	3.1	3.3	2.8	**8.5**
6	α-Phellandrene	MH	1003	1.1	0.2	0.8	0.7
7	α-Terpinene	MH	1017	0.4	5.5	1.2	0.4
8	*p*-Cymene	MH	1025	0.5	0.2	-	-
9	Limonene	MH	1029	0.2	0.1	-	-
10	(*Z*)-β-Ocimene	MH	1037	**10.4**	**12.8**	**6.5**	**9.2**
11	Camphor	OM [e]	1146	-	-	-	0.5
12	α-Terpineol	OM	1189	2.0	0.9	2.1	1.7
13	Piperitone	NH	1221	1.8	1.2	0.4	0.9
14	Bornyl acetate	OM	1289	0.3	0.1	-	0.1
15	4aα,7α,7aα-Nepetalactone	OM	1317	**28.1**	**18.0**	**25.7**	**7.6**
16	4aα,7α,7aβ-Nepetalactone	OM	1325	**7.4**	**4.6**	**16.1**	**20.3**
17	4aβ,7α,7aβ-Nepetalactone	OM	1357	**20.5**	**32.4**	**25.4**	**4.3**
18	α-Copaene	SH [f]	1377	0.2	0.5	0.1	0.3
19	β-Bourbonene	SH	1388	0.1	0.2	0.2	0.3
20	β-Caryophyllene	SH	1419	3.5	1.8	1.5	3.3
21	*trans*-β-Farnesene	SH	1457	0.5	0.5	0.4	0.6
22	*allo*-Aromadendrene	SH	1460	-	0.2	0.1	-
23	β-Selinene	SH	1490	-	0.2	-	-
24	α-Muurolene	SH	1500	1.4	0.3	0.5	-
25	β-Bisabolene	SH	1506	-	-	0.7	0.8
26	γ-Cadinene	SH	1514	0.5	0.4	0.4	0.4
27	δ-Cadinene	SH	1523	0.4	0.4	0.7	0.4
28	Spathulenol	OS [g]	1578	2.6	4.0	1.8	1.8
29	α-Cadinol	OS	1640	-	-	-	-
30	α-Bisabolol	OS	1685	0.2	0.2	0.3	0.8
	Total percentage			**98.1**	**96.6**	**97.7**	**96.4**
	MH (%)			28.0	30.2	20.1	**51.5**
	OM (%)			58.3	56.0	**69.3**	34.5
	SH (%)			**9.2**	4.5	4.6	6.1
	OS (%)			0.2	**4.2**	2.1	2.6
	NH (%)			**2.4**	1.7	1.6	1.7
	NIC [h]			**25**	**26**	**24**	**24**

[a] The compounds have been sorted according to their retention indices on an HP-5 MS capillary column.
[b] Kovatz retention indices given in the literature
[c] Nonterpene hydrocarbons
[d] Monoterpene hydrocarbons
[e] Oxygenated monoterpene
[f] Sesquiterpene hydrocarbons
[g] Oxygenated sesquiterpene;
[h] Number of the identified compounds

Specifically, the major components in the hydrodistilled oil of the *N. racemosa* aerial parts were found to be 4aα,7α,7aα-nepetalactone (28.1%),4aβ,7α,7aβ-nepetalactone (20.5%), (*Z*)-β-ocimene (10.4%), α-pinene (10.2%) and 4aα,7α,7aβ-nepetalactone (7.4%). The percentage yields of essential oils, in terms of the weight of the collected oil per gram of dried plant, were 0.17%, 0.16%, 0.13% and 0.14% (w/w) for four replicate distillations.

Using HS-SPME (Table 1), we were able to identify 26 volatile compounds, 4aβ,7α,7aβ-nepetalactone (32.4%), 4aα,7α,7aα-nepetalactone (18.0%), (*Z*)-β-ocimene (12.8%), α-pinene (7.4%) and 4aα,7α,7aβ-nepetalactone (4.6%). In terms of general categories, eight were monoterpene hydrocarbons (30.2%), five, oxygenated monoterpenes (56.0%), nine, sesquiterpene hydrocarbons (4.5%), two, oxygenated sesquiterpenes (4.2%) and two, non-terpene hydrocarbons (1.7%).

The SFME method allowed for the identification of 24 components in the isolated oil (see Table 1), of which seven were monoterpenes (20.1%), four, oxygenated monoterpenes (69.3%), nine, sesquiterpene hydrocarbons (4.6%), two, oxygenated sesquiterpenes (2.1%) and two, non-terpene hydrocarbon (1.6%). The main components included 4aα,7α,7aα-nepetalactone (25.7%), 4aβ,7α,7aβ-nepetalactone (25.4%),4aα,7α,7aβ-nepetalactone (16.1%) (*Z*)-β-ocimene (6.5%) and α-pinene (6.0%). The yields of four experiments done using this method were 0.21%, 0.20%, 0.18% and 0.30% (w/w).

Finally, 24 components were identified in the aerial parts oils using the MAHD method (Table 1).

The major components 4aα,7α,7aβ-nepetalactone (20.3%), α-pinene (18.9%), camphene (12.3%), (*Z*)-β-ocimene (9.2%) β-pinene (8.5%) and 4aα,7α,7aα-nepetalactone (7.6%), 4aβ,7α,7aβ-nepetalactone (4.3%), (See Table 1).

The names, retention indices and percentages of the constituents obtained from the aerial parts of *N. racemosa* by the aforementioned methods have been listed in Table 1. As can be seen, there are negligible differences in numerical values of Kovats retention indices between the calculated ones and those cited in the literature. Furthermore, a total of 30 components were identified, accounting for 96.4-98.1% of the components, depending on the profile.

Using the HD method (Table 1), 25 components could be identified in the oil from the aerial parts: Nine monoterpene hydrocarbons (28.0%), five oxygenated monoterpenes (58.3%), eight sesquiterpene hydrocarbons (9.2%), one oxygenated sesquiterpene (0.2%) and two non-terpene hydrocabons (2.4%).

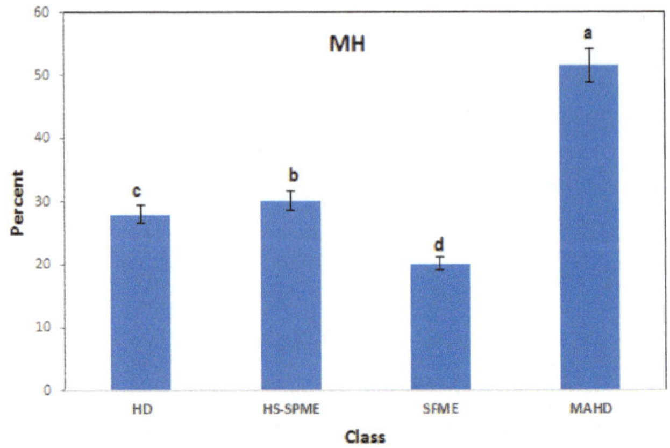

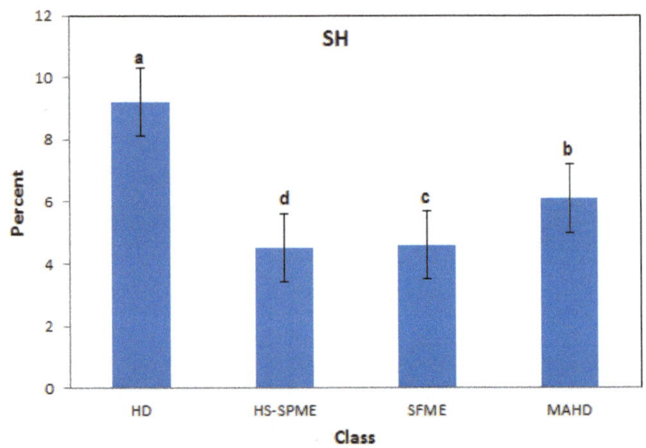

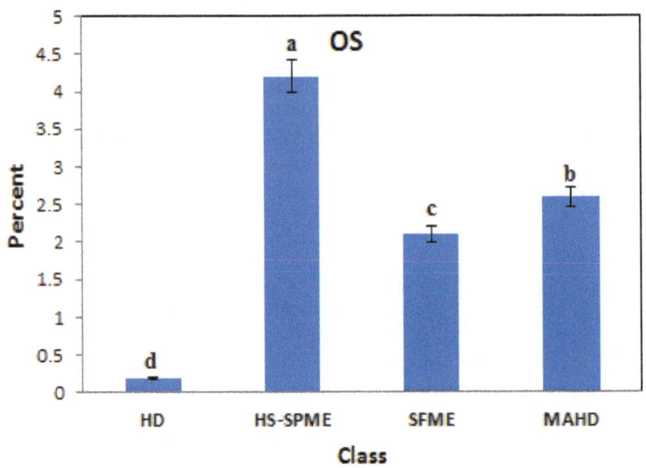

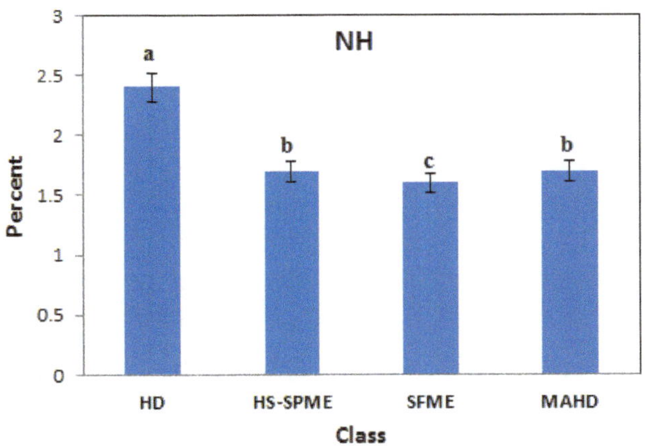

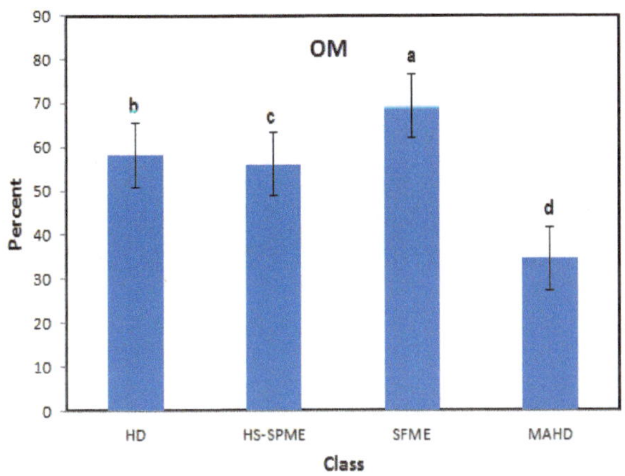

Fig 2. Comparative plots of different types of constituting class of the essential oils and volatiles from the aerial parts of *Nepeta racemosa* (As shown there are significant differences between the groups with the exception of relative percentage of non-terpene hydrocarbons in the HS-SPME and MAHD profiles regarding one-way ANOVA analysis; MH= Monoterpene hydrocarbons; OM= Oxygenated monoterpenes; SH= Sesquiterpene hydrocarbons; OS= Oxygenated sesquiterpenes; NH= Non-terpene hydrocarbons).

In terms of general categories, seven components were monoterpenes (51.5%), six, oxygenated monoterpenes (34.5%), seven, sesquiterpene hydrocarbons (6.1%), two, oxygenated sesquiterpenes (2.6%) and two, non-terpene hydrocarbons (1.7%). In addition, for three replicate extractions the yields were found to be 0.22%, 0.24% and 0.19% (w/w), respectively.

In Figure 2, the relative percentages of the various classes of the oils and volatile fractions constituting compounds are compared. From this figure, it is immediately evident that in the three the profiles (HD, HS-SPME and SFME), oxygenated monoterpenes constituted the main components, while the largest class being monoterpene hydrocarbons in that obtained using the MAHD approach.

3.2. Chemical composition of the Nepeta oils in similar reports

In the literature there are some reports concerning the constituents of the essential oils from a variety of the *Nepeta* genus plants in different parts of the world. In a related study, Ali *et al.* (2016) reported the water-distilled essential oils from the aerial parts of four ornamental species and hybrids of *Nepeta*: *N. racemosa* Lam. hybrid, Select., *N. sibirica* L., *N. subsessilis* Maxim, and *N. xfaassenii* Bergmans ex Stearn, 'Dropmore . In this report, *N. racemosa* hybrid, Select. and *N. xfaassenii*, Dropmore essential oils were rich in 1,8-cineole whereas *N. sibirica* and *N. subsessilis* essential oils mainly consisted of sesquiterpenes including (*Z*)-β-farnesene, β-bisabolene, δ-cadinene or β-caryophyllene, and caryophyllene oxide.

On the other hand, Baser *et al.* (2000) have reported a comprehensive report concerning the essential oils from 22 *Nepeta* species growing in Turkey. Accordingly, gas chromatography-mass spectrometric analyses of the essential oils revealed that four *Nepeta* species contain 4aα,7α,7aα-nepetalactone as the major constituent component. 4aα,7α,7aβ, Nepetalactone was the main constituent in *N. racemosa*. In addition, seven *Nepeta* species contained caryophyllene oxide as the main constituent in their essential oils. 1,8-Cineole/linalool were the major components in the essential oils of six species, as well. On the other hand, β-pinene, α-terpineol, germacrene-D and spathulenol were the main constituents in the essential oils from *N. phyllochlamys*, *N. viscida*, *N. sorgerae* and *N. trachonitica*, respectively.

In the work of Dabiri and Sefidkon (2003) on chemical composition of the essential oil of *N. racemosa* Lam. prepared by hydrodistillation, twenty-four components were identified constituting approximately 99.3% of the oil with major constituents being 4aβ,7α,7aβ-nepetalactone (33.6%), 4aα,7α,7aβ-nepetalactone (25.6%), 4aα,7α,7aα-nepetalactone (24.4%) and 1,8-cineole (9.0%) in the volatile essential oil. Kobaisy and coworkers (2005) have evaluated composition and phytotoxic activity of *N. pannonica* L. essential oil from Kazakhstan region. This study led to the characterization of sixty components from *N.*

pannonica with 1,8-cineole (28.9%), and 4α,7β,7aα-nepetalactone (14.3%) as the major constituents. Rustaiyan *et al.* (2000) have characterized chemical composition of the essential oil of *N. racemosa* Lam. from Iran in 2000. In this attempt, the main constituents of the oil were found to be 4aα,7α,7aα-nepetalactone (64.9%), (*Z*)-β-ocimene (9.5%), (*E*)-nerolidol (8.8%) and 4aα,7α,7aβ-nepetalactone (7.4%).

In the work of Safaei-Ghomi *et al.* (2006) on water distilled essential oil composition from the aerial parts of *N. gloeocephala* Rech. f. from Iran, 1,8-cineole (35.2%), β-pinene (21.8%), sabinene (7.8%), (*E*)-β-ocimene (7.1%), α-pinene (7.1%) and (*Z*)-β-ocimene (6.9%) were the major components of the oil. In another report of Safaei-Ghomi *et al.* (2009) dealing with the volatile constituents analysis of *N. cataria* from Central Iran, among the constituents of the volatile oil, 4aα,7α,7aα-nepetalactone (87.1%), 4aα,7α,7aβ-nepetalactone (3.1%), β-caryophyllene (2.5%), and β-pinene (1.7%) were the major ones while the other constituents were present in relatively small amounts representing only (3.6%) of the total oil. In the study of Shafaghat *et al.* (2008) on chemical composition of the essential oil isolated from flower, leaf, stem and root of *N. sintenisii* Bornm. growing in Khalkhal, North-West Iran: Fourteen compounds representing 98.7% of the flower oil were identified; among them 4aβ,7α,7aβ-nepetalactone (60.3%), germacrene D (12.7%) and 1,8-cineole (8.2%) were the major ones; twenty constituents accounting for 95.7% of the leaf oil were identified of which 4aβ,7α,7aβ-nepetalactone (34.6%), germacrene D (14.1%), 1,8-cineole (7.9%), α-cadinol (6.8%) and δ-cadinene (5.8%) were the main components. In this work, the stem oil of *N. sintenisii* was characterized by higher amount of 4aβ,7α,7aβ-nepetalactone (64.2%), α-cadinol (8.9%), α-pinene (6.7%), 4aα,7aα,7aβ-nepetalactone (5.2%) and 1,8-cineole (3.6%), among the eight components comprising 96.3% of the total oil detected. In addition, twelve compounds were characterized in the root oil representing 98.6% of the total profile with 4aβ,7α,7aβ-nepetalactone (61.2%), germacrene D (12.0%), 4aα,7aα,7aβ-nepetalactone (8.5%), 1,8-cineole (5.7%) and β-caryophyllene (4.5%) as the main constituents. In terms of general categories, the oil of flower, stem and root consisted mainly of monoterpenes, but monoterpenes and sesquiterpenes of leaf oil were approximately in equal amounts (48.2% and 47.5% respectively).

Sonboli *et al.* (2009) have also studied the antibacterial activity and composition of the essential oil of *N. menthoides* (Iran) leading to identification of twenty-nine compounds representing 97.6% of the total oil implying high frequency of oxygenated monoterpenes with 1,8-cineole (33.8%) and 4aα-7α-7aα-nepetalactone (23.2%) as the most abundant constituents. In a complimentary report of this research group, focusing on the essential oil composition of *N. involucrate*, forty-eight components were identified in the oil, accounting for 97.2% of the total oil including 1,8-cineole (23.1%), β-pinene (12.2%), sabinene (6.7%) and α-pinene (4.9%), germacrene-D (15.1%) and spathulenol (2.3%) (Sonboli *et al.*, 2005). Moreover, they have assessed antimicrobial activity and chemical composition of the essential oil of *N. crispa* Willd. in Iran consisting of twenty-three compounds and accounting for 99.8% of the total profile with the main constituents being 1,8-cineole (47.9%) and 4aα,7α,7αβ-nepetalactone (20.3%) (Sonboli *et al.*, 2004).

4. Conclusion

The main objective of this investigation was to evaluate the inherent capabilities of four different extraction techniques, namely, hydrodistillation (HD), solvent-free microwave extraction (SFME), microwave assisted hydrodistillation (MAHD) and headspace solid-phase micro-extraction (HS-SPME) in effective separation and trapping of the essential oils and volatile fractions from the aerial parts of *N. racemosa* in combination with the GC and GC-MS analyses. 25, 26, 24 and 24 components representing 98.1%, 96.6%, 97.7% and 96.4% of the total oil compositions and volatiles were recognized by using the HD, HS-SPME, SFME and MAHD methods, respectively. In most of the samples obtained by the aforementioned methods, oxygenated monoterpenes were found to be the dominant groups of constituents. On the other hand, the largest amounts of monoterpene hydrocarbons (51.5%), oxygenated monoterpenes (69.3%), sesquiterpene hydrocarbons (9.2%), oxygenated sesquiterpenes (4.2%) and non-terpene hydrocarbons (2.4%) were respectively observed in the MAHD, SFME, HD, HS-SPME and HD profiles. Among the whole identified compounds, 4aα,7α,7aα-nepetalactone was the major component of the chemical profiles of the HD, HS-SPME and SFME methods, while 4aα,7α,7aβ-nepetalactone was the dominant natural compound in the profile of the MAHD method

As a concluding remark, compared with the HD approach, green and environmentally friendly techniques based upon microwave beams (MAHD and SFME) permit prominent superiorities containing lower wastewater, energy and cost, and greater potential capability to separate volatile essential oils. However, the HS-SPME approach is the simplest method to use by far to trap the volatile fractions of the plant materials. The time required to obtain volatiles from a single specimen is shorter than the other methods. Moreover, it can be used to trap volatile fractions from several plant specimens simultaneously, which requires fewer samples.

5. Acknowledgements

Financial and technical support from the Office for Research Affairs of the Islamic Azad University, Shahrood Branch and Islamic Azad University is gratefully acknowledged.

6. References

Abad, M.J., Guerra, J.A., Bermejo, P., Irurzun, A., and Carrasco, L. 2000. Search for antiviral activity in higher plant extracts. *Phytotherapy Research*. 14: 604-607.

Adams, R.P. 2007. Identification of Essential Oil Components by Gas Chromatography/Mass Spectrometry. Allured Publishing Co., Carol Stream, IL., USA

Adiguzel, A., Ozer, H., Sokmen, M., Gulluce, M., Sokmen, A., Kilic, H., Sahin, F., and Baris, O. 2009. Antimicrobial and antioxidant activity of the essential oil and methanol extract of *Nepeta cataria*. *Polish Journal of Microbiology*. 58: 69-76.

Akhlaghi, H., Nekoei, M., Mohammadhosseini, M., and Motavalizadehkakhky, A. 2012. Chemical composition of the volatile oils from the flowers, stems and leaves of *Prangos latiloba* Korov. using the head space solid phase microextraction method prior to analysis by gas chromatography-mass spectrometry. *Journal of Essential Oil Bearing Plants*. 15: 328-335.

Akhlaghi, H., Shafaghat, A., and Mohammadhosseini, M. 2009. Chemical composition of the essential oil from leaves of *Biebersteinia multifida* DC. growing wild in Iran. *Journal of Essential Oil Bearing Plants*. 12: 365-368.

Ali, A., Tabanca, N., Demirci, B., Blythe, E.K., Baser, K.H.C., and Khan, I.A. 2016. Chemical composition and biological activity of essential oils from four *Nepeta* species and hybrids against *Aedes aegypti* (L.) (*Diptera*: *Culicidae*). *Records of Natural Products*. 10: 137-147.

Ali, T., Javan, M., Sonboli, A., and Semnanian, S. 2012a. Antinociceptive and anti-inflammatory activities of the essential oil of *Nepeta crispa* Willd. in experimental rat models. *Natural Product Research*. 26: 1529-1534.

Ali, T., Javan, M., Sonboli, A., and Semnanian, S. 2012b. Evaluation of the antinociceptive and anti-inflammatory effects of essential oil of *Nepeta pogonosperma* Jamzad et Assadi in rats. *Daru-Journal of Pharmaceutical Sciences*. 20.

Aloqail, M., Al-Sheddi, E., Siddiqui, M.A., Musarrat, J., Al-Khedhaity, A., and Farshori, N. 2014. Anticancer activity of sub-fractions of chloroform extracts of *Nepeta deflersianaon* on human breast and lung cancer cells: An *in vitro* cytotoxicity assessment. *Planta Medica*. 80: 1546-1546.

Arthur, C.L., and Pawliszyn, J. 1990. Solid-phase microextraction with thermal desorption using fused-silica optical fibers. *Analytical Chemistry*. 62: 2145-2148.

Asgarpanah, J., Sarabian, S., and Ziarati, P. 2014. Essential oil of *Nepeta* genus (Lamiaceae) from Iran: A review. *Journal of Essential Oil Research*. 26: 1-12.

Baser, K.H.C., Kirimer, N., Kurkcuoglu, M., and Demirci, B. 2000. Essential oils of *Nepeta* species growing in Turkey. *Chemistry of Natural Compounds*. 36: 356-359.

Bessada, S.M., Barreira, J.C., and Oliveira, M.B.P. 2015. Asteraceae species with most prominent bioactivity and their potential applications: A review. *Industrial Crops and Products*. 76: 604-615.

Bhat, J.U., Parray, S.A., Aslam, M., Ansari, S., Nizami, Q., Khanam, R., Siddiqui, A., and Ahmad, M.A. 2012. Anti-seizure activity of flower extracts of

Nepeta bractaeta in swiss albino mice. *EXCLI Journal*. 11: 531-537.

Calmasur, O., Aslan, I., and Sahin, F. 2006. Insecticidal and acaricidal effect of three Lamiaceae plant essential oils against *Tetranychus urticae* Koch and *Bemisia tabaci* Genn. *Industrial Crops and Products*. 23: 140-146.

Dabiri, M., and Sefidkon, F. 2003. Chemical composition of the essential oil of *Nepeta racemosa* Lam. from Iran. *Flavour and Fragrance Journal*. 18: 157-158.

Dua, V.K., Verma, G., Agarwal, D.D., Kaiser, M., and Brun, R. 2011. Antiprotozoal activities of traditional medicinal plants from the Garhwal region of North West Himalaya, India. *Journal of Ethnopharmacology*. 136: 123-128.

Formisano, C., Rigano, D., and Senatore, F. 2011. Chemical constituents and biological activities of *Nepeta* species. *Chemistry & Biodiversity*. 8: 1783-1818.

Galati, E.M., Miceli, N., Galluzzo, M., Taviano, M.F., and Tzakou, O. 2004. Neuropharmacological effects of epinepetalactone from *Nepeta sibthorpii* behavioral and anticonvulsant activity. *Pharmaceutical Biology*. 42: 391-395.

Hashemi-Moghaddam, H., Mohammadhosseini, M., and Basiri, M. 2015. Optimization of microwave assisted hydrodistillation on chemical compositions of the essential oils from the aerial parts of *Thymus pubescens* and comparison with conventional hydrodistllation. *Journal of Essential Oil Bearing Plants*. 18: 884-893.

Hashemi-Moghaddam, H., Mohammadhosseini, M., and Salar, M. 2014. Chemical composition of the essential oils from the hulls of *Pistacia vera* L. by using magnetic nanoparticle-assisted microwave (MW) distillation: Comparison with routine MW and conventional hydrodistillation. *Analytical Methods*. 6: 2572-2579.

Hussain, J., Khan, F.-u., Gilani, S.A., Abbas, G., Ahmed, S., Khan, A.-u., Ullah, W., and Choudhary, M.I. 2010. Antiglycation, antiplatelets aggregation, cytotoxic and phytotoxic activities of *Nepeta suavis*. *Latin American Journal of Pharmacy*. 29: 573-578.

Hussain, J., Rehman, N.U., Al-Harrasi, A., Khan, A.L., Rizvi, T.S., Mohammad, F.V., Mehjabeen, and Ali, L. 2015. *In vivo* evaluation of analgesic, anti-inflammatory, and neuropharmacological activities of the chemical constituent from *Nepeta clarkei*. *Archives of Pharmacal Research*. 38: 1188-1194.

Iscan, G., Kose, Y.B., Demirci, B., and Baser, K.H.C. 2011. Anticandidal activity of the essential oil of *Nepeta transcaucasica* Grossh. *Chemistry & Biodiversity*. 8: 2144-2148.

Jamzad, Z., Grayer, R.J., Kite, G.C., Simmonds, M.S., Ingrouille, M., and Jalili, A. 2003. Leaf surface flavonoids in Iranian species of *Nepeta* (Lamiaceae) and some related genera. *Biochemical Systematics and Ecology*. 31: 587-600.

Kobaisy, M., Tellez, M.R., Dayan, F.E., Mamonov, L.K., Mukanova, G.S., Sitpaeva, G.T., and Gemejieva, N.G. 2005. Composition and phytotoxic activity of *Nepeta pannonica* L. essential oil. *Journal of Essential Oil Research*. 17: 704-707.

Mohammadhosseini, M. 2015a. Chemical composition of the essential oils and volatile fractions from flowers, stems and roots of *Salvia multicaulis* Vahl. by using MAHD, SFME and HS-SPME methods. *Journal of Essential Oil Bearing Plants*. 18: 1360-1371.

Mohammadhosseini, M. 2015b. Chemical composition of the volatile fractions from flowers, leaves and stems of *Salvia mirzayanii* by HS-SPME-GC-MS. *Journal of Essential Oil Bearing Plants*. 18: 464-476.

Mohammadhosseini, M. 2016. A Comprehensive Review on New Methods for Processing, Separation and Identification of the Essential Oils. Islamic Azad University of Shahrood Press, Shahrood, Iran

Mohammadhosseini, M., Akbarzadeh, A., Hashemi-Moghaddam, H., Mohammadi Nafchi, A., Mashayekhi, H.A., and Aryanpour, A. 2016a. Chemical composition of the essential oils from the aerial parts of *Artemisia sieberi* by using conventional hydrodistillation and microwave assisted hydrodistillation: A comparative study. *Journal of Essential Oil Bearing Plants*. 19: 32-45.

Mohammadhosseini, M., Akbarzadeh, A., Hashemi-Moghaddam, H., Shahnama, M., Fahimi, B., and Azami, S. 2016b. Gas chromatographic-mass spectrometric analysis of volatiles obtained by HS-SPME-GC-MS technique from aerial parts of *Ziziphora capitata* L., and evaluation for biological activity. *Oriental Journal of Chemistry*. 32: 1439-1451.

Mohammadhosseini, M., Akbarzadeh, A., Shafaghat, A., Hashemi-Moghaddam, H., Mohammadi Nafchi, A., and Ashouri, H. 2016c. Chemical composition of the essential oils from flowers and leaves of *Marsdenia erecta* using microwave assisted hydrodistillation technique. *Journal of Essential Oil Bearing Plants*: In press.

Mohammadhosseini, M., and Beiranvand, M. 2013. Chemical composition of the essential oil from the aerial parts of *Satureja hortensis* as a potent medical plant using traditional hydrodistillation. *Journal of Chemical Health Risks*. 3: 49-60.

Mohammadhosseini, M., Mahdavi, B., and Akhlaghi, H. 2013. Characterization and chemical composition of the volatile oils from aerial parts of *Eryngium bungei* Bioss. (Apiaceae) by using traditional hydrodistillation, microwave assisted hydrodistillation and head space solid phase microextraction methods prior to GC and GC/MS analyses: A comparative approach. *Journal of Essential Oil Bearing Plants*. 16: 613-623.

Mohammadhosseini, M., Mahdavi, B., and Shahnama, M. 2015. Chemical composition of essential oils from aerial parts of *Ferula gummosa* (Apiaceae) in Jajarm Region, Iran using traditional hydrodistillation and solvent-free microwave extraction methods: A comparative approach. *Journal of Essential Oil Bearing Plants*. 18: 1321-1328.

Mohammadhosseini, M., and Nekoei, M. 2014. Chemical compositions of the essential oils and volatile compounds from the aerial parts of *Ferula ovina* using hydrodistillation, MAHD, SFME and HS-SPME methods. *Journal of Essential Oil Bearing Plants*. 17: 747-757.

Mohammadhosseini, M., Pazoki, A., and Akhlaghi, H. 2008. Chemical composition of the essential oils from flowers, stems, and roots of *Salvia multicaulis* growing wild in Iran. *Chemistry of Natural Compounds*. 44: 127-128.

Mohammadhosseini, M., Pazoki, A., Zamani, H.A., Akhlaghi, H., and Nekoei, M. 2010. Chemical composition of the essential oil from aerial parts of *Senicio gallicus* Chaix growing wild in Iran. *Journal of Essential Oil Bearing Plants*. 13: 704-709.

Mohammadhosseini, M., Zamani, H.A., Akhlaghi, H., and Nekoei, M. 2011. Hydrodistilled volatile oil constituents of the aerial parts of *Prangos serpentinica* (Rech.f., Aell. Esfand.) Hernnstadt and Heyn from Iran and quantitative structure-retention relationship simulation. *Journal of Essential Oil Bearing Plants*. 14: 559-573.

Mozaffarian, V. 1996. A Dictionary of Iranian Plant Names. Farhang Moaser Press, Iran

Nekoei, M., and Mohammadhosseini, M. 2014. Application of HS-SPME, SDME and cold-press coupled to GC/MS to analysis the essential oils of *Citrus sinensis* CV. Thomson Navel and QSRR study for prediction of retention indices by stepwise and genetic algorithm-multiple linear regression approaches. *Analytical Chemistry Letters*. 4: 93-103.

Nekoei, M., and Mohammadhosseini, M. 2016a. Chemical composition of essential oils of *Salvia leriifolia* by three different extraction methods prior to gas chromatographic-mass spectrometric determination: Comparison of HD with SFME and HS-SPME. *Journal of Essential Oil Bearing Plants*. 19: In press.

Nekoei, M., and Mohammadhosseini, M. 2016b. Chemical compositions of the essential oils from the aerial parts of *Achillea wilhelmsii* using traditional hydrodistillation, microwave assisted hydrodistillation and solvent-free microwave extraction methods: Comparison with the volatile compounds obtained by headspace solid-phase microextraction. *Journal of Essential Oil Bearing Plants*. 19: 59-75.

Pawliszyn, J. 1999. Applications of Solid Phase Microextraction. (Ed.) RSC, Cambridge, UK,

Pawliszyn, J. 2003. Sample preparation: Quo Vadis? *Analytical Chemistry*. 75: 2543-2558.

Rustaiyan, A., Khosravi, M., Larijany, K., and Masoudi, S. 2000. Compostion of the essential oil of *Nepeta racemosa* Lam. from Iran. *Journal of Essential Oil Research*. 12: 151-152.

Safaei-Ghomi, J., Bamoniri, A., Haghani, M., and Batooli, H. 2006. Essential oil composition of *Nepeta gloeocephala* Rech. f. from Iran. *Journal of Essential Oil Research*. 18: 635-637.

Safaei-Ghomi, J., Djafari-Bidgoli, Z., and Batooli, H. 2009. Volatile constituents analysis of *Nepeta cataria* from Central Iran. *Chemistry of Natural Compounds*. 45: 913-915.

Setkova, L., Risticevic, S., and Pawliszyn, J. 2007. Rapid headspace solid-phase microextraction-gas chromatographic-time-of-flight mass spectrometric method for qualitative profiling of ice wine volatile fraction - I. Method development and optimization. *Journal of Chromatography A*. 1147: 213-223.

Shafaghat, A., Salimi, F., and Akhlaghi, H. 2008. Chemical composition of the essential oil isolated from flower, leaf, stem and root of *Nepeta sintenisii* Bornm. from Iran. *Journal of Essential Oil Bearing Plants*. 11: 391-396.

Sharma, S.K., and Goyal, N. 2011. Biological studies of the plants from genus *Pluchea*. *Annals of Biological Research*. 2: 25-34.

Sonboli, A., Gholipour, A., Yousefzadi, M., and Mojarrad, M. 2009. Antibacterial activity and composition of the essential oil of *Nepeta menthoides* from Iran. *Natural Product Communications*. 4: 283-286.

Sonboli, A., Salehi, P., and Allahyari, L. 2005. Essential oil composition of *Nepeta involucrata* from Iran. *Chemistry of Natural Compounds*. 41: 683-685.

Sonboli, A., Salehi, P., and Yousefzadi, M. 2004. Antimicrobial activity and chemical composition of the essential oil of *Nepeta crispa* Willd. from Iran. *Zeitschrift Fur Naturforschung C-A Journal of Biosciences*. 59: 653-656.

Vuckovic, D., Zhang, X., Cudjoe, E., and Pawliszyn, J. 2010. Solid-phase microextraction in bioanalysis: New devices and directions. *Journal of Chromatography A*. 1217: 4041-4060.

Wu, Q.-X., Shi, Y.-P., and Jia, Z.-J. 2006. Eudesmane sesquiterpenoids from the Asteraceae family. *Natural Product Reports*. 23: 699-734.

Zargari, A. 1989. Medicinal Plants. University of Tehran Press, Tehran (In Persian).

18

Phytochemical investigation of the essential oils from the leaf and stem of *Dorema ammoniacum* D. Don. (Apiaceae) in Central Zagros, Iran

Fakhteh Zandpour[1], Mohammad Reza Vahabi[1*], Ali Reza Allafchian[2], Hamid Reza Farhang[3]

[1]*Department of Natural Resources, Isfahan University of Technology, Isfahan 84156–83111, Iran;*
***Email:** Vahabi@cc.iut.ac.ir*

[2]*Research Institute for Nanotechnology and Advanced Materials, Isfahan University of Technology, Isfahan 84156–83111, Iran;*

[3]*MSc of Range Management, Isfahan University of Technology, Isfahan 84156–83111, Iran;*

ARTICLE INFO

***Topic:** Medicinal Plants*

Key words:
- ✓ *Dorema ammoniacum D. Don.*
- ✓ *Essential oil*
- ✓ *GC/MS*
- ✓ *Isfahan province*
- ✓ *Iran*

ABSTRACT

Background & Aim: *Dorema ammoniacum* D. Don. (ammoniac plant) belongs to Apiaceae family and *Dorema* genus. It is one of the most important endemic medicinal plants in its family which grows in the arid and semi-arid areas in the regions of Iran and some of the Asian countries such as Turkmenistan, Afghanistan, Pakistan and India. This study was carried out with aim of the extraction and identification of constituents of *D. ammoniacum* D. Don. in the western areas of Isfahan province, Iran.
Experimental: For this purpose, after the plant collecting in the mentioned area its target organs namely stem and leaf were separated, air dried, milled and weighted in the certain amount. Then the essential oil of the plant was isolated by hydrodistillation method and analyzed by GC/MS device.
Results: The results indicated that major components were Limonene (49.18%), Neophytadiene (10.21%), beta Caryophyllene (3.54%), Phytol (2.61%) and Neryl acetone (1.46%).
Recommended applications/industries: Several therapeutic cases have been reported in traditional medicine and currently in contemporary medicine for *Dorema ammoniacum* D. Don. that some of them are include the treatment of cough, vasodilator, anti-flatulence and anti-microbial. Also, the mentioned plant has varied applications in the fields of foods, cosmetic and detergent industries.

1. Introduction

Essential oils have been used for thousands of years in various cultures for medicinal and health purposes. They have a widespread range of application from aromatherapy, household cleaning products, personal beauty care and natural medicine treatments (Worwood, 1991; Farhang *et al.*, 2015). The Apiaceae family has been distributed with 300 genera and 3000 plant species in the world approximately. The genus *Dorema* D. Don (Apiaceae) is represented in the flora of Iran by seven species, among which both *D. ammoniacum* D. Don. and *D. aucheri* Boiss. are endemic (Mozaffarian, 1996). *Dorema ammoniacum* D. Don. (ammoniac plant) is a perennial monocarpic plant grows to height about 1–3 m and in spring and early summer contains a milky juice. It is one of the most important endemic medicinal plants in its family which grows in the arid and semi-arid areas in the regions of Iran and some of the Asian countries such as Turkmenistan, Afghanistan, Pakistan and India (Rechinger, 1980). The mentioned species in the Iranian traditional medicinal has numerous names. Some of the most prevalent names include ushaq, vasha, kandal, koma-kandal and also as Persian ammuniacum in Greek and medicinal literatures (Amin, 1991; Mozaffarian, 1996; Rechinger, 1980; Howes, 1950). *Dorema ammoniacum* D. Don. produces a medicinal gum resin, commonly known as ammoniacum gum, which can be found in the holes of stems, roots, and petioles (Langenheim, 2003). Overall, the plants extract constituents and their secondary metabolisms are provided use to efficacious on human and animal health that can be used to cure maladies (Evans, 1996). The gum resin of *Dorema ammoniacum* D. Don. in the Iranian traditional medicine has been considered beneficial in treatment of spastic pains, gastric disorders, intestinal parasitic infections and skin inflammations and as analgesic, stimulant, expectorant and laxative (Amin, 1991; Parsa, 1959; Zarshenas *et al.*, 2013). In addition the existence resin in the stem of *Dorema ammoniacum* D. Don. are used as antimicrobial, vasodilator, a carminative, diaphoretic, mildly diuretic, expectorant and poultice (Irvani *et al.*, 2010). *Dorema ammoniacum* D. Don. in the British pharmacopeia as the plant with various therapeutic properties has been recognized that some of the most important of them are as follow: antispasmodic, sputum containing horny sputum, cough irritant, sudorific, the regulation of menstrual, reducer of blood fats, prevention of diabetes, hepatoprotective mechanism, sexual stimulus and sedative (British herbal pharmacopoeia, 1983; British pharmacopoeia, 1993). Several studies have been conducted in relation to identification of chemical compounds of the gum and volatile oil of different parts of *Dorema ammoniacum* D. Don. in some mentioned countries (Yassa *et al.*, 2014; Yousefzadi *et al.*, 2011a; Yousefzadi *et al.*, 2011b; Sajjadi *et al.*, 2007; Appendino *et al.*, 1991; and Arnone *et al.*, 1991). In all these studies miscellaneous chemical compositions were identified and the amount of the yields of essential oils was varied. The mentioned plant species in France are utilized in the factories producing of glues and cosmetic industry. Moreover, this plant has other varied uses such as food industry, confectionary products, paint industry, manufacturing, and production of the detergents and especially in production of special glues for jewelry (Bown, 1995; Grieve, 1971; Chevallier, 2001). Plants, with their wide variety of chemical constituents, offer a promising source of new antimicrobial agents with general as well as specific antimicrobial activity (Evans, 1996). In the previous studies the antimicrobial activity of the extract of *Dorema ammoniacum* D. Don. had been reported (Rajani, 2002). The purpose of the current study was to identify all chemical compositions of the essential oil of *Dorema ammoniacum* D. Don. in the western areas of Isfahan province which is situated in the section of the Central Zagros area, Iran; for the first time.

2. Materials and Methods

2.1. Plant materials

Dorema ammoniacum D. Don. (Apiaceae) is perennial endemic native herb plant that grows as high as three meters (around one to three meters) in Iran, between the months of March and June. Samples of *Dorema ammoniacum* D. Don. aerial parts consisted of the leaves and stems collected in the middle of March 2015 (in its natural habitat situated in the Bardasiab zone of the Fereydun Shahr county which is part of Central Zagros area, Iran), during the flowering period. The taxonomic identity of the plant was confirmed by comparing the collected voucher specimen with that of the known identity available in the herbarium of the Department of Natural Resources, Isfahan University of Technology (IUT), Iran **(Fig. 1)**.

2.2. Experimental procedure

At first, 1000g of the aerial parts of plant specifically stems and leaves were dried in the standard position so that they were protected from light, humidity and infection; also, the samples of suspected to pest and immature organs were separated. All of the samples were powdered using a mill (Model PX–MFC90D) with the mesh size of 1mm for the following analysis. Meanwhile, some of the ecological factors of the sampling area are as follows: the climate of the area is cold, the mean annual rainfall and temperature were 549 mm and 10.1 °C respectively. The average of altitude of area is between 2676–2716 m and the soil texture of area is moderate, semi heavy to heavy.

2.3. Isolation of the essential oils

The air dried of the aerial parts of the plant (100 g) was separated for hydrodistillation using a Clevenger-type apparatus (European pharmacopeia, 1998) .The distillation was done for 4 hours. The essential oil obtained was kept in a dark glass sealed vial at 4˚C for further analysis. The yields of the oils were calculated based on dried weight of the plant material.

2.4. Gas chromatography/mass spectrometry (GC/MS) analysis

The oils were examined by GC/MS, using Agilent Technologies GC/MS 7890A (built on the industry-leading Agilent GC platform, USA) in the central laboratory of Isfahan University of Technology (IUT), Iran. The injector temperature was set at 220 ˚C for 5 minutes with a split ratio of 1:10. A 1 µl and a volume of 1000 ppm of the obtained oil solution in a GC grade (*n*-hexane) were injected. To isolate different oil components, a linear temperature program was adjusted as described here: first of all, the column was kept at 50 ˚C for 2 minutes, ramped at a rate of 10 ˚C/min to 150 ˚C, and held isothermal for 5 minutes; then the ramp of 20 ˚C/min was applied up to 220 ˚C and held isothermal for 10 minutes. The mass spectrometry detector was taken at 70 eV and the mass range was 40–400 *m*/*z*. The identification of components was carried out using their recorded spectra by utilizing the spectrometric electronics libraries provided by the instrument software (Wiley, 1994; Adams, 2001). Also, the comparative amounts of the essential oil constituents were stated and recorded as percentage obtained via retention time (R_t) and peak area (Area%).

3. Results and discussion

The light yellowish essential oil of *Dorema ammoniacum* D. Don. was obtained with the yield of 0.31 % (v/w) based on the dried weight of the aerial parts. The major compounds of the essence in dried organs were formed about 67% of the total oils so that mentioned identified compounds were Limonene (49.18%), Neophytadiene (10.21%), beta Caryophyllene (3.54%), Phytol (2.61%) and Neryl acetone (1.46%). In this study, 89 compounds belonged to seven main chemical groups consists of nitrogen containing compounds such as terpenes, hydrocarbons, alcohols, ketones and others compounds were identified in the essence of *Dorema ammoniacum* D. Don. Some of these groups were divided to more minor chemical functional groups for example: nitrogen containing compounds including (amines, alkaloids and amides), terpenoieds (monoterpens, sesquiterpens and diterpens), hydrocarbons (aliphatic, aromatic and cyclic hydrocarbons) and the others of remaining groups were assigned in the next levels. The quantitative amounts of mentioned compounds in order of priorities were as follows: nitrogen containing compounds including amines (73.5 %), alkaloids (17.2 %) and amides (9.3 %), terpenoieds consists of monoterpens (82.88 %), sesquiterpens (12.97 %) and diterpens (4.14 %), hydrocarbons involving aliphatic hydrocarbons (88.66 %), aromatic hydrocarbons (7.5 %), cyclic hydrocarbons (3.83 %), alcohols (2.76 %), ketones (3.95 %) and miscellaneous coumpounds (2.22 %). The specifications of the entire identified constituents of the essential oils of *Dorema ammoniacum* D. Don. along with their retention time and also GC/MS chromatogram of it are shown in Table 1 and figure 2 **(Table 1** and **Fig 2).**

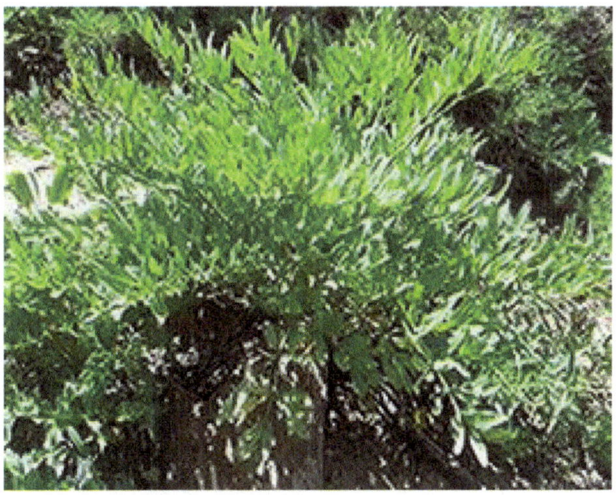

Fig 1. *Dorema ammoniacum* D. Don.

In the current research, two major groups of constituents namely nitrogen containing compounds and terpens were reported more than the other compounds. Overall, nitrogen compounds play an important role in many aspects of life and commercial processes. Nitrogen is a molecule in every major drug class in pharmacology and medicine (Bussau, 1999; Tamras, 1995). On the other hand, terpenes are one of the large group of chemical compounds with more minor divisions which sometimes called isoprenoides. These compounds are used extensively for their aromatic qualities and play a role in traditional herbal remedies (Connolly and Hill, 1996; Mann *et al.,* 1994). In this regard, a set of concise studies in relation to identification of constituents of *Dorema ammoniacum* D. Don. were carried out around the world. In most of which existence of different Terpenoieds compounds have been confirmed and some of the mentioned compounds were similar to the ones identified in this report (Mansouji Avval *et al.*, 2013; Yousefzadi *et al.*, 2011b; Yassa *et al.*, 2014; Batooli *et al.*, 2014). In spite of the reported constituents in the previous studies, there were a wide range of new identified compounds which were not reported in any of the previous research.

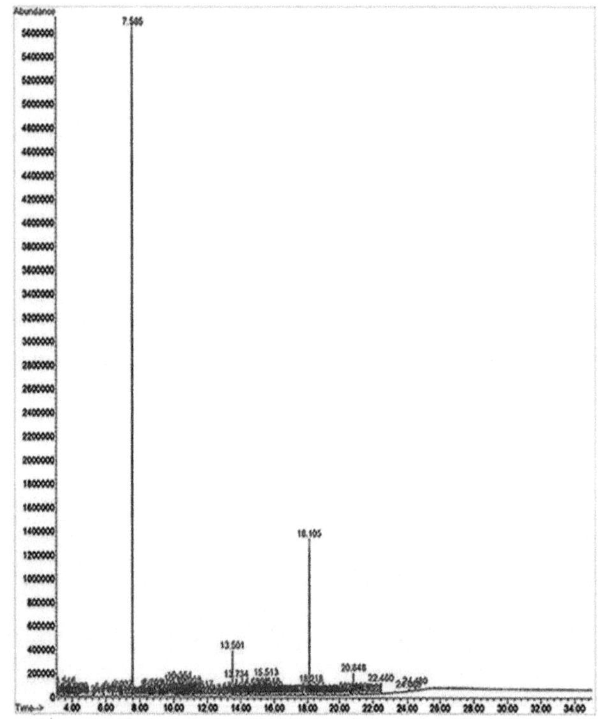

Fig 2. GC/MS chromatogram of *Dorema ammoniacum* D. Don.

The findings of the present research shows similarities and differences of essence constituents in mentioned organs of *Dorema ammoniacum* D. Don. compared to the previous conducted research. There are two significant reasons for such variances including, genetic characteristics (different genotypes of plants) and special environmental conditions (Omidbeigi, 2000).

Table 1. The specifications of the entire identified constituents of the essential oils of *Dorema ammoniacum* D. Don.

No.	Compounds[a]	Rt[b]	%
1	2,5-Dimethyltetrahydrofuran	3.162	0.25
2	Methylbenzene	3.222	0.10
3	Cyclohexane, 1,3-dimethyl, *trans*	3.351	0.3
4	Valeraldehyde	3.456	0.12
5	Octane	3.546	0.65
6	Imidazole-5-carboxylic acid, 2-amino	3.652	0.11
7	Butyl acetate	3.848	0.33
8	Cyclohexane, 1,2-dimethyl, *cis*	4.149	0.36
9	N,N-dimethyl cyclobutane-1,1-bis(methylamine)	4.194	0.06
10	Furfural	4.300	0.44
11	Deuteroacetone	4.353	0.18
12	Styrene	5.249	0.18
13	1-Methyldodecylamine	5.317	0.11
14	α-Pinene	5.882	0.32
15	Aziridine, 1-(2-buten-2-yl)	6.402	0.47
16	Sabinene	6.541	0.24
17	β-Myrcene	6.824	0.26
18	Decane	6.937	0.52
19	Acetamide, 2-chloro	7.209	0.08
20	**Limonene**	**7.585**	**49.18**
21	2-Butylamine	7.751	0.31
22	2-Pyridinepropanoic acid, α-methyl- β-oxo- ethyl ester	7.819	0.24
23	Phenyl Acetaldehyde	8.007	0.15
24	2-Amino-4-hydroxypteridine-6-carboxylic acid	8.520	0.07
25	Benzenamine, N-methyl-2-(2-propenyl)	8.572	0.17
26	Undecane	8.610	0.5
27	α-Terpinolene	8.723	0.61
28	Aramine	9.175	0.29
29	Limonene oxide	9.409	1.26
30	Isopropyl isocyanate	9.718	0.45
31	2-Hexanamine, 4-methyl	9.914	0.63
32	2,6-Dimethyl-4-pyrone	10.095	0.27
33	Dodecane	10.162	0.97
34	2,4-Hexadiene, 3-methyl	10.275	0.07
35	β-Fenchyl alcohol	10.351	1.27
36	Homarine	10.404	0.48
37	2-(N,N-dimethyl hydrazino) cyclohexane carbonitrile	10.494	0.19
38	Phenol, 4-(2-aminopropyl)	10.554	0.5
39	2-Oxo-3-methyl-cis-perhydro-1,3-be nzoxazine	10.607	0.35
40	*trans*-Carveol	10.697	0.58
41	Benzene, (2-fluoro-2-methoxycyclopropyl)	10.826	0.35
42	2(1H)-Naphthalenone, octahydro-8a-methyl, *trans*	10.908	1.14
43	p-Methoxyamphetamine	11.044	0.57
44	2-Cyclohexen-1-one, 2-methyl-5-(1-methylethenyl)	11.127	0.32
45	2-Methyl amphetamine	11.255	0.13

46	Tridecane	11.617	0.55
47	1-(3,5-Dimethyl-1-adamantanoyl) semi carbazide	11.767	0.52
48	Benzenemethanol, alpha-(1-aminoethyl)	12.084	0.05
49	Naphthalene, 1,2-dihydro-1,1,6-trimethyl	12.672	0.25
50	Rimantadine	12.853	0.1
51	Heptadecane	12.981	0.36
52	**β-Caryophyllene**	**13.501**	**3.54**
53	2-Amino-1-(O-methoxyphenyl) propane	13.591	0.35
54	Calarene	13.651	0.43
55	**Neryl acetone**	**13.734**	**1.46**
56	2-Methoxy amphetamine	14.164	0.63
57	1-[a-(1-Adamantyl) benzylidene] thiosemicarbazide	14.405	0.23
58	Benzenemethanol, 3-hydroxy-alpha-[(methylamino) methyl]	14.465	0.2
59	delta-Cadinene	14.699	1.11
60	1 S-*cis*-Calamenene	14.797	0.16
61	Aptrol	14.857	0.35
62	Benzenemethanol, 4-hydroxy-alpha-[(methylamino) methyl]	14.925	0.31
63	Nerolidol	15.128	0.36
64	N-Methyl-propylamine	15.384	0.11
65	Pentadecane	15.475	0.32
66	Farnesol 2	15.513	1.37
67	Caryophyllene oxide	15.618	1.36
68	2-Hexanamine, 5-methyl	16.145	0.1
69	Benzenemethanol, 2-(2-aminopropoxy)-3-methyl	16.274	0.22
70	2-Propanamine	16.703	0.1
71	2-Aminononadecane	16.922	0.27
72	Methanimidamide, N,N-dimethyl-N-phenyl	17.035	0.34
73	Methylpent-4-enylamine	17.713	0.7
74	Cyclobutanol	18.014	0.3
75	**Neophytadiene**	**18.105**	**10.21**
76	Hexahydro farnesyl acetone	18.218	0.86
77	n-Hexylmethylamine	18.293	0.06
78	Ethylene bromohydrin	18.361	0.46
79	Didodecyl phthalate	18.549	0.21
80	3-Propoxyamphetamine	18.836	0.09
81	Glycine, N-(N-acetyl-L-alanyl) butyl ester	19.069	0.2
82	2-Propenamide	19.250	0.13
83	2-Heptanol, 6-amino-2-methyl	19.348	0.05
84	Benzene ethanamine, 4-fluoro-beta,3-dihydroxy-N-methyl	19.484	0.08
85	1H-Indole-3-ethanamine, 6-fluoro-beta-methyl	19.529	0.05
86	Nonadecane	20.689	0.27
87	**Phytol**	**20.848**	**2.61**
88	Eicosane	22.460	0.83
89	Cyclotrisiloxane, hexamethyl	24.480	0.62
	Total identified		99.01

[a] Compounds listed in order of elution on the DB5 column.
[b] Retention time (as min)

Nevertheless, other factors such as phenology stages, the period of growing season and different organs of plants have been taken into consideration. It should be noted, our efforts have been focused on investigation and introduction of the new major chemical compounds which would be concisely described by the end of this study. The molecular structure of the major chemical compounds from the essential oil of *Dorema ammoniacum* D. Don. is shown in figure 3 **(Fig. 3)**.

Limonene is the first compound that is widely used in the process of manufacturing and production of various cosmetic products. Numerous applications are mentioned for this compound in literatures. Some of them are as follows: air care products, cleaning and furnishing care products, laundry and dishwashing products, personal care products and it has been considered as biofuel (Connolly and Hill, 1996; Mann *et al.,* 1994; Bauer, et al., 2001; Ming Lin *et al.,* 2015).

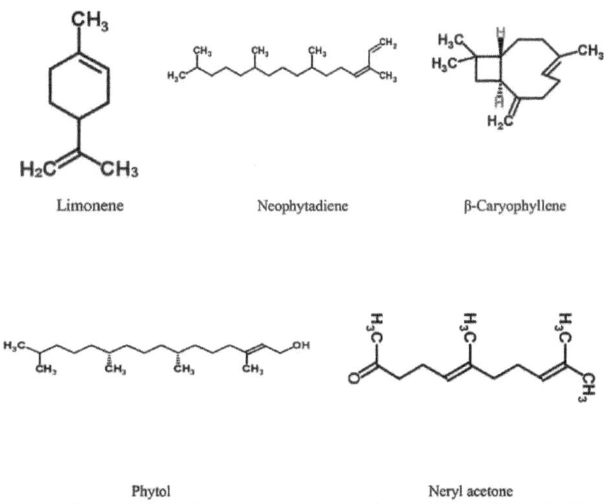

Fig 3. The molecular structure of the major chemical compounds from the essential oil of *Dorema ammoniacum* D. Don.

Neophytadiene is the second compound. It is one of the major compounds of *Nicotiana tobacum* L. that exists in leaves, stems and wastes of mentioned plant or is created by the hydration of phytol. It is a potent antimicrobial and anti-inflammatory compound and in some of literatures reviews it is identified as an antifungal terpenoid in the red alga, *Centroceras clavulatum* (C. Agardh) and Montagn. Other applications are as listed: antipyretic, analgesic and vermifugic, which cures sores and inflammation (Stojanovic *et al.*, 2000; Mendiola *et al.*, 2008; Carretero *et al.*, 2008). The third compound is beta Caryophyllene. This compound is extensively seen in the essential oils of various plants since it has several biomedical properties. The mentioned compounds contributes in the odor and flavor of the plants and also is used in lotions, creams and soaps (Skold *et al.*, 2006). Moreover, several therapeutic features of this compound have been reported in literatures. Some of the most important of them are as follows: anti-anemic effect, anti-inflammatory agent and anti-mutagen, a protector of gastric injury and oxidative stress and finally anti-carcinogen (Legault and Pichette, 2007; Di Sotto *et al.*, 2008; Da Silva *et al.*, 2007). Phytol is the fourth compound that like limonene are used in the fragrance industry and it could be used for manufacturing combined forms of the vitamins E and K_1 (Daines *et al.*, 2003; Mc Ginty *et al.*, 2010). The latest major compound is beta Neryl acetone. This compound has been reported as one of the major combination in some angiosperm (flowering plant) families such as Rutaceae, Burceraceae, Poaceae, Lamiaceae, Lauraceae, Verbenaceae, Asteraceae, Cuppressaceae and Hypericaceae (Pengely, 1996). It is classified in the group of flavor and fragrance agent and participates in the manufacture of various solvents. Additionally, therapeutics effects of the mentioned compound in some studies related to medical field has been proven (Curtis and Williams, 2001; Curzons *et al.*, 1999; Huttenlocher *et al.*, 1971; Gilbert *et al.*, 2000).

4. Conclusion

In this study, we have investigated existing constituents in the extract of *Dorema ammoniacum* D. Don. in one of its habitats in the Central Zagros, Iran. It led to discovery of some new constituents for the first time which were not reported in the previous studies. As discussed in the results section two major factors namely genetic features and environmental conditions have a significant contribution in shaping up and appearance of the various constituents. However, there are some habitats of the mentioned plant on earth that no phytochemical studies have been done on them and it needs to be further researched. *Dorema ammoniacum* D. Don. due to therapeutic properties is used in Iran folk medicine and it has various applications in cosmetics, detergent industries and food industry. Also, in the contemporary medicine the resin of mentioned plant has been utilized for the treatment of asthma and its case study is still ongoing. Finally, Iran due to its abundant species richness and particular climate conditions can be regarded as a unique country in the world in terms of medicinal species.

5. Acknowledgments

The authors appreciatively acknowledge from Department of Natural Resources and Nanotechnology and Advanced Materials Institute at Isfahan University of Technology for providing facilities and equipment required for the research. Authors are also thankful to the central laboratory of the University for helping to conduct of GC/MS analysis.

6. References

Adams, R.P. 2007. *Identification of Essential oils Components by Gas Chromatography/Mass Spectroscopy*, fourth ed. Allured Publishing Corporation, Carol Stream, IL, USA.

Amin, G.R. 1991. *Popular medicinal plants of Iran. Iranian* Research Institute of Medicinal Plants Iran. PP 262.

Appendino, G., Nano, G.M., Viterbo, D., Munno, G.D., Cisero, M., Palmisano, G. and Aragno, M. 1991. Ammodoremin, a epimeric mixture of prenylated chromandiones from ammoniacum. *Helvetica Chimica Acta*, 74: 495–500.

Arnone, A., Nasini, G., De Pava., O.V. and Cammarda, L. 1991. Isolation and structure elucidation of doremine A, a new spiro-sesquiterpenoidic chroman-2,4-dione from ammoniac gum resin. *Gazzetta Chimica Italiana Journal*, 121: 383–386.

Batooli, H., Haghir Ebrahimabadi, A., Mahmodi, B. and Mazochi, A. 2014. Comparison of essential oil chemical composition of vegetative and reproductive organs of *Dorema ammoniacum* D. Don. in Shahsavaran Kashan, *Iranian Journal of Medicinal and Aromatic Plants*, 30: 746–755.

Bauer, K., Garbe, D., and Surburg, H. 2001. *Common fragrance and flavor materials*, 4th Ed.

Wiley–VCH verlag GmbH, Germany.

Bown, D. 1995. *Encyclopedia of Herbs and Their Uses*. Dorling Kindersley, UK.

British Herbal Pharmacopoeia. 1983. The British Herbal and Medical Association, West Yorkshire, UK. PP 24.

British Pharmacopoeia. 1993. Vol. 2, HMSO, London. UK, PP. A165–169.

Bussau, A. 1999. *Soluble Nitrogen Containing Compounds in Eucalyptus Globulus (Labill.) Foliage: Effect of Site, Season and Nutrient Addition.* University of Melbourne, Australia. PP 244.

Carretero, M.E., Lopez Perez, J.L., Abad, M.J., Bermejo, P., Tillet, S., Israel, A. and Noguera, P.B. 2008. Preliminary study of the anti-inflammatory activity of hexane extract and fractions from *Bursera simaruba* (Linneo) Sarg, (Burseraceae) leaves. *Journal of Ethnopharmacology*, 116: 11–15.

Chevallier, A. 2001. *Encyclopedia of Medicinal Plants*. Dorling Kindersley, UK. PP 285.

Connolly, J.D., and Hill, R.A. 1996, *Terpenoids*. Chappman and Hall Company, UK, PP. 291–356.

Convention on the Elaboration of a European Pharmacopoeia. 1998. European Pharmacopoeia: Supplement. Council of Europe.

Curtis, T., and Williams, D.G. 2001. *Introduction to Perfumery*. Micelle Press, USA.

Curzons, A.D., Constable, D.C. and Cunningham, V.L. 1999. Solvent selection guide: a guide to the integration of environmental, health and safety criteria into the selection of solvents. *Clean Products and Processes*, 1: 82–90.

Daines, A., Payne, R., Humphries, M. and Abell, A. 2003. The Synthesis of Naturally Occurring Vitamin K and Vitamin K Analogues. *Current Organic Chemistry,* 7: 1625–1634.

Da Silva, S.L., Figueiredo, P.M. and Yano, T. 2007. Chemotherapeutic potential of the volatile oils from *Zanthoxylum rhoifolium* Lam leaves. *European Journal of Pharmacology*, 576: 180–188.

Di Sotto, A., Evandri, M.G. and Mazzanti, G. 2008. Antimutagenic and mutagenic activities of some terpenes in the bacterial reverse mutation assay. *Mutation Research*, 635: 130–133.

Evans, W.C. 1996. *Trease and Evans' Pharmacognosy*. 14th ed.; W.B. Saunders Company, UK.

Farhang, H.R., Vahabi, M.R. and Allafchian, A.R. 2015. Chemical compositions of the essential oil of *Gundelia tournefortii* L.(Asteraceae) from Central Zagros, Iran, *Journal of Herbal Drugs*, 6: 227–233.

Gilbert, D.L., Pyzik, P.L. and Freeman, J.M. 2000. The ketogenic diet: seizure control correlates better with serum beta-hydroxybutyrate than urine ketones. *Journal of Child Neurology*, 15: 787–790.

Grieve, M. 1971. *A Modern Herbal.* Vol. 1, Peter Smith Publisher, USA.

Howes, F. 1950. Age-old resins of the Mediterranean region and their uses. *Economic Botany,* 4: 307–316.

Huttenlocher, P.R., Wilbourn, A.J. and Signore, J.M. 1971. Medium chain triglyceride as a therapy for intractable childhood epilepsy. *Neurology*, 21: 1097–1103.

Irvani, N., Solouki, M., Omidi, M., Zare, A.Z. and Shahnazi, S. 2010. Callus induction and plant regeneration in *Dorem ammoniacum* D. an endangered medicinal plant. *Plant Cell Tissue and Organ Culture*, 100: 293-300.

Langenheim, J.H. 2003. *Plant resins: chemistry, evolution, ecology, and ethnobotany*. Timber Press, USA.

Legault, J. and Pichette, A. 2007. Potentiating effect of β-caryophyllene on anticancer activity of α-humulene, isocaryophyllene and paclitaxel. *Journal of Pharmacy and Pharmacology*, 59: 1643–1647.

Mann, J., Davidson, R.S., Hobbs, J.B., Banthorpe, D.V. and Harborne, J.b. 1994. *Natural products: Their Chemistry and Biological Significance.* Longman Group, UK.

Mansouji Avval, M., Sajjadifar, S. and Sadeghei Takallo, M. 2013. Chemical Composition of the Essential Oils from Flowers, Stems and Roots of *Dorema ammoniacum* D.Don. from Iran. *Research Journal of Pharmaceutical, Biological and Chemical Sciences*, 4: 640–644.

Mc Ginty, D., Letizia, C.S. and Api, A.M. 2010. Fragrance material review on phytol. *Food and Chemical Toxicology*, 48: 59–63.

Mc Lafferty, F.W. 2013. *Wiley registry of mass spectral data.* tenth ed. Mass Spectrometry Library Search System Bench-Top/PBM, New York, USA.

Mendiola, J.A., Santoyo, S., Cifuentes, A., Reglero, G., Ibanez, E. and Senorans, F.J. 2008. Antimicrobial activity of sub- and supercritical CO2 extracts of the green alga *Dunaliella salina*. *Journal of Food Protection*, 71: 2138–2143.

Ming Lin, F., Neil, E., Marsh, G. and Nina Lin, X. 2015. Recent progress in hydrocarbon biofuel synthesis:

pathways and enzymes. *Chinese chemical letters*, 26: 431–434.

Mozaffarian, V.A. 1996. *Dictionary of Iranian Plant Names*. Farhang Moaser Publication Iran, PP. 145.

Omid Beigi, R. 2000. *The production and processing of medicinal plants*. Fekr Ruose Publication, Iran.

Parsa, A. 1959. Medicinal plants and drugs of plant origin in Iran III. *Plant Food for Human Nutrition*, 6: 137–156.

Pengely, A. 1996. *The constituents of medicinal plants*. Allen and Unwin, Australia.

Rajani, M., Saxena, M.N., Ravishankara, N., Desai, N. and Padh, H. 2002. Evaluation of the Antimicrobial Activity of Ammoniacum Gum from *Dorema ammoniacum*. *Pharmaceutical Biology*, 40: 534–541.

Rechinger, K. H. 1980. *Flora Iranica*. Umbelliferae; Akademische Drucku. Verlags Antalt Graz, Austria. PP. 234.

Sajjadi, S.E., Ghassemi, N. and Mohammadzamani, P. 2007. Chemical Constituents of the Essential Oil of *Dorema ammoniacum* D. Don. Leaf, an Iranian Resinous Plant. *Revue des regions Arides*, 1: 194–197.

Skold, M., Karlberg, A.T., Matura, M. and Borge, A. 2006. The fragrance chemical β-caryophyllene air oxidation and skin sensitization. *Food and Chemical Toxicology*, 44: 538–545.

Stojanovic, G., Palic, R., Alagic, S. and Zekovic, Z. 2000. Chemical composition and antimicrobial activity of the essential oil and CO2 extracts of semi-oriental tobacco *Otlja*. *Flavour and Fragrance Journal*, 15: 335–338.

Tarmas, S. 1995. *Electrophilic Aromatic Thallation of Nitrogen containing Compounds*. California State University, Fresno, USA.

Worwood, V.A. 1991. *The Complete Book of Essential Oils and Aromatherapy*. New World Library Publication California, USA.

Yassa, N., Rustaie, A., Tavakoli, S., Delnavazi, M.R. and Batooli, H. 2014. Antioxidant and antibacterial activities of the essential oils and extracts of *Dorema ammoniacum* roots and aerial parts, *Research Journal of Pharmacognosy*, 1: 11–18.

Yousefzadi, M., Heidari, M., Akbarpour, M., Mirjalili, M.H., Zeinali, A. and Parsa, M. 2011a. In vitro Cytotoxic Activity of the Essential Oil of *Dorema ammoniacum* D. Don. *Middle East Journal of Scientific Research*, 7: 511–514.

Yousefzadi, M., Mirjalili, M.H., Alnajar, N., Zeinali, A. and Parsa, M. 2011b. Composition and *in vitro* antimicrobial activity of the essential oil of *Dorema ammoniacum* D. Don. fruit from Iran. *Journal of Serbian Chemical Society*, 76: 857–863.

Zarshenas, M.M., Arabzadeh, A., Tafti, M.A., Kordafshari, G., Zargaran, A. and Mohagheghzadeh, A. 2013. Application of Herbal Exudates in Traditional Persian Medicine. *Galen Medical Journal*, 1: 78–83.

Influence of chitosan concentration on morpho-physiological traits, essential oil and phenolic content under different fertilizers application in *Thymus daenensis*

Zohreh Emami Bistgani[1*], Seyed Ata Siadat[1], Abdolmehdi Bakhshandeh[1], Abdollah Ghasemi Pirbaluti[2], Masoud Hashemi[3]

[1]*Department of Agronomy (Physiology of Crop Plants). Ramin Agriculture and Natural Resources University of Khozestan, Iran;*

***Email:** *zohreemami66@gmail.com*

[2]*Department of Medicinal and Aromatic Plants, Research Center for Medicinal Plants and Ethnoveterinary, Shahrekord, Iran;*

[3]*Stockbridge School of Agriculture, University of Massachusetts, Amherst, MA 01003-9294. U.S.A.*

ARTICLE INFO

Topic: *Medicinal Plants*

Key words:
- ✓ *Chitosan*
- ✓ *Thymus daenensis*
- ✓ *Fertilizers*

ABSTRACT

Background & Aim: *Thymus daenensis* is recognized as aromatic herbs, which used in food, flavoring, pharmaceutical, and perfumery industries. This study was conducted to investigate the response of *T.daenensis* to different fertilizers (chemical and organic) along with chitosan.

Experimental: Treatments consisted of different fertilizers including: F1 =C (control without manure and fertilizer); F2 = CF (chemical fertilizers 100-150-100 kg ha^{-1}NPK, respectively), F3= CM (cow manure, 20 $tonha^{-1}$), F4= VC (vermicompost, 10 $tonha^{-1}$), F5=CF+CM+VC (chemical fertilizers + cow manure + vermicompost) and three chitosan levels (0, 0.2%, 0.4%) and acetic acid. This experiment conducted in split plot based on randomized complete block design with three replications during the period from 2014 to 2015 in Shahrekord, Iran. Morphological traits, essential oil yield from aerial parts and phenolic content were studied.

Results: Results indicated that canopy diameter, lateral branches, number of flower and leaf area index increased by CF+CM+VC treatment as compared to the control in 2014 and 2015. Chitosan increased biomass yield in both of growing year. Phenolic content increased in CF+CM+VC treatment in 2015 and it was also affected by application of 0.4% chitosan.

Recommended applications/industries: Since essential oil of *T. daenensis*, especially thymol and carvacrol, have a lot of applications in pharmacological and also has antimicrobial and antioxidant activities, the use of integrated fertilizer along with chitosan as a elicitor is recommended to obtain more essential oil yield and phenolic content.

1. Introduction

Thymus daenensis Celak. is a perennial herb distributed in many regions of Iran, (Nickavar *et al.* 2005; Ghasemi Pirbalouti *et al.* 2011). This herb is an endemic species of Iran and grows in the regions in Zagros Mountains chain, western and south western of Iran (Ghasemi Pirbalouti *et al.*, 2014; Ghasemi Pirbalouti *et al.*, 2013;

Nickavar *et al.,* 2005). It is widely used as a flavoring in meat products, salads, soups, and sauces but is also commonly used in traditional medicine to treat various diseases such as cold, cough, and digestive disorders (Nickavar *et al.* 2005; Ghasemi Pirbalouti, 2009).

*T. daenensis*is known for its powerful antimicrobial and antioxidant activity, which may to some extent explain its use in traditional medicine. The culinary function of this herb is due to its relatively high concentration of essential oils, which normally consist of the monoterpenes, thymol and carvacrol accompanied by their biosynthetic precursor's p-cymene and γ-terpinene as the primary components. These compounds are responsible for the aroma and flavor of this herb but also significantly contribute to its antimicrobial activity (Ghasemi Pirbalouti, 2014).

The major challenge for agriculture is to enhance crop production in a manner that is sustainable for present and future as well. The agricultural production and sustainable intensification goals in commercially important crops over both short and long terms demand proper plant nutrient and soil management. In arid and semi-arid areas, organic matter level of the soil is often very low. Thus, conservation and improvement of the soil organic matter is crucial for maintaining soil health and sustainability of farming in these regions. Moreover, successful crop production requires replacing adequate nutrients that have been removed by crops from the soil or lost to the environment one way or another. It is generally accepted that continuous application of chemical fertilizers may have negative impacts on soil health and environment (Yadav, 2003). Soil organic amendments therefore are considered as sustainable alternative sources of nutrients compared with synthesized fertilizers. Reports indicated that poultry manure and vermicompost are amongst efficient soil organic amendments for crop production (Keshavarzafshar *et al.,* 2014).

Elicitors are extensively used to enhance the yield of secondary metabolites in medicinal plants (Yin *et al.,* 2012) The most widely used elicitors are fungal carbohydrates, yeast extracts, and chitosan (Karuppusamy *et al.,* 2009) Chitosan is frequently used in cell cultures of medicinal plants as well as plant organs for inducing the accumulation of bioactive secondary metabolites. For example, it has been demonstrated that the total amounts of phenolics and terpenoids in sweet basil (*Ocimumbasilicum* L.) increased after chitosan treatment (Shetty et al., 1997).

The hypothesis of this study is that chitosan may be used as an additional method to the purely agronomic approaches to enhance the content of bioactive secondary metabolites in *T. daenensis*. In this study, we used chitosan levels and fertilizers in different kinds to treat *T. daenensis* plants and to study the effect of chitosan on plant growth, essential oil yield and phenolic content in aerial parts under different fertilizers.

2. Materials and Methods

2.1. Site description

A 2-year (2013 and 2014) experiment was conducted at the Research Farm of Shahrekord (latitude 32° 20′ N, longitude 50° 51′ E, altitude 2061 m above sea level), southwestern Iran. Type of study area climate by Emberger's climatology method is cold and semiarid and semi humid with temperate summer and very cold winter by Karimi's climatology method (IRIMO, 2012).

2.2. Experimental details

The experiment was laid out with a split plot pattern in randomized complete block design with three replicates. Five kinds of fertilizers treatment including F_1 =C (control without manure and fertilizer); F_2 = CF (chemical fertilizers 100-150-100 kg ha^{-1}NPK, respectively), F_3= CM (cow manure 20 tonha^{-1}), F_4= VC (vermi compost 10 tonha^{-1}), F_5=CF+CM+VC (chemical fertilizers + cow manure + vermicompost) and three chitosan levels (0, 0.2%, 0.4%) and acetic acid were studied.

2.3. Soil amendments

Prior to planting, soil samples were taken from 0 to 30 cm depth and were analyzed for selected physical and chemical characteristics The soil was classified as silt clay, pH=7.6, OC=0.42%, EC=0.43 ds m^{-1}, total nitrogen = 200 mg kg $^{-1}$, available phosphorus = 5.1 mg kg $^{-1}$, potassium = 189 mg kg $^{-1}$.

Accordingly, vermicompost was applied at the rate of 10000 kg ha^{-1} and manure fertilizer was used at the rate of 20000 kg ha^{-1}in the experiment. Before planting, organic amendments were evenly spread on the soil surface and incorporated manually into the top 20 cm of the soil.

2.4. Plant Material

T. daenensis Seeds were purchased from the seed company (Esfahan, Iran). In Apil 2014, transplants were produced in a green house in the pot (20 × 35 cm), and in June 2014, the seedlings were transplanted in the farm system (Sandy loam soil). Experiment conducted in split plot based on randomized complete block design with three replications, during the period from 2014 and 2015 in the research farm of Islamic Azad University of Shahrekord. (latitude 32° 20′ N, longitude 50° 51′ E, altitude 2061 m above sea level). The distance between plants in each row was 30 cm, each experimental plot size was 2.5×2 m.

2.5. Measurements

Plant height, canopy diameter, number of lateral branches, number of flowers, leaf area, as well as dry matter were determined at harvesting time (full flowering stage, on July 20, 2014 and June 30, 2015).

2.6. Essential oil isolation

Fifty g of dried plant materials was subjected to hydro-distillation for 3 h using a Clevenger-type apparatus. Anhydrous sodium sulphate was used to dry essential oil and oil samples were saved in sealed vials at 4 °C prior to analyses.

2.7. Leaf phenol content

Leaf total phenol content was measured according to the Folin–Ciocalteu method (Spanos and wrostand, 1990). Sample extract (10 μ lit) was mixed with distillation water (490 μ lit) and Folin–Ciocalteu reagent, (500 μl) of saturated sodium carbonate (1%) was added, and then tubes were vortexed for 1 min.After incubation at room temperature for 2 h, absorbance of the solution was measured at 765 nm, UV spectrometry. Gallic acid (0.015 and 0.5 mg ml−1) was used to create a calibration curve (r2= 0.998) and the concentration of total phenolic compounds was calculated as mg gallic acid equivalents (GAE) per g dry weight (DW).

2.8. Leaf flavonoid content

Total flavonoid content of leaf in the extracts was determined by the method of (Quettier-Deleu *et al.*, 2000). Fresh leaf sample (0.1 g) were mixed with 10 ml of ethanol (96%). Two ml of aluminum chloride and 6ml of acetate potassium were added to the extract which were subsequently incubated in the dark for 40 min. Absorbance was measured at 450 nm using UV-1800-Shimatzo (UV-spectrometry. Rutin (0.011and 0.370 mg ml−1) was used for calibration (r2= 0.999). All tests were done in triplicate and total flavonoid content was expressed as mg quercetin equivalent (QE) per g dry weight (DW).

2.9. Statistical analysis

For statistical analysis an ANOVA method for factorial design was conducted using SAS software (version9.1). Mean comparisons were applied using least significant difference (LSD) tests at 5% level of probability.

3. Results and discussion

3.1. Effect of different fertilizers and chitosan on plant morphology

Plant height, increased under different fertilizers in both years and this effect was more pronounced with the chemical fertilizer (Table 1). Except plant height, other traits were higher in second year. That was expected since plants were produced more biomass and the plant roots were deeper in the second year. The highest values for canopy diameter, lateral branches, number of flower, Leaf area index were observed under chemical and integrated fertilizer in 2014 and 2015 respectively (Table 1). The most of morphological traits were unaffected by the application of chitosan (Table 1).

Fertilization is the main factor affecting plant growth of active substances per unit area in herbaceous plants (Kozera *et al.,* 2013). According to Koeduka *et al.* (2006) nitrogen plays a key role in the biosynthesis of many organic compounds such as amino acids, proteins, enzymes, and nucleic acid. This phenomenon boosts nutrient availability resulting in higher nutrient content leading to higher plant growth. Nitrogen is the essential constituents of the chlorophyll molecule. The higher levels of N resulted in enhanced chlorophyll concentration leading to higher photosynthesis activity and plant growth. Further, organic amendments increased the availability of nutrients for plant growth and simultaneously decreased the nitrogen leaching. The combined phenomenon boosted nutrient availability resulting in higher nutrient content and plant growth (Pandry *et al.,* 2015).

Table 1. The effect of different fertilizers and application of chitosan on morpho-physiological, essential oil, ssential oil yield and phenolic content in *T. daenensis*.

Year	Treatments	PH	CD	NF	NS	LAI	DW	OC	OY	Phenol	Flavonoid
2014	**Fertilizers**										
	Control	21.25^{b}	105.58d^{c}	144.25^{d}	253.8^{d}	0.78^{a}	1355.42^{d}	1.50^{d}	20.57^{d}	97.35^{a}	39.69^{a}
	CF	33.58^{a}	119.66a^{b}	267.5^{b}	340.8^{b}	0.94^{b}	2635.16^{a}	2.00^{c}	52.77^{a}	97.07^{a}	37.78^{b}
	CM	23.00^{b}	103.16^{d}	147.4^{d}	263^{cd}	0.81^{dc}	1794.17^{c}	2.28^{b}	41.27^{c}	97.37^{a}	40.1^{a}
	VC	24.75^{b}	113.75^{bc}	163.75^{c}	274.9^{c}	0.87^{c}	835.17^{e}	1.41^{e}	12.07^{e}	97.23^{b}	36.90^{b}
	CF+CM+VC	30.66^{a}	124.58^{a}	284.9^{a}	362.5^{a}	1.43^{a}	2023.33^{b}	2.40^{a}	50.35^{b}	97.1^{c}	39.69^{b}
	LSD	4.08	9.23	10.2	18.36	0.06	153.54	0.05	1.58	0.005	0.69
	ANOVA	P≤0.01	P≤0.01	P≤0.01	P≤0.01	P≤0.01	P ≤0.01.	P≤0.01	P≤0.01	ns	P≤0.01
	Chitosan										
	AA	26.40^{a}	114.2^{a}	200.86^{a}	298.3^{a}	0.94^{b}	1506.33^{c}	1.79^{d}	28.74^{d}	96.62^{b}	38.25^{a}
	0.0	26.46^{a}	113.8^{a}	200.80^{a}	298.5^{a}	0.96^{ab}	1552.67^{c}	1.86^{c}	30.46^{c}	96.62^{b}	38.63^{a}
	0.2	26.86^{a}	112.7^{a}	201.80^{a}	300.4^{a}	0.97^{ab}	1842.8^{b}	1.96^{b}	38.14^{b}	96.74^{b}	38.77^{a}
	0.4	26.93^{a}	112.73^{a}	202.80^{a}	298.8^{a}	0.99^{a}	2012.79^{a}	2.05^{a}	44.26^{a}	98.90^{a}	39.40^{a}
	LSD	1.46	4.85	7.60	10.34	0.03	94.57	0.05	1.27	2.20	1.5
	ANOVA	ns	ns	ns	ns	ns	P ≤ 0.01	P≤0.01	P≤0.01	P≤0.01	ns
2015	**Fertilizers**										
	Control	21.25^{b}	105.58^{dc}	144.25^{d}	253.83^{d}	0.78^{d}	2013.33^{e}	1.72^{e}	34.97^{e}	97.08^{b}	24.16^{c}
	CF	33.58^{a}	119.66^{ab}	267.50^{b}	340.83^{b}	0.94^{b}	2826.67^{c}	2.55^{c}	72.47^{c}	97.87^{b}	21.79^{d}
	CM	23.00^{b}	103.16^{d}	147.41^{b}	263^{cd}	0.81^{dc}	2154.17^{d}	2.43^{d}	52.78^{d}	88.45^{c}	26.58^{b}
	VC	24.75^{b}	113.75^{bc}	163.75^{c}	274.91^{c}	0.87^{c}	2916.67^{b}	3.00^{b}	87.77^{b}	98.79^{b}	26.83^{b}
	CF+CM+VC	30.66^{a}	124.58^{a}	284.91^{a}	362.50^{a}	1.43^{a}	3334.17 ^{a}	3.33^{a}	111.45^{a}	107.87^{a}	34.83^{a}
	LSD	4.08	9.23	10.20	18.36	0.06	57.67	0.1	4.20	7.78	1.81
	ANOVA	P≤0.01	P≤0.01	P ≤ 0.01	P ≤ 0.01	P ≤ 0.01	P ≤ 0.01	P≤0.01	P≤0.01	P≤0.01	P≤0.01
	Chitosan										
	AA	26.40^{a}	114.30^{a}	200.86^{a}	298.33^{a}	0.94^{b}	2445.33^{d}	2.44^{d}	62.21^{d}	96.53^{c}	25.16^{c}
	0.0	26.46^{a}	113.80^{a}	200.80^{a}	298.53^{a}	0.96^{ab}	2588.67^{c}	2.52^{c}	67.86^{c}	97.36^{bc}	26.20^{bc}
	0.2	26.86^{a}	112.66^{a}	201.80^{a}	300.40^{a}	0.97^{ab}	2708.67^{b}	2.67^{b}	74.96^{b}	97.76^{ab}	27.50^{ab}
	0.4	26.93^{a}	112.73^{a}	202.80^{a}	298.80^{a}	0.99^{a}	2853.33^{a}	2.80^{a}	82.53^{a}	99.40^{a}	28.50^{a}
	LSD	1.46	4.85	7.60	0.06	0.03	31.69	0.05	1.73	2.01	1
	ANOVA	ns	ns	ns	ns	P≤0.01	P≤0.01	P≤0.01	62.21d	P≤0.01	P≤0.01

Similar letter (s) in each column are not significantly different at 5% probability level using LSD test PH: plant height (cm); CD: canopy diameter (mm); NLB: number of lateral branches; NF: number of flowers ; LAI: leaf area index; DW: dry weight (kg ha^{-1}); OC: oil content (%); OY: oil yield (kg ha^{-1}); PHE: phenol (mg g-1);FL: flavonoid (mg g-1): AA: acetic acid.

Table 2. Interactive effect of different fertilizers and application of chitosan on morpho-physiological, essential oil, essential oil yield and phenolic content of *T. daenensis* in 2014.

Year	Treatments	PH	CD	NF	NS	LAI	BY	OC	OY	Phenol	Flavonoid
2014	C×AA	27.33^{f}	78.66^{g}	99.33^{efg}	158.66^{m}	0.55^{h}	1174.66^{d-g}	1.40^{jk}	16.41^{m}	39.73^{abc}	96.80^{c}
	C×0.0	30.30^{bcd}	79.00^{g}	99.00^{fgh}	159.331^{m}	0.73^{def}	1333.33^{c-g}	1.40^{jk}	19.44^{l}	39.00^{a-d}	96.90^{c}
	C×0.2	28.00^{ef}	80.00^{fg}	98.33^{efg}	161.33^{kl}	0.74^{c-f}	1463.33^{c-g}	1.50^{hij}	22.39^{k}	39.70^{a-c}	98.10^{ab}
	C×0.4	29.00^{c-f}	80.00^{fg}	100.3^{ef}	163.00^{jk}	0.53^{h}	1450.33^{c-g}	1.60^{h}	24.03^{k}	40.31^{a}	96.76^{c}
	CF×AA	36.00^{a}	123.33^{b}	132.66^{a}	259.66^{c}	0.77^{cd}	2450.3^{abc}	1.90^{g}	46.20^{ef}	37.60^{def}	96.73^{c}
	CF×0.0	36.33^{a}	124.3^{ab}	133.33^{a}	260.66^{c}	0.82^{ab}	2490^{abc}	1.90^{g}	48.74^{de}	36.81^{f}	96.83^{c}
	CF×0.2	36.66^{a}	126.00^{a}	133.66^{a}	262.66^{a}	0.84^{a}	2700^{ab}	2.00^{fg}	54.40^{cd}	38.74^{a-e}	98.00^{a}
	CF×0.4	37.66^{a}	126.00^{a}	134^{a}	265.00^{b}	0.75^{c-f}	2900.29^{a}	2.13^{ef}	61.73^{a}	37.96^{c-f}	96.73^{c}
	CM×AA	31.00^{bc}	102.33^{c}	97.33^{h}	197.66^{f}	0.75^{c-f}	1553.3^{b-g}	2.18^{e}	33.89^{i}	40.12^{ab}	96.63^{c}
	CM×0.0	30.30^{bcd}	102.66^{c}	98.00^{gh}	198.33^{f}	0.78^{bc}	1390^{c-g}	2.20^{de}	30.99^{j}	40.16^{a}	96.73^{c}
	CM×0.2	29.30^{c-f}	103^{c}	98.6^{fgh}	201.00^{e}	0.83^{a}	1800^{a-d}	2.30^{cd}	41.54^{gh}	40.00^{ab}	99.50^{a}
	CM×0.4	30.00 $^{b-e}$	104.33^{c}	101.00^{e}	204.00^{d}	0.74^{c-f}	2433.33^{abc}	2.40^{bc}	58.55^{bc}	40.00^{ab}	96.63^{c}
	VC×AA	28.33^{d-f}	81.33^{f}	99.33^{efg}	160.00^{lm}	0.67^{g}	536.66^{g}	1.26^{l}	7.01^{n}	36.70^{f}	96.53^{c}
	VC×0.0	27.66^{f}	81.33^{f}	99.66^{efg}	161.00^{klm}	0.73^{d-f}	690.0f^{g}	1.36^{kl}	8.84^{n}	37.00^{ef}	96.70^{c}
	VC×0.2	30.66^{bc}	81.66^{f}	99.66^{efg}	164.00^{ij}	0.76$_{cde}$	1050.6^{efg}	1.50^{ijk}	15.62^{m}	37.00$_{ef}$	99.13^{a}
	VC×0.4	28.50^{d-f}	82.0^{f}	100.00^{ef}	166.00^{i}	0.72$_{ef}$	1063.33^{defg}	1.57^{hi}	16.82^{lm}	37.20$_{ef}$	96.56^{c}
	CF+CM+VC ×AA	31.00^{b-e}	85.66^{e}	110.33^{d}	178.00^{h}	0.71$_{fg}$	1816.7^{a-d}	2.20^{e}	40.19^{n}	37.14$_{ef}$	96.43^{c}
	CF+CM+VC ×0.0	32.00^{b}	87.66^{de}	111.6^{cd}	178.00^{h}	0.75$_{c-f}$	1860.00$_{a-d}$	2.40^{bc}	44.27^{fg}	40.00$_{ab}$	96.60^{c}
	CF+CM+VC ×0.2	32.00^{b}	87.66^{de}	112.3^{b}	181.00^{g}	0.72^{e-f}	2200^{a-e}	2.50^{ab}	56.77^{c}	38.34$_{b-f}$	98.93^{ab}
	CF+CM+VC ×0.4	31.00^{b-e}	88.66^{d}	113.6^{b}	182.66^{g}	0.72^{ef}	2216.66^{a-d}	2.57^{a}	60.16^{ab}	36.68$_{f}$	96.46^{c}
	LSD	2.08	2.01	1.90	2.35	0.04	211.5	0.12	2.84	1.78	0.97
	ANOVA	ns	ns	ns	ns	ns	P≤ 0.01	ns	P ≤0.01	ns	ns

Similar letter (s) in each column are not significantly different at 5% probability level using LSD test

PH: plant height (cm); CD: canopy diameter (mm); NLB: number of lateral branches; NF: number of flowers ; LAI: leaf area index; DW: dry weight (kg ha^{-1}); OC: oil content (%); OY: oil yield (kg ha^{-1}); PHE: phenol (mg g-1);FL: flavonoid (mg g-1): AA: acetic acid.

Table 3. Interactive effect of different fertilizers and application of chitosan on morpho-physiological, essential oil, essential oil yield and phenolic content in *T. daenensis* in 201

Year	Treatments	PH	CD	NF	NS	LAI	BY	OC	OY	Phenol	Flavonoid
2015											
	C×AA	21.33^{e}	108.66^{d} ef	144.00^{d}	252.33^{g}	0.75^{b}	1753.33^{i}	1.58^{l}	27.82^{n}	96.66^{b}	22.33^{ghi}
	C×0.0	21.00^{e}	104.00^{e} f	144.00^{d}	250.66^{g}	0.79^{b}	2006.66^{j}	1.69^{kl}	33.91^{m}	96.33^{b}	22.00^{hi}
	C×0.2	21.33^{e}	104.66^{e} f	144.00^{d}	260.00^{f}	0.79^{b}	2076.66^{j}	1.79^{jk}	37.16^{lm}	97.66^{b}	26.00$^{c\text{-}h}$
	C×0.4	21.33^{e}	105.00^{e} f	144.00^{d}	252.33^{g}	0.81^{b}	2216.66^{i}	1.85^{j}	40.99^{kl}	97.66^{b}	26.33$^{c\text{-}h}$
	CF×AA	32.70^{abc}	122.33^{abc}	266.66^{b}	340.00^{b}	1.41^{a}	2690.00^{g}	2.36^{hi}	63.68^{h}	96.66^{b}	32.50^{ab}
	CF×0.0	33.70^{ab}	122.66$^{a\text{-}d}$	266.00^{b}	341.66^{b}	1.41^{a}	2750.00^{g}	2.41^{hi}	66.43^{h}	96.83^{b}	34.50^{a}
	CF×0.2	34.00^{a}	117.00$^{a\text{-}d}$	267.3 3^{b}	341.66^{b}	1.44^{a}	2866.66^{f}	2.69^{fg}	77.10^{g}	98.66^{b}	36.50^{a}
	CF×0.4	34.0^{a}	116.66$^{a\text{-}d}$	270.00^{b}	340.00^{b}	1.46^{a}	3000.00^{e}	2.75^{ef}	82.71^{f}	99.33^{b}	35.83^{a}
	CM×AA	23.0^{de}	102.00^{f}	146.33^{d}	261.66^{ef}	0.82^{b}	1883.33^{k}	2.31^{i}	43.57^{k}	86.66^{c}	23.16^{fghi}
	CM×0.0	22.33d^{e}	102.00^{f}	146.33^{d}	263.00^{de}	0.81^{b}	2033.33^{j}	2.36^{hi}	48.02^{j}	87.16^{c}	20.66$^{e\text{-}h}$
	CM×0.2	23.33d^{e}	104.00^{ef}	148.33^{d}	264.33^{d}	0.80^{b}	2266.66^{i}	2.46^{h}	55.92^{i}	89.83^{c}	21.00^{i}
	CM×0.4	23.66^{de}	104.00^{ef}	148.66^{c}	263.00^{de}	0.81^{b}	2433.33^{h}	2.61^{g}	63.61^{h}	90.16^{c}	22.33^{i}
	VC×AA	24.66^{d}	114.33$^{b\text{-}e}$	163.66^{c}	275.00^{c}	0.83^{b}	2733.33^{g}	2.76^{ef}	75.50^{g}	97.00^{b}	23.66$^{e\text{-}i}$
	VC×0.0	24.66^{d}	113.66$^{c\text{-}e}$	163.33^{c}	275.00^{c}	0.85^{b}	2883.33^{f}	2.87^{e}	82.84^{f}	99.00^{b}	28.66$^{b\text{-}d}$
	VC×0.2	24.66^{d}	113.00$^{c\text{-}e}$	163.33^{c}	274.33^{c}	0.88^{b}	2933.3^{ef}	3.08^{d}	90.51^{c}	98.83^{b}	26.83$^{c\text{-}g}$
	VC×0.4	25.00^{d}	114.00$^{b\text{-}e}$	164.66^{c}	275.33^{c}	0.90^{b}	3116.66^{d}	3.28^{bc}	102.24^{d}	100.33^{b}	28.16$^{b\text{-}e}$
	CF+CM+VC ×AA	30.33^{c}	123.66$^{a\text{-}c}$	283.66^{a}	362.66^{a}	0.92^{b}	3166.66^{d}	3.17^{cd}	100.48^{d}	105.66^{a}	24.16$^{d\text{-}i}$
	CF+CM+VC ×0.0	30.66^{bc}	126.66^{a}	284.33^{a}	362.33^{a}	0.94^{b}	3270.0^{c}	3.30^{b}	108.12^{c}	107.50^{a}	25.16$^{d\text{-}i}$
	CF+CM+VC ×0.2	31.0^{abc}	124.66a^{b}	285.66^{a}	361.66^{a}	0.94^{b}	3400^{b}	3.35^{b}	114.12$^{.b}$	108.83^{a}	27.16$^{c\text{-}f}$
	CF+CM+VC ×0.4	30.66^{bc}	123.33a^{b} c	286.00^{a}	363.33^{a}	0.96^{b}	3500^{a}	3.51^{a}	12309.16^{a}	109.50^{a}	29.83^{bc}
	LSD	3.28	10.85	5.32	2.35	0.23	70.88	0.12	3.88	4.51	4.33
	ANOV A	ns	ns	ns	ns	ns	$P \leq 0.01$.	ns	$P \leq 0.01$.	ns	ns

Similar letter (s) in each column are not significantly different at 5% probability level using LSD test

PH: plant height (cm); CD: canopy diameter (mm); NLB: number of lateral branches; NF: number of flowers; LAI: leaf area index; DW: dry weight (kg ha^{-1}); OC: oil content (%); OY: oil yield (kg ha^{-1}); PHE: phenol (mg g-1); FL: flavonoid (mg g-1): AA: acetic acid.

3.2. Effect of different fertilizers and chitosan on biomass of thyme

Biomass of thyme plants were higher in 2015 compared to 2014. This was not a surprise since plants sowed in 2014, extended their growth in 2015 in all treatments (Table 1). The results presented in Table 1 showed that the amount of dry matter yield was enhanced progressively by chemical fertilizers in 2014, but in 2015, combination of organic manures and chemical fertilizer significantly increased thc crop biomass. The biomass yield increased by 64.5 % and 46.2% in CF and CF+CM+VC treatments, in 2014 and 2015 respectively. Increasing in biomass yield in CF in 2014 can be attributed to applying nitrogen in different growths stage has stimulating effects in organic compounds of the plant system. Moreover, the increasing effect of N fertilization on plant biomass may be due to the positive effects of nitrogen on activation of photosynthesis and metabolic processes of organic compounds in plants. According to Baranauskienne *et al.* (2003) found that N fertilizer increased biomass yield of *Thymus vulgaris*.

In 2015, when thyme plants were exposed to integrated fertilizers, an increase in biomass yield was observed which may be due to integration of organic manures and chemical fertilizers that can increase the organic matter level of metabolic processes in plant. This event increases nutrient availability resulting in more nutrient content leading to higher biomass yield. Only use of organic manures or chemical fertilizer indicated lower nutrient uptake leading to lower biomass yield. Organic manure and chemical fertilizer alone need to more complex compound in the soil for development and growth in each plant cell for its proper functioning (Pandey *et al.,* 2015).

Application of 0.4% chitosan improved biomass yield by approximately 25.8% and 25.3% in 2014 and 2015, respectively. (Table 1). Results also showed that suitable chitosan oligomer concentration for the growth of thyme was 0.4%.

3.4 Effect of different fertilizers and chitosan on essential oil and oil yield of thyme

Data presented in Table 1 indicated, essential oil percentage and oil yield were higher in 2015 than in 2014. The highest essential oil percentage was found in plants under integrated fertilizer sprayed with 0.4% in both of growing year (Table 3), However, in 2014 due to substantial enhancement in dry matter yield of plants that under application of chemical fertilizer, the highest oil yield (5958.24 kg ha $^{-1}$ in 2014) was obtained from plants grown in cow manure, sprayed with 0.2% chitosan (Table 2). CF+CM+VC treatment resulted in maximum essential oil yield sprayed with 0.4% with (12309.16 kg ha $^{-1}$in 2015) (Table 3). Other fertilizers treatments also indicated significant difference as compared to the control (Table 1).

The enhance in essential oil yield by using of integrated fertilizer (CF+CM+VC) may be due the higher supply of N from cow manure, vermicompost and chemical fertilizer, which could lead to higher essential oil yield and dry matter (Pandey and Patra, 2015). The synthesis of essential oils is dependent on photosynthetic activity. Providing of photosynthetic nutrient boost and metabolic processes correlated to cell division and elongation (Hatwar *et al.,* 2003). According to Pandey *et al.* (2015) nitrogen plays a key role in the division, growth and development of cells that stimulate essential oil accumulation via higher density of oil glands due to the improvement in biomass yield. Thus, it is useful to combine organic fertilizer with chemical fertilizer for optimum thyme productivity and essential oil yield.

Spraying chitosan increased essential oil content, possibly it acted as a potent inducer for increasing the biosynthesis of secondary metabolites. Chitosan is also considering as an elicitor of signaling molecule which increase essential oil. Yin *et al.* (2014) indicated that 0.4% chitosan significantly increased the biomass and essential oil yield of *Origanum vulgare*.

3.5. Effect of different fertilizers and chitosan on phenol and **flavonoid content**

It was found that the phenolic contents of aerial parts of *T. daenensis* increased under integrated fertilizer in 2015, but the effect of fertilizers wan not significant on this trait. The effect of foliar application of chitosan on phenol content of *T. daenensis* was affected by different fertilizers (Table 2, 3). The highest phenol content was obtained by foliar application of 0.4% chitosan in 2014 and 2015, respectively. (Table 1).

According to table 2 and table 3, phenol content was not affected by fertilizers and application of chitosan in both of growing years (2014 and 2015). The highest flavonoid content was obtained from plants which received manure fertilizer in 2014, however the highest flavonoid content was obtained from integrated fertilizer in 2015 (Table 1). Among different levels of chitosan, concentration of 0.4% improved flavonoid content (Table 1).

In our results, phenol and flavonoid content increased when thyme plants exposed to organic manure and integrated fertilizer. Thus, application of organic amendments remarkably improved phenolic content. The improvement in phenolic content in case of organic manure treatments may be due to the presence of easily available water-soluble carbon, which acts as a source of energy for soil microorganisms (Pandry and Patra, 2015). Organic fertilizers enhance plant growth by providing nutrients and improving the effectiveness of the soil by favorably modifying its water retention and aeration. The results support the previous findings of beneficial effects of combined application of organic and inorganic nutrients on soil fertility and productivity in menthol mint (Patra *et al.,* 2000).

Foliar application of chitosan resulted in the highest phenolic content, in both years (Table 1). Yin *et al* (2011) indicated that chitosan is a significant secondary signal messenger, which can play a key role in many plants activities such as plant growth and secondary metabolite production. Also they indicated that chitosan has the potential to induce the accumulation of polyphenol in *Origanum vulgare*. Kim (2005) reported that application of chitosan solution improved the total phenolic and terpenoids content in sweet basil.

4. Conclusion

The results recommended that combination of organic manure and chemical fertilizer gave higher canopy diameter, lateral branches, number of flower, leaf area index, essential oil and also increased phenolic content in *T. daenensis*. Combination of organic manure and chemical fertilizers was the most suited combination for improving the crop productivity, oil yield and overall profitability and economics of cultivation of the *T. daenensis*. Moreover, cow manure or vermicompost had potential to reduce the application of chemical fertilizers with improvement in the essential oil yield. Foliar application of chitosan increased essential oil content and oil yield in *T. daenensis* by up-regulating the biomass. Thus, foliar application of chitosan for improving oil yield was of great practical value and could be an effective method to reduce the costs associated with essential oil production.

5. References

Ghasemi Pirbalouti, A. 2009. Medicinal plants used in Chaharmahal and Bakhtyari districts Iran. *HerbaPolon*, 55:69–75.

Ghasemi Pirbalouti, A., Hashemi, M., TaherianGhahfarokhi, F. 2013. Essential oil and chemical compositions of wild and cultivated (*Thymus daenensis*Celak) and (*Thymus vulgaris* L.) *Industrial Crops and Products*, 48:43–48.

Ghasemi Pirbalouti, A., Rahimmalek, M., Malekpoor, F., Karimi, A. 2011. Variation in antibacterial activity, thymol and carvacrol contents of wild populations of (*Thymus daenensis*) subsp. daenensisCelak. *Plant Omics. Journal,* 4:209–214.

Ghasemi Pirbaloti, A., Samani, M., Hashemi, M., Zeinali, H., 2014. Salicylic acid affects growth, essential oil and chemical compositions of thyme (*Thymus daenensis*Celak) under reduced irrigation. *Plant Growth Regulation*, 72:289-301.

Hatwar, G.P., Gondane, S.U., Urkude, S.M., Gahukar, O.V. 2003. Effect of micronutrients on growth and yield of chili. Soils Crops, 13:123–125.

IRIMO, 2012. (Islamic Republic of Iran Meteorological Organization). Climatology methods. http://www.irimo.ir.

Karuppusamy, S. 2009. A review on trends in production of secondary metabolites from higher plants by in vitro tissue, organ and cell cultures. *Journal of Medicinal Plants Research*, 3:1222–1239.

KeshavarzAfshar, R., Chaichi, M.R., Assareh, M.H., Hashemi, M. Liaghat, A. 2014. Interactive effect of deficit irrigation and soil organic amendments on seed yield and flavonolignan production of milk thistle (*Silybummarianum* L. Gaertn.) *Industrial Crops and Products.*58:166–172.

Kim, H. J., Chen, F., Wang, X., Rajapakse, N. C. 2005. Effect of chitosan on the biological properties of sweet basil (*Ocimumbasilicum* L.). *Journal of Agricultural and Food Chemistry,* 53: 3696–3701.

Koeduka, T., Fridman, E., Gang, D.R., Vassao, D.G., Jackson, B.L., KoshChM.Orlova, I., Spassova, S.M., Lewis, N.G., Noel, J.P., Baiga, T.J., Dudareva, N., Pichersky, E. 2006. Eugenol and isoeugenol, characteristic aromatic constituents of spices, are biosynthesized via reduction of a coniferyl alcohol ester. PNAS 103, 10128–10133.

Kozera, W., Majcherczak, E., Barczak, B. 2013. Effect of varied NPK fertilisation on the yield size, content of essential oil and mineral composition of caraway fruit(*Carumcarvi* L.). *Journal of Elementary,* 18: 255–267

Nickavar, B., Mojab, F., Dolat-Abadi, R. 2005. Analysis of the essential oils of two Thymus species from Iran. *Food Chemistry*, 90: 609–611.

Pandey, V., Patra, D. 2015. Crop productivity, aroma profile and antioxidant activity in Pelargonium graveolens L. Her. under integrated supply of various organic and chemical fertilizers. *Industrial Crops and Products*, 67:257–263.

Pandey, V., Patel, A., Patra D.D. 2015. Amelioration of mineral nutrition, productivity, antioxidant activity and aroma profile in marigold (*Tagetesminuta* L.) with organic and chemical fertilization. *Industrial Crops and Products*, 76: 378–385.

Patra, D.D., Anwar, M., Chand, S. 2000. Integrated nutrient management and waste water for restoring soil fertility and productivity of Japanese mint and mustard sequence in Uttar Pradesh, *Indian Journal of Agricultural and Environmental Science*, 80:267-275.

Quettier-Deleu, C., Gressier, B., Vasseur, J., Dine, T., Brunet, J., Luyck, M., Cazin, M., Cazin, J.C., Bailleul, F., Trotin, F. 2000. Phenolic compounds and antioxidant activities of buckwheat (*Fagopyrumesculentum*Moench) hulls and flour. *Journal of Ethnopharmacology*,72: 35-40.

Shetty, K. 1997. Biotechnology to harness the benefits of dietary phenolics: Focus on Lamiaceae. *Asia Pacific Journal of Clinical Nutrition,*6:162–171.

Spanos, G. A., Wrolstad, R. E. 1990. Influence of processing and storage on the phenolic composition of Thompson seedless grape juice. *Journal of Agricultural and Food Chemistry*, 38:1565–1571.

Yadav, J.S.P. 2003. Managing soil health for sustained high productivity. Journal of the *Indian Society of Soil Science*,51 (4): 448–465.

Yin, H., Xavier, F., Chrestensen, L.P., Grevsen, K. 2012. Chitosan Oligosaccharides promote the Content of polyphenols in Greek Oregano (Oreganumvulgaressp.hirtum). *Journal of Agricultural and Food Chemistry*, 60: 136-143.

Anti-inflammatory activity of leaf extract of *Solanum anomalum*

Jude E Okokon[1]*, Koofreh O. Davies[2], Louis U. Amazu[3], Emem E. Umoh[1]

[1]*Department of pharmacology and toxicology, Faculty of pharmacy, University of Uyo, Uyo, Nigeria;*
***Email: judeefiom@yahoo.com**

[2]*Department of Physiology, Faculty of Basic Medical Sciences, University of Uyo, Uyo, Nigeria;*

[3]*Department of Pharmacology and Therapeutics, College of Medicine, Evans Enwerem University, Orlu Campus, Imo State;*

ARTICLE INFO

Topic: *Medicinal Plants*

Key words:
- ✓ *Solanum anomalum*
- ✓ *Antiinflammatory*
- ✓ *Oedema*

ABSTRACT

Background & Aim: *Solanum anomalum* Thonn. ex Schumach. (family Solanaceae) is a shrub growing up to 2 metres tall. The edible fruits are gathered from the wild and consumed locally and the leaves are used locally in the treatment of various diseases. Evaluation of anti-inflammatory activity of leaf extract of *Solanum anomalum* was carried out to ascertain its uses in traditional medicine.
Experimental: The crude leaf extract (70 – 210 mg/kg) of *Solanum anomalum* was investigated for anti-inflammatory activity using various experimental models; carragenin, egg albumin and xylene induced oedema.
Results: The extract (70 -210 mg/kg) caused a significant ($p<0.05 - 0.001$) dose-dependent reduction of inflammations caused by carragennin, egg albumin and xylene. The anti-inflammatory effect of this plant may in part be mediated through the chemical constituents of the plant.
Recommended applications/industries: The plant, *Breynia nivosa,* possesses antiinflammatory property which can be exploited in the treatment of inflammatory diseases.

1. Introduction

Solanum anomalum Thonn. ex Schumach. (family Solanaceae) is a shrub growing up to 2 metres tall. The stem, branches and midribs of the leaves are usually armed with prickles up to 5 mm long. The edible fruits are gathered from the wild and consumed locally. Both the fruits and the leaves are used medicinally. The plant is sometimes cultivated or semi-cultivated for its fruits. It is found in West tropical Africa - Sierra Leone to southern Nigeria, Cameroon and DR Congo. It is Known as 'childrens' tomatoes', they are more commonly used as a condiment in soups and sauces and the fruits are eaten raw or cooked (Burkill, 2000). The sap from the leaves and fruits is drunk, or taken by enema 1 - 2 times daily, as a treatment for leprosy and gonorrhoea (Burkill, 2000). The fruits are used as a laxative and digestive (Burkill, 2000). They are also served ground up in soups and sauces as an appetizer for sick persons, sometimes mixed with fruits of Parkia (Burkill, 2000). The crushed fruits are applied to maturate inflammations on fingers or toes (Burkill, 2000) The fruit juice is applied to sores on the ears to alleviate pain (Bukenya and Hall, 1988). Offor and Ubengama (2015) reported the antidiabetic activity of the fruit of this plant. Although there is a little information on the fruit of this plant, there is no report of phytochemical constituents and biological activity of the leaf of *S. anomalum*. We report in this study the phytochemical composition and antiinflammatory activity of the leaf extract of the plant.

2. Materials and Methods

2.1. Plants collection

The plant material *Solanum anomalum* (leaves) were collected in compounds in Uruan area, Akwa Ibom State, Nigeria in August, 2015. The plant was identified and authenticated by a taxonomist in the Department of Botany and Ecological Studies, University of Uyo, Uyo, Nigeria. Hebarium specimen was deposited at Department of Pharmacognosy and Natural Medicine Herbarium.

2.2. Extraction

The plant parts (leaves) were washed and shade-dried for two weeks. The dried plants' materials were reduced to powder using mortar and pistle. The powdered material was soaked in 50% ethanol. The liquid filtrate was concentrated and evaporated to dryness in vacuo 40°C using rotary evaporator and stored in a refrigerator at - 4°C.

2.3. Phytochemical Screening

Phytochemical screening of the crude extract was carried out employing standard procedures and tests (Trease and Evans, 1989; Sofowora, 1993), to reveal the presence of chemical constituents such as alkaloids, flavonoids, tannins, terpenes, saponins, anthraquinones, reducing sugars, cardiac glycosides among others.

2.4. Animals

Albino Swiss mice (19 – 28g) of either sex were obtained from the University of Uyo animal house. They were maintained on standard animal pellets and water *ad libitum*. Permission and approval for animal studies were obtained from the College of Health Sciences Animal Ethics committee, University of Uyo.

2.5. Determination of median lethal dose (LD_{50})

The median lethal dose (LD_{50}) of the extract was estimated using albino mice by intraperitoneal (i.p) route using the method of Lorke (1983). This involved intraperitoneal administration of different doses of the extract (100 -1000 mg/kg) to groups of three mice each. The animals were observed for manifestation of physical signs of toxicity such as writhing, decreased motor activity, decreased body/limb tone, decreased respiration and death. The number of deaths in each group within 24 hours was recorded. The LD_{50} was calculated as geometrical means of the maximum dose producing 0% (a) and the minimum dose producing 100% mortality (b).

$$LD_{50} = \sqrt{ab}$$

2.6. Evaluation of antiinflammatory activity of the extract

2.6.1. Carrageenin – induced mice hind paw oedema. Adult albino male mice were used after 24 hours fast and deprived of water only during experiment. Inflammation of the hind paw was induced by injection of 0.1 ml of freshly prepared carrageenin suspension in normal saline into the sub planar surface of the hind paw. The linear circumference of the injected paw was measured before and 0.5, 1, 2, 3, 4 and 5 hrs after administration of phlogistic agent. The increase in paw circumference post administration of phlogistic agent was adopted as the parameter for measuring inflammation (Winter *et al.,* 1962; Akah and Nwambie, 1994; Ekpendu *et al*., 1994, Besra *et al*., 1996; Nwafor *et al.,* 2010). The difference in paw circumference between the control and 0.5, 1, 2, 3, 4 and 5 hrs after administration of phlogistic agent was used to assess inflammation (Hess and Milonig, 1992). The extract (70, 140 and 210 mg/kg i.p) was administered to various groups of 6 mice each, 1h before inducing inflammation. Control mice received carrageenin while reference group received ASA (100 mg/kg). The average (mean) oedema was assessed by measuring with vernier calipers. Average inflammation/oedema ($C_t - C_0$) was calculated for each dose (Oriowo, 1982; Akah and Njike, 1990).

2.6.2. Egg-albumin induced inflammation. Inflammation was induced in mice by the injection of egg albumin (0.1ml, 1% in normal saline) into the sub planar tissue of the right hind paw (Akah and Nwambie, 1994; Okokon and Nwafor, 2010). The linear circumference of the injected paw was measured before and 0.5, 1, 2, 3, 4 and 5 hrs after the administration of the phlogistic agent. The leaf extract (70, 140 and 210 mg/kg i.p) and ASA (100 mg/kg orally) were administered to groups (n=6) of 24 h fasted mice 1 h before the induction of inflammation. Control group received 10 ml/kg of distilled water orally. Edema (inflammation) was assessed as the difference in paw circumference between the control and 0.5, 1, 2, 3, 4 and 5 hrs post administration of the phlogistic agent (Hess and Milonig, 1972). The average (mean) edema was assessed by measuring with vernier calipers. Average inflammation/oedema ($C_t - C_0$) was calculated for each dose (Oriowo, 1982; Akah and Njike, 1990).

2.6.3. Xylene – induced ear oedema. Inflammation was induced in mice by topical administration of 2 drops of xylene at the inner surface of the right ear. The xylene was left to act for 15 mins. *Solanum anomalum* leaf extract (70, 140 and 210 mg/kg i.p), dexamethasone (4 mg/kg) and distilled water (0.2 ml/kg) were orally administered to various groups (n=6) of mice 1 h before the induction of inflammation. The animals were sacrificed under light anaesthesia and the left ears cut off. The difference between the ear weights was taken as the oedema induced by the xylene (Tjolsen *et al.*, 1992; Okokon and Nwafor, 2010).

2.7. Statistical analysis and data evaluation

Data obtained from this work were analyzed statistically using Students't-test and ANOVA (One-way) followed by a post test (Tukey-Kramer multiple comparison test). Differences between means were considered significant at 1% and 5% level of significance i.e $P \leq 0.01$and 0.05.

3. Results and discussion

3.1. Phytochemical screening

The phytochemical screening of the ethanol extract of the leaf of *Solanum anomalum* revealed the presence of alkaloids, cardiac glycosides, tannins, saponins, terpenes and flavonoids .

3.2. Determination of Median lethal dose (LD_{50})

The median lethal dose (LD_{50}) was calculated to be 724.56 mg/kg. The physical signs of toxicity included excitation, paw licking, increased respiratory rate, decreased motor activity, gasping and coma which was followed by death.

3.3. Carragenin-induced oedema in mice

The effect of ethanol leaf extract of *Solanum anomalum* on carragenin-induced oedema is as shown in Table 1. The extract (70 - 210 mg/kg) exerted a significant ($P<0.05 – 0.001$) anti-inflammatory effect in a dose –dependent manner. The activity of the highest dose was more than that of the standard drug, ASA, 100 mg/kg (Table 1a and 1b).

3.4. Egg albumin- induced oedema

Administration of extract of *Solanum anomalum* (70 - 210 mg/kg) on egg albumin - induced oedema in mice caused a significant ($p<0.05 – 0.001$) dose-dependent anti-inflammatory effect against oedema caused by egg albumin. The effect was incomparable to that of standard drug, ASA (100 mg/kg) (Table 2a and 2b).

3.5. Xylene- induced ear edema

Anti-inflammatory effect of crude extract of *Solanum anomalum* against xylene-induced ear oedema in mice is shown in Table 3. The extract exerted a dose-dependent anti-inflammatory effects that were significant ($P<0.05 - 0.01$) but incomparable to that of the standard drug, dexamethasone (4.0 mg/kg).

In this study, the ethanol leaf extract of *Solanum anomalum* was evaluated for anti-inflammatory activity using various experimental models.

In the carragenin-induced oedema, the extract (70 - 210 mg/kg) was observed to have exerted significant effect at the early stage of inflammation (1-2 hr) indicating effect probably on histamine, serotonin and kinnins that are involved in the early stage of carragenin-induced oedema (Vane and Booting, 1987). The extract further reduction of the later stage of the oedema maybe due to its ability to inhibit prostaglandin which is known to mediate the second phase of carragenin induced inflammation (Vane and Booting, 1987). However, ASA (100 mg/kg) a prototype NSAID, a cyclooxygenase inhibitor whose mechanism of action involves inhibition of prostaglandin, produced a considerable inhibition of the paw swelling induced by carragenin injection.

The extract also inhibited egg albumin-induced oedema demonstrating that it can inhibit inflammation by blocking the release of histamine and 5-HT, two mediators that are released by egg albumin (Nwafor *et al.,* 2007). However, ASA, a cyclooxygenase inhibitor reduced significantly oedema produced by egg albumin.

The extract exerted a significant ($P<0.01$) inhibition of ear oedema caused by xylene only at all doses of the extract, suggesting the inhibition of phospholipase A_2 which is involve in the pathophysiology of inflammation due to xylene (Lin *et al.,*1992).

Table 1a. Effect of *Solanum anomalum* leaf extract on carrageenin- induced oedema in rats.

Treatment/ Dose (mg/kg)	Time intervals (hr) 0	0.5	1	2	3	4	5
Control	2.49 ± 0.01	3.94 ± 0.22	4.17 ± 0.23	4.00 ± 0.12	3.87 ± 0.03	3.87 ± 0.19	3.82 ± 0.02
Extract 70	2.27 ± 0.03	3.45 ± 0.28	3.28 ± 0.61	3.29 ± 0.25	3.06 ± 0.31	2.81 ± 0.30	2.80 ± 0.33
140	2.24 ± 0.04	3.51 ± 0.22	3.34± 0.16	3.06 ± 0.05	3.01 ± 0.15	2.74 ± 0.13	2.66 ± 0.14
210	2.32 ± 0.03	3.57 ± 0.26	3.27± 0.14	3.22 ± 0.08	3.13 ± 0.15	2.79 ± 0.21	2.62 ± 0.16
ASA 100	2.41 ± 0.06	2.89±0.04	2.59 ± 0.05^{b}	2.75 ± 0.02^{a}	2.60 ± 0.02^{a}	2.57 ± 0.08	2.51 ± 0.09

Data are expressed as mean ± SEM. Significant at $^{a}p<0.05$; $^{b}p< 0.01$ when compared to control. n = 6.

Table 1b. Effect of *Solanum anomalum* leaf extract on carrageenin induced oedema in rats.

Treatment/ Dose (mg/kg)	Average inflammation/oedema (mm) ± SEM 0.5hr	1hr	2hr	3hr	4hr	5hr
Control	1.45 ± 0.02	1.68 ± 0.04	1.51 ± 0.03	1.30 ± 0.11	1.25 ± 0.17	1.33 ± 0.02
Extract 70	1.18 ± 0.18	1.04 ± 0.10	1.02 ± 0.12	0.79 ± 0.21	0.54 ± 0.18^{a}	0.53 ± 0.21
140	1.27± 0.05	1.10 ± 0.06	1.03 ± 0.07	0.77 ± 0.15^{a}	0.50 ± 0.09^{a}	0.42 ± 0.03^{c}
210	1.25± 0.02	0.95 ± 0.05	0.90 ± 0.04	0.81 ± 0.06^{a}	0.47 ± 0.06^{a}	0.30 ± 0.03^{c}
ASA 100	0.68±0.01	0.38 ± 0.01^{C}	0.54 ± 0.01^{C}	0.39 ± 0.01^{C}	0.36 ± 0.01^{C}	0.30 ± 0.01^{C}

Data are expressed as mean ± SEM. Significant at $^{c}P < 0.001$ when compared to control. n = 6.

Table 2a. Effect of *Solanum anomalum* leaf extract on egg- albumin induced oedema in mice.

Treatment/ Dose (mg/kg)	Time intervals (hr) 0	0.5	1	2	3	4	5
Control	2.65 ± 0.07	3.55± 0.25	3.50 ± 0.06	3.45 ± 0.11	3.41 ± 0.07	3.35 ± 0.07	3.25 ± 0.06
Extract 70	2.38 ± 0.03	3.24 ± 0.53	3.06 ± 0.29	2.82 ± 0.30	2.70 ± 0.25	2.59 ± 0.33	2.56 ± 0.41
140	2.34 ± 0.08	3.44 ± 0.12	3.30 ± 0.20	3.16 ± 0.20	2.93 ± 0.27	2.71 ± 0.19	2.58 ± 0.24
210	2.33 ± 0.01	3.37 ± 0.12	3.09 ± 0.11	2.87 ± 0.11	2.80 ± 0.18	2.67 ± 0.13	2.57 ± 0.10
ASA 100	2.61 ± 0.06	2.99 ±0.16^{a}	2.89 ± 0.02^{a}	2.84 ± 0.02^{c}	2.76 ± 0.03^{c}	2.64 ± 0.05^{b}	2.64 ± 0.05^{c}

Data are expressed as mean ± SEM. Significant at ap<0.05; $^{b}p< 0.01$, $^{C}p< 0.001$ when compared to control. n = 6.

Table 2b. Effect of *Solanum anomalum* leaf extract on egg-albumin induced oedema in rats.

Treatment/ Dose (mg/kg)	Average inflammation/oedema (mm) ± sem 0.5hr	1hr	2hr	3hr	4hr	5hr
Control	1.68 ± 0.05	1.68 ± 0.04	1.52 ± 0.04	1.30 ± 0.11	1.25 ± 0.17	1.33 ± 0.02
Extract						
70	0.86± 0.21	0.68 ± 0.15	0.44 ± 0.15	0.32 ± 0.12	0.21 ± 0.04^{a}	0.18 ± 0.03
140	1.10± 0.12	0.96 ± 0.05	0.78 ± 0.05	0.59 ± 0.10^{a}	0.37 ± 0.05^{a}	0.24 ± 0.11^{c}
210	1.04± 0.03	0.76 ± 0.07	0.54 ± 0.03	0.47 ± 0.02^{a}	0.34 ± 0.06^{a}	0.24 ± 0.01^{c}
ASA 100	0.83±0.05	0.62 ± 0.07	0.50 ± 0.04^{a}	0.40 ± 0.01^{a}	0.24 ± 0.07^{b}	0.20 ± 0.29^{C}

Data are expressed as mean ± SEM. Significant at $^{c}P < 0.001$ when compared to control. n = 6.

Table 3. Effect of *Solanum anomalum* leaf extract on xylene-induced ear oedema in mice.

Treatment/ Dose (mg/kg)	weight of right ear (g)	weight of left ear (g)	Increase in ear weight (g)	% inhibition
Control (normal saline) 0.2ml	0.032 ± 0.002	0.090 ± 0.002	(181.25) 0.058 ± 0.002	
Extract 70	0.044 ± 0.002	0.071 ± 0.00	(61.36) 0.027 ± 0.002[a]	53.44
140	0.042 ± 0.003	0.065 ± 0.004	(71.42) 0.030 ± 0.006[b]	48.27
210	0.035± 0.003	0.063 ± 0.005	(80.00) 0.028 ± 0.002[c]	51.72
Dexamethasone 4.0	0.036 ± 0.003	0.054 ± 0.003	(24.52) 0.018 ± 0.003[c]	68.96

Figures in parenthesis indicate % increase in ear weight.*significant at ap<0.05, bp < 0.01, cp < 0.001 when compared with ontrol. n = 6.

However, dexamethasone, a steroid antiinflammatory agent produced significant reduction in the mean right ear weight of positive control rats indicating an inhibition of PLA_2.

The phytochemical screening shows that the leaf extract contains alkaloids, cardiac glycosides, tannins, saponins, terpenes and flavonoids.

Flavonoids are known anti-inflammatory compounds acting through inhibition of the cyclo-oxygenase pathway (Liang *et al.,* 1999). Some flavonoids are reported to block both the cyclooxygenase and lipoxygenase pathways of the arachidonate cascade at relatively high concentrations, while at lower concentrations they only block lipoxygenase pathway (Carlo *et al*., 1999). Some flavonoids exert their antinociception via opioid receptor activation activity (Suh *et al.,* 1996; Rajendran *et al*., 2000; Otuki *et al*., 2005). Flavonoids also exhibit inhibitory effects against phospholipase A2 and phospholipase C (Middleton *et al.,* 2000), and cyclooxygenase and/or lipoxygenase pathways (Robak *et al.,* 1998).

Triterpenes have been implicated in anti-inflammatory activity of plants (Huss et al., 2002; Suh et al., 1998) and reports on their analgesic activities have also been published (Liu, 1995; Krogh et al., 1999; Tapondjou et al., 2003; Maia et al., 2006). Ursolic acid is a selective inhibitor of cyclooxygenase-2 (Ringbom et al., 1998). Oleanolic acid is known to exert its analgesic action through an opioid mechanism, and possibly, a modulatory influence on vanilliod receptors (Maia *et al.,* 2006).

In conclusion, the results of this study demonstrated that *Solanum anomalum* leaf possess antinflammatory property and this confirms its usage in traditional medicine to treat inflammatory diseases.

4. Conclusion

The results of this study demonstrated that *Solanum anomalum* leaf possess antinflammatory property and this confirms its usage in traditional medicine to treat inflammatory diseases

5. Acknowledgement

Authors are grateful to Mr Aniefiok Ukpong of Department of Pharmacology and Toxicology, University of Uyo, Uyo, for his technical assistance.

6. References

Akah PA, Njike HA. (1990). Some pharmacological effects of rhizome aqueous extract of *Anchomanes diformis. Fitoterapia* 60: 368-370.

Akah PA, Nwanbie A. (1994). Evaluation of Nigerian traditional medicines plants used for rheumatic (inflammatory) disorder. *Journal of Ethnopharmacology* 42: 179 – 182.

Besra SE, Sharma RM, Gomes A. (1996). Antiinflammatory effect of petroleum ether extract of leaves of *Litchi chinensis*. Caertn (sapindaceae). *Journal of Ethnopharmacology*. 54:1-6.

Bukenya ZR, Hall JB. (1988). Solanum (Solanaceae) in Ghana. Bothalia 18(1): 79–88.

Burkill HM. (2000). The useful plants of West Tropical Africa. 2nd Edition. Volume 5, Families S–Z, Addenda. Royal Botanic Gardens, Kew, United Kingdom. 686 pp.

Carlo Di G, Mascolo N, Izzo AA, Capasso F. (1999). Flavonoids, old and new aspects of a class of natural therapeutic drugs. *Life Science* 65:337–353.

Ekpendu TO, Akah PA, Adesomoju AA, Okogun JI. (1994). Antinflammatory and antimicrobial activities of *Mitracarpus scaber* extracts. *International Journal of Pharmacology*. 32:191-195.

Hess SM, Milonig RC. (1972). Inflammation In: Lepow LH, Ward PS. (Eds). Inflammation, Mechanism and control. Academic Press, New-York, USA. pp.1-2.

Huss U, Ringbom T, Perera P, Bohlin L, Vasange M. (2002). Screening of ubiquitous plant constituents for COX-2 inhibition with a scintillation proximity based assay. *Journal Natural Products* 65: 1517-1521.

Krogh R, Kroth R, Berti C, Madereira AO, Souza MM, Cechinel-Filho V, Delle-Monache F, Yunes RA. (1999). Isolation and identification of compounds with antinociceptive action from *Ipomoea pes-caprae*. *Pharmazie* 54: 464 – 466.

Liang YC, Huang YT, Tsau SH, Lin-Shiau SY, Chen CF, Lin JK. (1999). Suppression of inducible cyclo-oxygenase and inducible nitric acid synthase by apigenia and related flavonoid in mouse macrophages. *Carcinogenesis*. 20: 1945-52.

Lin LL, Lin AY, Knopt JL. (1992). Cytosolic phospholipase A_2 is coupled to hormonally regulated release of arachidonic acid. *Proceeding of National Academy of Science, U. S. A*. 89:6147-6157.

Liu J. (1995). Pharmacology of oleanolic acid and ursolic acid. *Journal of Ethnopharmacology* 49: 57-68.

Lorke, D. (1983). A new approach to practical acute toxicity testing. *Achieves of Toxicology*. 54:275-286.

Maia JL, Lima-Junior RC, David JP, David JM, Santos FA, Rao VS. (2006). Oleanolic acid, a pentacyclic triterpene attenuates the mustard oil induced colonic nociception in mice. *Biological and Pharmaceutical Bulletin* 29: 82–85.

Middleton E Jr, Kandaswami C, Theoharides TC. (2000). The effects of plant flavonoids on mammalian cells: Implications for inflammation, heart disease, and cancer. *Pharmacological Reviews*. 52: 673–751.

Nwafor PA, Jacks TW, Ekanem AU. (2007). Analgesic and anti-inflammatory effects of methanolic extract of *Pausinystalia mecroceras* stem bark in rodents. *Journal of Pharmacology* 3: 86-90.

Nwafor PA, Nwajiobi N, Uko IE, Obot JS. (2010). Analgesic and anti-inflammatory activities of an ethanol extract of *Smilax krausiana* leaf in mice. *African Journal of Biomedical and Research 13: 141 -148.*

Offor SJ, Ubengama EE. (2015) Phytochemical and antidiabetic studies of ethanolic extracts and fractions of the fruits of *Solanum* anomalum Thonn. Ex. Schumach. *International Journal of Scientific Research and Education.*3 (9):4343-4350.

Okokon JE, Nwafor PA. (2010). Antiinflammatory, analgesic and antipyretic activities of ethanolic root extract of *Croton zambesicus*. *Pakistan Journal of Pharmaceutical sciences*. 23(4): 383 - 390.

Oriowo MA.(1982). Anti-inflammatory activity of piperonyl,-4-acrylic isobutyl amide, an extractive from *Zanthoxylum zanthoxyloids. Planta Medica* 44: 54 - 56

Otuki MF, Ferreira J, Lima FV, Meyre-Silva C, Malheiros Â, Muller LA, Cani GS, Santos ARS, Yunes RA, Calixto JB (2005). Antinociceptive properties of mixture of α-amyrin and β-amyrin triterpenes: Evidence for participation of protein kinase C and protein kinase A pathways. *Journal of Pharmacology and Experimental Therapeutics* 313: 310–318.

Rajendran NN, Thirugnanasambandam P, Viswanathan S, Parvathavarthini S, Ramaswamy S. (2000). Antinociceptive pattern of flavone and its mechanism as tested by formalin assay. *Indian Journal of Experimental Biologiocal* 38: 182–185.

Ringbom T, Segura L, Noreen Y, Perera P, Bohlin L. (1998). Ursolic acid from *Plantago major*, a selective inhibitor of cyclooxygenase-2 catalysed prostaglandin biosynthesis. *Journal of Natural Products* 61: 1212–1215.

Robak J, Shridi F, Wolbis M, Krolikowska M (1998). Screening of the influence of flavonoids on lipoxygenase and cyclooxygenase activity, as well as on nonenzymic lipid oxidation. *Polish Journal of Pharmacology and Pharmacy* 40: 451–458.

Santos AR, Cechinel Filho V, Niero R, Viana AM, Moreno FN, Campos MM, Yunes RA, Calixto JB. (1994). Analgesic effects of callus culture from selected species of *Phyllanthus. Journal of Pharmacy and Pharmacology*. 46 : 755 – 759.

Sofowora, A. Medicinal Plants and Traditional Medicine in Africa. 2nd edn, Spectrum Book Ltd, Ibadan, Nigeria. 1993.

Suh HW, Song DK, Son KH, Wie MB, Lee KH, Jung KY, Do JC, Kim YH (1996). Antinociceptive mechanisms of dipsacus saponin C administered intracerebroventricularly in the mouse. *General Pharmacology* 27: 1167–1172.

Suh N, Honda T, Finaly HJ, Barchowsky A, Williams C, Benoit NE. (1998). Novel triterpenoids suppress inducible nitric oxide synthase (iNOS) and inducible cyclooxygenase (COX-2) in mouse macrophages. *Cancer Resesearch* 58: 717-723.

Trease, G.E., Evans, W. C. Pharmacognosy, 13th ed. Bailliere Tindal, London. 1989.

Tapondjou LA, Lontsi D, Sondengam BL, Choi J, Lee KT, Jung HJ, Park HJ. (2003). In vivo antinociceptive and antiinflammatory effect of the two triterpenes, ursolic acid and 23-hydroxyursolic acid, from *Cussonia bancoensis*. *Archives of Pharmacal Research* 26: 143–146.

Tjolsen A, Berge OG, Hunskaar S, Rosland JH, Hole K. (1992). The formalin test: An evaluation of the method. *Pain* 51:5-17.

Vane T, Booting R. (1987). Inflammation and mechanism of action of anti- inflammatory drugs. *FASSEB J.* 1:89-96.

Winter CA, Risley EA, Nuss GW. (1962). Carrageenin-induced oedema in hind paw of the rats as an assay of anti-inflammatory drugs. *Proceeding of Society for Experimental Biology Medicine* 111:544 -547.

Qualitative and quantitative changes in the essential oil of sage (*Salvia hydrangea* DC exBenth.) as affected by different drying methods

Forugh Mahdiyan, Abdollah Ghasemi Pirbalouti*

Medicinal Plants Department, Shahrekord Branch, Islamic Azad University, Shahrekord, 88146, Iran;

***Email:** ghasemi@iaushk.ac.ir

ARTICLE INFO

***Topic:** Medicinal Plants*

Key words:
- ✓ *Salvia hydrangea*
- ✓ *Essential oil*
- ✓ *a-pinene*

ABSTRACT

Background & Aim: *Salvia hydrangea* is one of the medicinal plants belonging to Lamiaceae family. Medicinal plants can be marketed as fresh or dried products; however aromatic plants are often dried before extraction to reduce moisture content. The aim of this study was to evaluate the impact of different drying methods on qualitative and quantitative changes in essential oil of sage.

Experimental: To determine the effect of drying methods on qualitative and quantitative characteristics of the plant essential oil, samples were dried in sunlight, shade, mechanical oven at 65°C and then compared with fresh samples. The essential oils of all samples were extracted by hydrodistillation and analyzed using GC and GC–MS.

Results: The results showed that different drying methods had significant effects on essential oil content. According to results fresh herbs had the highest essential oil content followed by shade drying, sun drying and oven drying samples, respectively. Significant changes in chemical compound amount of the essential oils were observed which associated with the drying methods. Significant differences occurred among several constituents in the extracted essential oils, including a-pinene, camphene, phellandrene, 1,8-cineole and bornylacetate.

Recommended applications/industries: Drying of *Salvia hydrangea* aerial parts in the shade is more suitable for obtaining higher amount of oil yield and percentage of a-pinene and 1,8-cineole. Therefore, shade drying could be recommended for extraction of essential oil from this plant on an industrial scale.

1. Introduction

The genus *Salvia* (common name: sage) is the largest and the most important aromatic and medicinal member of the Lamiaceae family and includes about 1000 species of shrubs, herbaceous perennials and annuals (Farimani *et al.*, 2011). Salvia has radiated extensively in three regions of the world: Central and South America, western Asia and eastern Asia (Alziar, 1988–1993).

The pharmacological effects of *Salvia* essential oils are based on the presence of more than 100 active elements which can be categorized into Monoterpene hydrocarbons, Oxygenated monoterpenes, Sesquiterpene hydrocarbons, Diterpenes, isoprenoid compounds and Oxygenated sesquiterpenes. Salvia species are also rich sources of polyphenolic flavonoids and phenolic acids. The major components contain 1,8-cineole, camphor, borneol, β-pinene, α- pinene, camphene and α-thujene and each of them has their own outstanding medicinal effects (Zhiming *et al.*, 2013).

Medicinal plants can be marketed as fresh or dried products, according to their use, howere aromatic plants are often dried before extraction to reduce moisture content. Fresh herbs (especially Lamiaceae) usually contain 75–80% water, and these water levels need to be lowered to less than 15% for preservation (Ghasemi Pirbalouti *et al.*, 2013a; Diaz-Maroto, *et al.*, 2002). Dehydration of herbs can be performed using different methods. The aim of this study was to evaluate the effect of various drying conditions (sun, shade and oven at 65°C) on essential oil content and oil composition in *S. hydrangea*.

2. Materials and Methods

2.1. Plant materials

The arial parts of sage (*S. hydrangea*) were collected from Tang-e-sayad (Shahrekord), Southwest Iran (3563716 N and 0510449E) about 2430m above sea level. The plants were identified by taxonomic references (Rechinger, 1969) and specimens that have been placed in the Herbarium of the Research Center of Medicinal Plants, Shahrekord Branch, I.A.U., Iran (Voucher specimen no. 2316). The collected samples were randomly divided into four batches containing four sets of 300 g. One set was used for analysis of the fresh tissue and the remaining batches were dried using one of the following methods: air drying in shade at ambient temperature (20 ± 5 °C); air drying in full sunlight at ambient temperatures (20–37°C); oven drying in hot air at 65 °C. All drying methods were replicated three times, the final moisture content of dried samples was determined after drying at 72 h in a lab oven at 75 °C. Dried (100 g) and fresh plant (200 g) materials were subjected to hydrodistillation (1000 ml distillated water) for 3 h using a Clevenger- type apparatus. Oil samples were kept in amber glass vials at 4 °C until analysis.

2.2. Gas chromatography/mass spectrometry (GC–MS) analysis

GC analysis was done on an Agilent Technologies 7890 gas chromatograph equipped with Flame Ionization Detector (FID) and a HP-5MS 5% capillary column (30 m × 0.25 mm, 0.25 μm film thicknesses). Oven temperature was kept at 60 °C for 4 min initially, and then raised at the rate of 4 °C/min to 280 °C. Injector and detector temperatures were set at 290 °C and 300 °C, respectively. Helium was used as carrier gas at a flow rate of 2 ml/min, and 0.1 μl samples were injected manually in the split mode(1:40). Peak areas were used for quantifying the constituent percentage in total oil. The gas chromatograph was coupled to an Agilent 5975 C (Agilent Technologies, Palo Alto, CA, USA) mass selective detector (MSD) and quadrupole EI mass analyzer (Agilent Technologies, Palo Alto, CA, USA). Operating parameters for the EI-MS were: ionization voltage, 70 eV and ion source temperature, 250 °C. Retention indices were calculated for all components using a homologous series of n-alkanes (C5–C24) injected in conditions equal to the oil samples. Identification of oil components was accomplished based on comparison of retention times with those of authentic standards, and by comparison of their mass spectral fragmentation patterns (WILLEY/ChemStation data system) (Adams, 2007). Area percent was obtained electronically from the GC–FID responses without the use of an internal standard or correction factors.

2.3. Statistical analyses

The data was statistically analyzed using one-way ANOVA by SPSS (19.0), and comparison of the means of main constituents for essential oils was evaluated by Duncan's multiple range test at $p < 0.05$ level. Analytical data for hierarchical cluster analysis were treated by means of the SPSS statistical software.

3. Results and discussion

3.1. Effect of drying methods on the essential oil yield

All essential oils extracted from the aerial parts of *S. hydrangea* dried under different conditions produced a clear, yellow liquid. An analysis of variance indicated that the drying method had a significant effect on oil yield. In accordance with our results, there are similar reports from other researchers about other medicinal plants (GhasemipirbaloutI *et al.,* 2013 a, b; Ahmadi *et al.,* 2008). Fresh herbs had the highest essential oil contents (0.40ml/100g) followed by shade drying (0.20ml/100g), sun drying (0.15ml/100g) and oven drying (0.025ml/100g) respectively (Fig. 1). In total, the results showed that drying methods brought about significant losses of the essential oil content compared with fresh state and dried samples in shade had the higher essential oil as compared to samples that dried in sun and oven. In agreement with our results, the oil content of shade-dried *Roman chamomile* flowers was found to be larger (1.9% w/w) than there of sun-dried (0.4%) and oven-dried at 40°C (0.9%) (Omidbaigi *et al,* 2004).

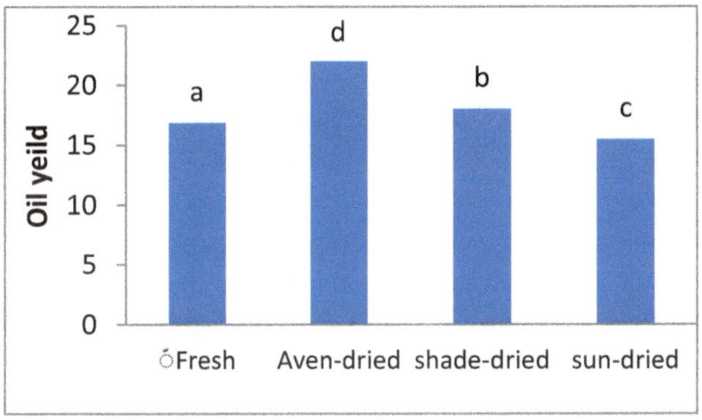

Fig. 1. Comparison of essential oil yield of fresh sample and dry samples of the drying methods. (Significant different at $p < 0.05$ have been indicated with different letters.).

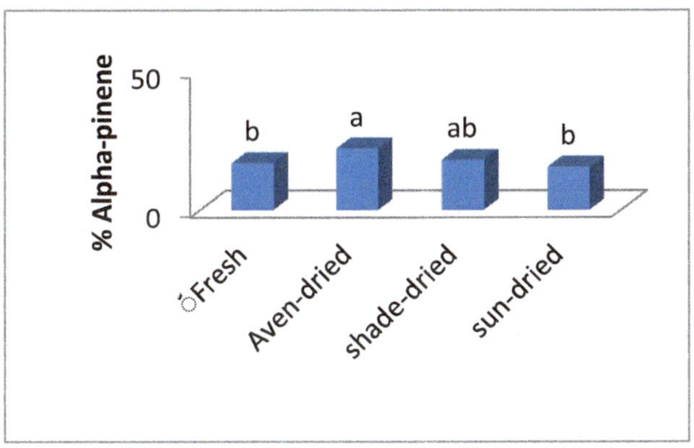

Fig. 2. Comparison of Alpha-pinene of fresh sample and dry samples of the drying methods. (Significant different at $p < 0.05$ have been indicated with different letters.)

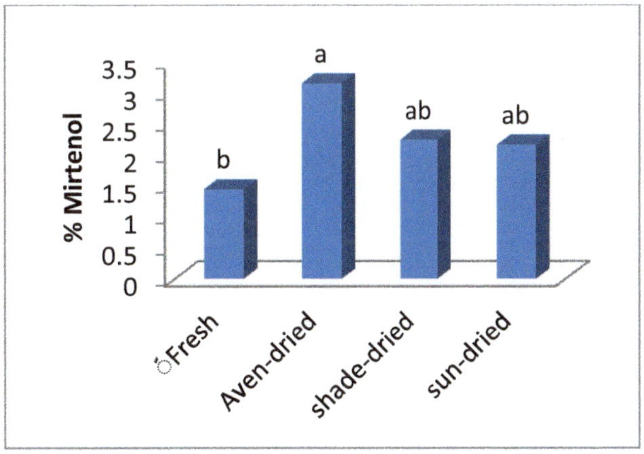

Fig 3. Comparison of Mirtenol of fresh sample and dry samples of the drying methods. (Significant different at $p < 0.05$ have been indicated with different letters.)

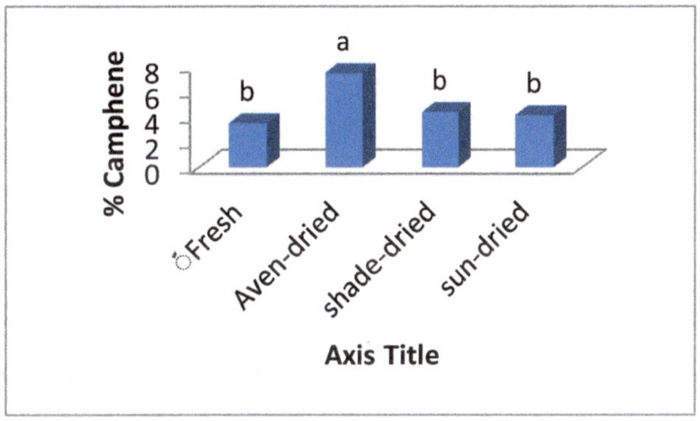

Fig. 4. Comparison of Camphene fresh sample and dry samples of the drying methods. (Significant different at $p < 0.05$ have been indicated with different letters.)

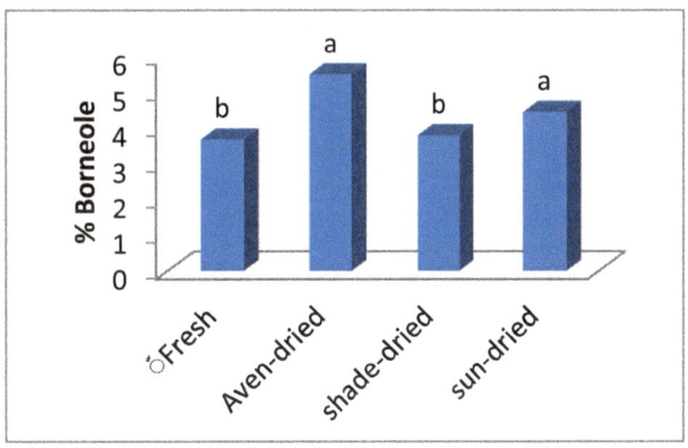

Fig. 5. Comparison of Borneole of fresh sample and dry samples of the drying methods. (Significant different at $p < 0.05$ have been indicated with different letters.).

Increasing in drying temperature significantly decreased the essential oil content, indicating that the biological structure of the oil glands of sage was collapsed, resulting in a loss of essential oils. In anatomical studies of fresh and dried leaves of spearmint (*Menthaspicata*), Diaz-Maroto *et al.* (2003) observed that epithelial cells in the dried samples can collapse and split open. A decrease in essential oil content with higher drying temperatures has been also reported by Venskutonis (1997) in thyme (*Thymusvulgaris*) when they were oven-dried at 60 °C.

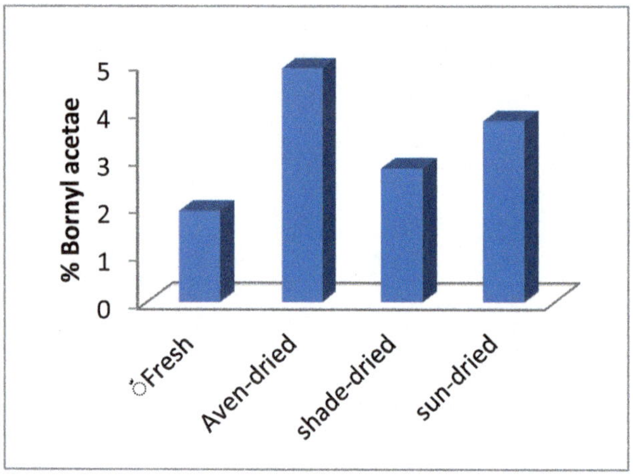

Fig. 6. Comparison Bornyl acetae of fresh sample and dry samples of the drying methods. (Significant different at $p < 0.05$ have been indicated with different letters.).

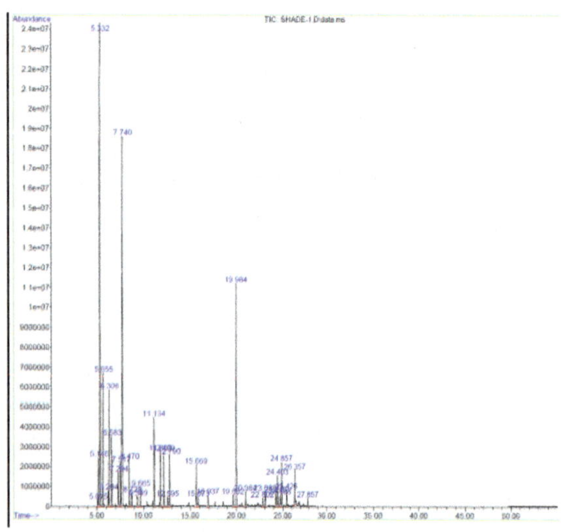

Fig. 7. Example of the chromatograms found in Shade-dried *S. hydrangea* samples.

3.1. Effect of drying methods on the essential oil composition

In general 33 components were identified in the essential oil of dried and fresh samples represented 86–96% of the oils. GC-Ms results showed that different drying methods had no effect on the main components of the oil but had a significant effect on their percentage. This result was in agreement with results of some studies on other essential oil-bearing plants (Omidbaigi *et al.,* 2004). In fresh aerial parts, the major components of the oil were 1,8-cineole (18.22%), α-pinene (15.58%), trans-caryophyllene (12.97%), camphore (5.34%) and camphene (4.60%). The main components of the oil of shade-dried aerial parts were α-pinene (18.4%), 1,8- cineole (18.08%), trans-caryophyllene (17.38%) and camphene (4.30%). The major components of the oil of sun-dried aerial parts were α-pinene (22.02%), 1,8-cineole (15.52%), trans-caryophyllene (10.13%), camphene (7.04%) and borneol (5.50%). The main components of the oil of oven-dried aerial parts were trans-caryophyllene (19.05%), α-pinene (16.88%), 1,8-cineole (11.38%), β-pinene (4.28%), borneol (3.68%) and camphore (3.51%). Therefore, the drying method caused some variation of the relative proportions of the components (Fig. 2-6).

Some studies (Hamrouni-Sellami *et al.,* 2011; Rahimmalek and Goli, 2013) showed presence of some components in essential oil of dried samples which were not present in essential oil of the fresh samples. Yuan and Zhezhi (2007) reported that different drying methods caused some variation of the relative proportions of the components in *Glechoma longituba* and the higher amount of germacrene D (19.0%) was obtained by shade-drying method. In the *Mentha longifolia* L. only oven drying caused significant losses of the major compounds (menthone, pulegone and 1,8-cineole) in essential oil when compared to the fresh samples (Asekun*et al.,* 2007). These variations in oil constituents can be related to formation of new compounds by oxidation, glycoside hydrolysis, esterification, and/or other processes (Diaz-Maroto*et al.,* 2004). Results of the present study showed that 1,8-Cineole was decreased in higher temperatures. Among medicinal and aromatic plants, the extensive decrease in the majority of essential oil constituents of dried samples at higher temperatures were reported in sage and thyme (Venskutonis, 1997) and basil (Yousif *et al.*, 1999). At high temperatures, the biological structure of the oil glands of medicinal and aromatic plants can be affected and subsequently the epithelial cells in the dried samples especially some sensible plants can collapse (Venskutonis, 1997). In the present study, trans-caryophyllene content increased at higher temperatures and oven drying at 65 °C led to higher amounts of trans-caryophyllene content in comparison to other drying methods. In other studies, thymol and β-caryophyllene contents increased at higher temperatures in essential oil of *Thymus vulgaris* L. and *Thymus daenensis* Celak. under different drying methods (Venskutonis, 1997; Rahimmalek and Goli, 2013).

Generally results showed that oven drying method had no effect on trans-caryophyllen, myrtenol, borneol, camphor, β-pinene, β-phellandrene and alpha-thujene compared to fresh sample. Sangwan *et al.* (2012) reported a non-significant difference ($p < 0.05$) in β-carotene, polyphenol and ascorbic acid contents of ginger powder prepared using different drying methods. Moreover, different drying methods do not influenced pyrethrins content of pyrethrum plants under customary drying conditions (Morris *et al.*, 2006). Overall, the results obtained from the present experiment and also reports of other researchers showed that there was a contradictory viewpoint on the effects of different drying methods on the essential oil profile of different plants.

4. Conclusion

Drying methods have a great importance in preparation of plants to extraction of essential oil and can affect the quantity and quality of essential oil. Higher drying temperature significantly reduced the essential oil obtained from aerial parts of *S. hydrangea*, especially when dried at 65°C. Thirty three components were identified in the essential oil of *S. hydrangea* which main constituents were α-pinene, 1,8- cineole and trans-caryophyllene. Significant differences were observed in the some volatile constituents as affected by drying methods. Finally, concerning the volatile oil content, it could be concluded that shade drying method is suitable for highest essential oil quantity and durability.

5. References

Adams, R.P. (2007). Identification of Essential Oil Components by Gas Chromatog-raphy/Quadrupole Mass Spectroscopy. Allured Publishing Corporation, CarolStream, IL, USA.

Ahmadi, K., Sefidkon, F. and Assareh, M. H. (2008). Effect of drying methods on quantity and quality of essential oil three genotype of *Rosa damascene* Mill. Iranian Journal of Medicinal and Aromatic Plant, 24(2),162-176.

Alziar, G. 1988–1993. Catalogue synonymique des Salvia L. du monde (Lamiaceae). I.–VI. BiocosmeMesogeen 5 (3–4): 87–136; 6 (1–2, 4): 79–115, 163–204; 7 (1–2): 59–109; 9 (2–3): 413–497; 10 (3–4): 33–117.

Asekun, O. T., Grierson, D. S., Afolayan, A. J. (2007). Effects of drying methods on the quality and quantity of the essential oil of *Menthalongifolia* L. subsp. *capensis*. Food Chemistry, 101(3), 995–998

Diaz-Maroto, M. C., Perez-Coello, M. S., Cabezudo, M. D. (2002). Effect of drying method on the volatiles in bay leaf (*Laurusnobilis* L.). Journal of Agricultural and Food Chemistry, 50(16): 4520–4524.

Diaz-Maroto, M. C., Perez-Coello, M. S., Vias, M. G., Cabezudo, M. D. (2003). Influence of drying on the flavor quality of spearmint (*Menthaspicata* L.). Journal of Agricultural and Food Chemistry, 51(5): 1265–1269.

Diaz-Maroto, M. C., Sanchez Palomo, E., Castro, L., Vias, G., Perez-Coello, M. S. (2004). Changes produced in the aroma compounds and structural integrity of basil (*Ocimumbasilicum* L.) during drying. Journal of the Science of Food and Agriculture, 84(15): 2070–2076.

Farimani, M.M., Bahadori, M.B., Taheri, S., Ebrahimi, S.N., Zimmermann, S., Brun, R., Amin, G., Hamburger, M. (2011). Triterpenoids with rare carbon skeletons from Salvia hydrangea: antiprotozoal activity and absolute configurations. Journal of Natural Products. 74: 2200- 2205.

GhasemiPirbalouti, A., Mahdad, E. and Craker, L., (2013a). Effects of drying methods on qualitative and quantitative properties of essential oil of two basil landraces. *Food Chemistry*., 141(3): 2440-2449.

GhasemiPirbalouti, A., Oraie, M., Pouriamehr, M., &Babadi, E. S. (2013b). Effects of drying methods on qualitative and quantitative of the essential oil of

Bakhtiari savory (*SaturejabachtiaricaBunge.*). *Industrial Crops and Products.*, 46, 324-327.

Hamrouni-Sellami, I., Wannes, W. A., Bettaieb, I., Berrima, S., Chahed, T., Marzouk, B., et al. (2011). Qualitative and quantitative changes in the essential oil of *Laurusnobilis* L. leaves as affected by different drying methods. Food Chemistry, 126(2): 691–697.

Morris, S.E., Davies, N.W., Brown, P.H., Groom, T. (2006). Effect of drying conditions on pyrethrins content. Industrial Crops and Products, 23: 9-14.

Omidbaigi, R., Sefidkon, F. and Kazem, F., (2004). Influence of drying methods on the essential oil content and composition of *Roman chamomile*. Flavor and Fragrance Journal. 19, 196-198.

Rahimmalek, M., &Goli, S. A. H. (2013). Evaluation of six drying treatments with respect to essential oil yield, composition and color characteristics of *Thymysdaenensis* subsp. *daenensis*Celak leaves. Industrial Crops and Products, 42, 613–619.

Rechinger, K.H. (Ed.), (1963–2005). Flora Iranica. Lfg. 1-176. Graz. AkademischeDrucku.-Verlagsanstalt. Graz.

Sangwan, A., Kawatra, A., Sehgal, S. (2012). Nutritional composition of gin-ger powder prepared using various drying methods. Journal of Food Science and Technology. 51(9): 2260-2262.

Venskutonis, P., (1997). Effect of drying on the volatile constituents of thym (*Thymus vulgaris* L.) and sage (*Salvia officinalis* L.). Food Chem. 59, 219–227.

Yousif, A.N., Scaman, C.H., Durance, T.D., Girard, B., (1999). Flavor volatiles and physical properties of vacuum-microwave- and air-dried sweet basil (*Ocimumbasilicum* L.). J. Agric. Food Chem. 47, 4777–4781.

Yuan, Z., Zhezhi, W. (2007). Influenced of drying methods on chemical composition of the essential oil of Glechoma longitude. Chemistry of Natural Compounds; 43 (5): 625-628.

Zhiming F., Hang W., Xiaofei H., Zhaolin S., Chunchao H. (2013). The Pharmacological Properties of Salvia Essential Oils, Journal of Applied Pharmaceutical Science. 3 (7): 122-127.

Traditional and local use of medicinal plants by local communities in Hezar Jerib summer area, north of Iran

Isa Jafari Footami[*1], **Moosa Akbarlou**[2]

[1]*Ph.D student of Gorgan University of agriculture and natural resources, Gorgan, Iran;*
***Email:** *Isa.jafari84@gmail.com*
[2]*Associate professor of Rangeland management, Gorgan University of agriculture and natural resources, Gorgan, Iran;*

ARTICLE INFO

Topic: *Medicinal Plants*

Key words:
- ✓ *Ethnobotany*
- ✓ *Traditional medicine*
- ✓ *Essential oil*
- ✓ *Hezar Jerib area*
- ✓ *Iran*

ABSTRACT

Background & Aim: Some knowledge about medicinal plants is available in old references or books. But important point is the information of traditional usage of medicinal plants from different parts of Iran will be worthwhile and in addition to encouraging people to it provides a good background for future examination about medicinal plants. The objectives of this study is to identify the medicinal plants along with local names, utilized parts, administration route, ailments treated, therapeutic effect and preparation methods.
Experimental: So to get this information, we use semi-structured interviews. This research was conducted in the summer and spring of 2016. During this period around 150 individuals (75 men, 75 women; in an age group between 20 and 95 years) were interviewed in 6 villages. Number of questions in this survey was 15 questions. Ethno botanical data were analyzed by use-reports. In addition important indices like Informant Agreement Ratio (IAR), Relative Frequency of Citation (RFC) and Cultural Importance (CI) were calculated. Furthermore, a traditional null hypothesis testing was adopted. These are the most popular indices in quantitative ethno botany.
Results: A total of 54 medicinal plants belonging to 22 families were identified. The most common families are Lamiaceae, Asteraceae, Apiaceae and Rosaceae, with 22, 17, 5 and 4%, respectively. The most common preparations methods were infusion (52%), eaten raw and decoction (13%). Also, between different parts of the plant, the leaves are mostly used. According to RFC and CI indices, the most important plant is *Gallium verum*. Nervous disease has the highest Informant Consensus Factor value with the rate of 0.80.
Recommended applications/industries: Introduction of medicinal plants in each region, along with their use can be a great help to create jobs and Encouraging people to cultivate these plants.

1. Introduction

Ethnobotanical studies are very important to tell the past and present culture about plants in the world (Bulut & Tuzlaci, 2013). About 80% of human in the world use plants to treat several diseases (UICN, OMS, WWF, 1993). Medicinal plants were main source of treatment but now, after advances in medical science, they are an important source of current drugs and around 25 % of the drugs prescribed worldwide come from plants (Rates, 2001). Tetik *et al.,* (2013), Communities like, Ayurvedic, Kampo, Unani, Jamu, Iranian, Aztec are known as prominent examples of ethnobotany in medicinal plants. However, in unknown communities, there are not historical document in Traditional knowledge of medicinal plants, so our information is based on investigators efforts to document these knowledge (Heinrich, 2010).

In rural and poor societies, the use of medicinal plants is a valuable resource and necessity, and furthermore they provide some real alternatives for primary health care systems (Hayta *et al.*, 2014). According to WHO, the international market of herbal products is estimated to be US $62 billion which is poised to grow to US $5 trillion by the year 2050 (WHO, 2002).

Historical document illustrate the fact that Iranian have depth knowledge in using the medicinal plants (Zargari, 1989–1992). Khajoei Nasab & Khosravi (2014) concluded that Lamiaceae is the largest family that is used to treat various ailments and these plants are often used as decoction.

Ethnobotanical surveys were done in the Turkmens of Golestan and Khorasan Province for the first time and in this study, 136 species from 51 families were documented by Ghorbani (2005). After that, several researchers conducted survey about medicinal plants in other parts of the country (Ghollassimood, 2008; Dolat khahi *et al.*, 2010; Iran manesh, 2010; Sharifi far *et al.*, 2010; Mosaddegh *et al.,* 2012; Safa *et al.*,2013). Naghibi *et al.,* (2005) represented 46 genus and 410 species from Labiatae family in Iran that many members of this family were used in traditional and folk medicine.

Naghibi *et al.*, (2014), fulfilled their research by semi-structured interview and concluded that Asteraceae and Fabaceae were the dominant locally used families. Mosaddegh *et al.* (2016), conducted a study in the highland of Alvand and Tuyserkan, and concluded that the most treated ailments were digestive problems and *Stachys lavandulifolia* and Thymus *lancifolius* have the highest indices of RFC and CI.

Although the present study is not the first ethnobotanical survey in Hezar Jerib area, but there are gaps in ethnobotanical knowledge in this region. The aim of this study is to document and investigate the traditional use of medicinal plants by local people and keeping this type of information in mind and Databases to study further on the other applications of plants, this study was conducted from December 2014 to September 2015. According to the gathered information from local people, there were more medicinal plants in Hezar Jerib region which extinct due to Land Use change and excessive harvesting and this study seems to be useful in identifying the helpful plants and keeping their records for the future investigations.

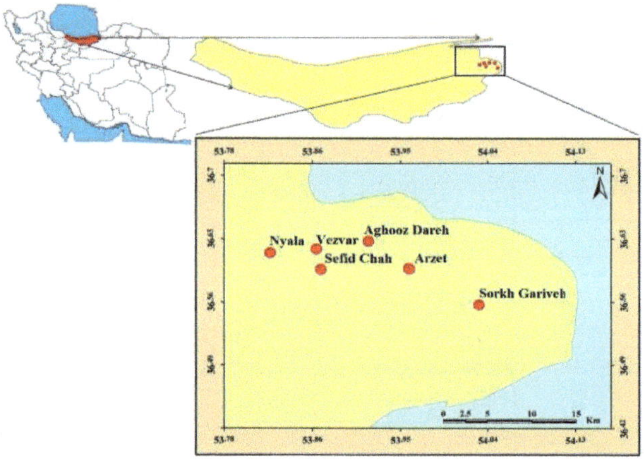

Fig. 1. Map of Iran showing Mazandaran Province and Hezar Jerib Summer area

2. Materials and Methods

2.1. Study area

Hezar Jerib district consists of 6 villages, encompasses an area of 14528 ha, and has a total population of 11017 inhabitants. Hezar Jerib Summer Rangeland is located (36°24'18"– 36°34'22" N, 53°58'16"– 54°03'48" E) in the North part of Iran and Its altitudinal range is between 1600-2800 MASL, and Including; Nyala, Vezvar, Sefid Chah, Aghooz Dareh, Arzet, Sorkh Geriveh villages (Fig. 1). Hezar Jerib

Summer Rangeland has a semi-arid climate with dry and cold winter and moderate and dry summer. The average annual temperature, average humidity and average rainfall in this city are about 12.44 ° C, 185 mm and 383 mm, respectively. Soil pH is about 7.

2.2. Field survey and data collection

In our study, we used semi-structured interviews (Rehecho *et al.,* 2011) in order to collect information about how they use medicinal plants, and for which disease treatment. During this period (about 8 months) around 150 individuals (75 men, 75 women; in an age group between 20 and 95 years) were interviewed in 6 villages. Interviewees were shepherds, Farmers and other people, also we asked detailed questions on medicinal uses of plants in places like farmlands, gardens and Mosques. Interviews and questionnaires in this study continued until the duplicate answers were heard, and then the interview would not add a new point to the notes. During the interviews, demographic characteristics of the study participants, and local names, utilized parts, administration route and preparation methods of the plants were recorded. In this study, Use report, Number of use, Frequency of Citation, Relative frequency of citation and Cultural Importance Index were recorded for each plant.

2.3. Data analysis

Indices such as IAR, RFC and CI which are the most popular indices in quantitative ethno botany (Albuquerque & Lucena, 2005) were used in this study. Informant consensus factor was calculated according to the following formula (Trotter & Logan, 1986):

$$IAR = \frac{NUR - NT}{NUR - 1}$$

Nur and NT indicate the number of use reports for each ailment and the number of species that are used, respectively. IAR value ranges from 0 to 1.1 indicates more informants use the same species for treatment of the same diseases while 0 indicates informants do not exchange information about their use (Inta *et al.,* 2013).

Relative Frequency of Citation (RFC) calculated by the following formula: FC is the number of informants mentioning the use of the species and N is the total number of informants (Tardio & Santayana, 2008):

$$RFC = \frac{FC}{N}$$

The Cultural Importance Index (CI), calculated by the following formula (Tardio and Santayana, 2008). This index is based on diversity of use.

$$CI = \sum_{u=u1}^{uNC} \sum_{i=i1}^{iN} URui/_N$$

3. Results and discussion

150 people were interviewed in this survey and 54 specimens belonging to 22 families were collected in the research area. The experiences of the study participants were recorded during the interviews. Information about the local names of the plants, their uses and parts of the plants that used to treat ailment are listed in table 1.

Most of the medicinal plants used in this area belong to the Lamiaceae with 15 species and the most commonly used plant species are *Achillea* and *Apium* with 3 species (Fig. 2). Hosseini *et al.,* (2009) conducted a similar study in Golestan province and Stated that Lamiaceae have highest number of medicinal plants species that used by local people.

Other researchers such as Dolatkhahi *et al.,* (2010), Mosaddegh *et al.,* (2012-2016), Safa *et al.,* (2013), Rajaei *et al.,* (2012), Sharififar *et al.,* (2014) and Naghibi *et al.,* (2014) indicated Asteraceae and Lamiaceae were the most used families.

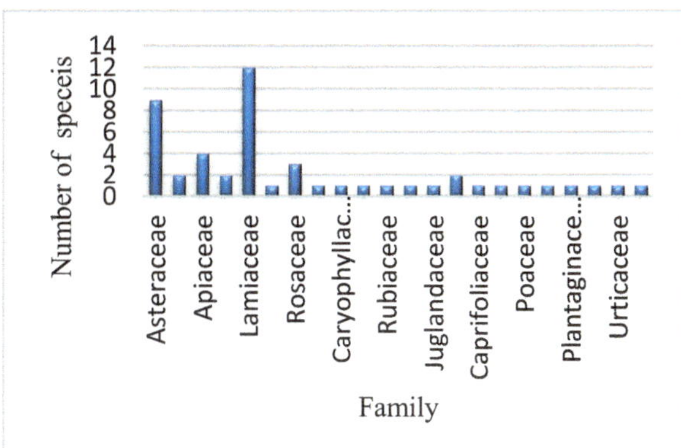

Fig. 2. The Number of medicinal species in each family

Table1. Folk medicinal plants of Hezar Jerib area

Family/botanical name/ voucher number	Local name	Plant part used	Preparation	Administration route	Ailments treated, therapeutic effect
Asteraceae *Achillea wilhelmsii* C. Koch HJ-101	Bomadaran alborzi	Flowering branches	Infusion	Oral	flatulence, carminative, pyretic
Asteraceae *Achillea biebersteinii* Afan HJ-102	Bomadaran (Parcham javan)	Flowering branches	Infusion	Oral	flatulence, stomachache and skin wound healer
Asteraceae *Achillea millefolium* L. HJ-103	Bomadaran	Flowering branches	Infusion	Oral	Carminative, Cold, expectorant, Urinary tract
Asteraceae *Anthemis persica* Boiss. HJ-107	Babooneh	Flowers	Infusion	Oral	Increased immunity, expectorant
Asteraceae *Artemisia vulgaris* L. HJ-109	Darmaneh	Leaves, Flowering branches	Infusion	Oral	Appetizer, digestion, regulate menstruation and disinfectants.
Asteraceae *Artemisia annua* L. HJ-110	Darmaneh (Gandevash)	Young branches	New water plant, Leaf poultice	Oral	Relieve Children ear pain and leg pain
Asteraceae *Cichorium intybus* L. HJ-113	Kasni	Root	Infusion, Poultice	Oral	Disinfection of the digestive system
Asteraceae *Tanacetum parthenium* (L.) Sch.Bip. HJ-144	Babooneh	Leaves, Flowers	Infusion, Decoction	Oral, Inhalation	Nourishing effect, stomach tonic, convulsion, diarrhea, Febrifuge, disinfectants
Asteraceae *Traxacum vulgare* (Lam.) Scrk HJ-145	kangar	Aerial parts, Roots	Infusion, Decoction	Oral	Blood purifier
Apiaceae *Apium graveolens* Cham. HJ-108	Karafs koohi	Leaves	Eaten raw	Oral	Febrifuge
Amaryllidaceae *Allium paradoxum* (M.Bieb.) G.Don HJ-104	Piaz zangulehi	Fruit	Eaten raw	Oral	Regulators of cholesterol and high blood fats, Power increasing for body and digestive system and circulatory system
Amaryllidaceae *Allium Akaka* S.G.Gmel. ex Schult. & Schult.f. HJ-105	Piaz zangulehi (Elleh zi)	Bulbs and Leaves	The leaves are crushed	Oral	Blood purifier, Blood pressure
Amaryllidaceae *Allium sativum* L. HJ-106	Piaz zangulehi	Bulbs and Leaves	Eaten raw, Decoction	Oral	Blood cholesterol, digesting food, regulating the digestive system

Apiaceae *Eryngium caucasicum* Trautv HJ-121	Zoleng (Sisketeli)	leaves	Eaten raw	Oral	Pain killers, appetizer
Apiaceae *Ferula persica* Willd. HJ-122	Barijeh (Ashteghaz)	Gum and resin	latex	Topical	expectorant, spasmodic, carminative
Apiaceae *Heracleum persicum* Desf. HJ-125	Golpar (Kolek par)	leaves, Seed	Decoction, Infusion	Inhalation	Diuretic
Berberidaceae *Berberis vulgaris* L. HJ-112	Zereshk	Root, Shoot, Leaves, flower, Fruit	Eaten raw, Dry plant, Decoction, Infusion	Oral	Febrifuge and laxative
Brassicaceae *Descurainia Sophia* (L,) Schur HJ-118	Khakeshir	Seed	Infusion	Oral	Febrifuge, constipation, sunstroke
Boraginaceae *Echium amoenum* Fisch. & Mey. HJ-120	Gol gavzaban (Eshko)	Flowers	Infusion	Oral	Stress pressure, expectorant, Febrifuge
Caryophyllaceae *Dianthus orientalis* Adams HJ-119	Mikhak	Bud	Infusion, Additive to foods and eaten raw	Oral, Inhalation	Headache, asthma, liver and kidney, Hiccup and appetizing
Caprifoliaceae *Lonicera floribunda Boiss et Buhse* HJ-131	Pich aminodole (Peche)	Leaves, Flowers, stem skin	Fruit, Leaves, Flower	Oral	Constipation, Bronchitis, Flu
Cornaceae *Cornus australis* C.A.Mey. HJ-115	Zoghal Akhteh	Fruit and stem skin	Eaten raw	Oral	Febrifuge
Cupressaceae *Juniperus communis* L. HJ-128	Ors (balesh khers)	Leaves, fruits, Twigs and wood	Decoction, Infusion	Oral	Blood purifier, Diuretic
Cupressaceae *Juniperus Sabina* L. HJ-129	Ors (May maraz)	Leaves, fruits, Twigs	Leaves and Fruits are crushed	Inhalation	Wart
Guttiferae *Hypericum perforatum* L. HJ-126	Metameti	Flowering branches	Infusion	Oral	Stress pressure
Juglandaceae *Juglans regia* L. HJ-127	Gerdo	Leaves, Fruits	Infusion	Oral, Inhalation	Diabetes, Hair protects, Lipid-lowering
Lamiaceae *Mentha persica* Benth. HJ-135	Pooneh (petenek)	Leaves	Infusion	Oral	flatulence, Stomachache
Lamiaceae *Nepeta pungens* (Bunge.) Benth HJ-137	Naana	Flowers	Decoction, Infusion, Waiting in olive oil	Oral	Stress pressure

Lamiaceae *Nepeta cataria* L. HJ-138	Naana	Leaves	Infusion	Oral	Cold, Antipyretic
Lamiaceae *Origanum vulgare* L. HJ-139	Marzanjoosh, Mardghoosh	Aerial parts	Infusion, Gargle	Oral, Inhalation	Appetite stimulants, painkillers, cough and pertussis, asthma and nerve pain, convulsion
Lamiaceae *Salvia sclarea* L. HJ-141	Mayam goli	Leaves	Infusion	Oral	Energy Provider
Lamiaceae *Stachys lavandulaefolia* Vahl HJ-142	Chai koohi	leaves	Infusion	Oral	flatulence, Headaches, Cough,
Lamiaceae *Stachys laxa* Boiss. & Buhse HJ-143	Chai koohi	leaves	Infusion	Oral	Fever and sedatives
Lamiaceae *Teucrium chamaedrys* L HJ-145	Maryam nekhodi (Hizvash alaf)	Young branches	Infusion	Oral	Help for digestion, Relieve constipation
Lamiaceae *Teucrium polium* L. HJ-146	Maryam nekhodi (Hizvash alaf)	Flowering branches	Incense, Infusion, crushed	Oral, Inhalation	Antiseptic, analgesic and inflammation, jaundice, Diabetes
Lamiaceae *Thymus kotschyanus* Boiss. & Hohen. HJ-147	Avishan (oshmak)	leaves	Infusion	Oral	flatulence, expectorant,, cough, headaches and nerve stimulation
Lamiaceae *Ziziphora sp.* HJ-150	Kakooti (Chai choopan)	Inflorescence	Infusion	Oral	Stress pressure
Malvaceae *Malva neglecta* Wallr. HJ-132	Panirak (Melki, Anchelek)	Leaves	Infusion	Oral	Diabetes and high blood pressure
Poaceae *Melica persica Kunth.* HJ-134	Baderanj booye (varengeboo)	Leaves	Infusion	Oral	Stress pressure, heart disease, Gastrointestinal and exhilarating
Plantaginaceae *Plantago lanceolate* L. HJ-141	Barhang koohi (Bartang)	Seeds, Leaves	Infusion	Topical	Cramps
Polygonaceae *Polygonum sp.* HJ-140	Haft band	Aerial parts	Powder, Infusion	Topical	Soothing contusion, Blisters and scorch, Purulent wounds
Rosaceae *Fragria vesca* L. HJ-123	Toot Franagi vahsi	Fruits, leaves and roots	Raw, decoction, jams, syrup	Oral	Diarrhea and diuretic

			and ice cream		
Rubiaceae *Gallium verum* L. HJ-124	Piyaz	Flowering plants, roots	Infusion	Topical, Oral	Diuretic, Nutritious, blood purifier, Anti-toxins, sedative, astringent, Anti-convulsion
Rosaceae *Mespilus germanica* L. HJ-136	Azgil	Fruits, leaves, and stem skin	Infusion, Marinated	Oral	Diarrhea, Diabetes, Vomit
Urticaceae *Urtica diocia* L. HJ-149	Gazaneh	Shoot, roots, seeds	Decoction, Infusion, vapors	Oral	kidney stones, Febrifuge, hypoglycemic, blood pressure
Violaceae *Viola odorata* L. HJ-148	Banafsheh	Flowers, leaves, roots and seeds	Infusion	Oral, Inhalation	Insomnia, cough, asthma and bronchitis
Zygophyllaceae *Peganum harmala* L. HJ-140	Espand	Flowers, Seeds, Stems, Leaves	Leaves and Fruits are crushed	Inhalation	Hypnotics

Table 3. Species ranking based on each index.

Scientific name	Family name	RFC ranking	CI ranking
Gallium verum	Rubiaceae	1	1
Thymus kotschyanus	Lamiaceae	1	2
Achillea wilhelmsii C. Koch	Asteraceae	1	3
Ziziphora sp.	Lamiaceae	1	4
Mespilus germanica L.	Rosaceae	1	4
Achillea biebersteinii	Asteraceae	1	4
Achillea millefolium	Asteraceae	1	5
Allium Akaka	Amaryllidaceae	1	5
Apium graveolens	Apiaceae	1	5
Dianthus orientalis	Caryophyllaceae	1	6
Echium amoenum Fisch. & Mey.	Boraginaceae	1	6
Eryngium caucasicum Trautv	Apiaceae	1	6
Hypericum perforatum	Guttiferae	1	7
Lonicera floribunda Boiss et Buhse	Caprifoliaceae	1	7
Mentha longifolia	Lamiaceae	1	8
Nepeta cataria	Lamiaceae	1	9
Traxacum vulgare (Lam.) Scrk	Asteraceae	1	10
Anthemis persica	Asteraceae	2	10
Berberis integerima	Berberidaceae	2	11

Cornus australis	Cornaceae	2	12
Cydonia Ablonga Mill.	Rosaceae	2	13
Ferula persica	Apiaceae	2	13
Fragria vesca	Rosaceae	2	13
Heracleum persicum Desf.	Apiaceae	2	13
Juglans redia L.	Juglandaceae	2	14
Juniperus communis	Cupressaceae	2	15
Mentha persica Benth.	Lamiaceae	2	16
Nepeta pungens (Bunge.) Benth	Lamiaceae	2	17
Plantago lanceolate	Plantaginaceae	2	18
Polygonum sp.	Polygonaceae	2	19
Stachys laxa	Lamiaceae	2	19
Teucrium polium	Lamiaceae	2	19
Urtica diocia	Urticaceae	2	20
Allium paradoxum	Amaryllidaceae	3	20
Allium sativum	Amaryllidaceae	3	20
Berberis vulgaris	Berberidaceae	3	21
Crataegus microphylla c. Koch	Rosaceae	3	21
Juniperus Sabina	Cupressaceae	3	22
Lamium album (Lam)	Lamiaceae	3	23
Malva neglecta	Malvaceae	3	23
Origanum vulgare	Lamiaceae	3	24
Peganum harmala	Zygophyllaceae	3	25
Stachys lavandulaefolia	Lamiaceae	3	26
Cichorium intybus L.	Asteraceae	4	27
Calamintha grandiflora	Lamiaceae	4	27
Descurainia Sophia (L,) Schur	Brassicaceae	4	27
Marrubium vulgare	Lamiaceae	4	27
Melica persica Kunth.	Poaceae	4	27
Salvia sclarea L.	Lamiaceae	4	27
Tanacetum parthenium	Asteraceae	4	27
Teucrium chamaedrys L	Lamiaceae	4	27
Viola odorata	Violaceae	4	27
Artemisia vulgaris	Asteraceae	5	27
Artemisia annua L,	Asteraceae	5	27

Table 2. IAR values of category of ailments.

No	Ailments	IAR
1	Endocrine, nutritional and metabolic diseases	0.50
2	Diabetes	0.73
3	Urinary disease	0.62
4	Respiratory disease	0.60
5	Cardiovascular disease	0.66
6	Cold	0.62
7	Nervous disease	0.80
8	Gastrointestinal disease	0.62

3.1. Utilization method

The preparation methods are presented in Fig. 3. There are many approaches in the use of medicinal plants, based on the type of plant and the type of pains; most common preparations were decoction, eaten raw and infusion.

Local people were recorded to make medicinal preparations by using wild plants for curative purposes via simple methods. The most frequently reported mode is infusion (52%) followed by decoction and eaten raw (13%). Dry mode (6%) is in fourth place and people use it in cold seasons. Naghibi *et al.,* (2014) indicated that decoction is the most common utilization methods in Hamedan. Mosaddegh *et al.,* (2016) reported that infusion and decoction are the most method of preparation in Alvand and Tuyserkan.

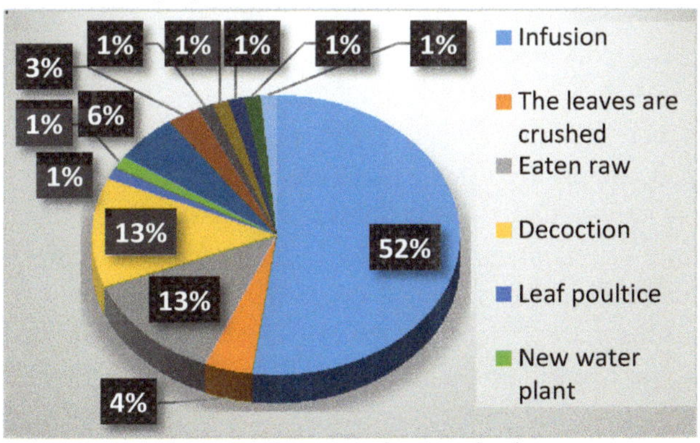

Fig. 3. Percentage of preparation methods.

3.2. Plant parts used as medicine

Informants were recorded to use the aerial parts, branches, bulb, inflorescence, flowers, fruits, gum, latex, resin, leaves, roots, seeds, bud, bark, flowering branches, twigs and woods of plants. Results showed that the most common parts of plants are their leaves (34%) (Fig. 4), and this is admitted by many ethnobotanical studies conducted elsewhere in Iran showed the dominance of leaves in the preparation of medicine.

Ghorbani *et al.,* (2005) conducted a study in Turkman sahra region, Iran, say leaves are dominant. The reasons is that because of their easily accessible, contain more easily extractable phytochemicals. Naghibi *et al.,* (2014) conducted similar study like our survey and their result showed that leaves are used more than other parts and their reason was accumulation of tannins and alkaloids in leaves. Hosseini *et al.,* (2009) showed leaves are used more than other parts.

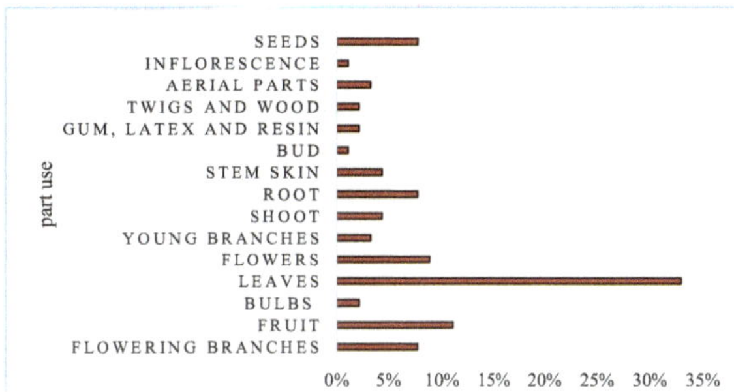

Fig. 4. Parts of the plants that commonly used (%).

The ailments of headache, stomachache upset, stress pressure, diarrhea, diabetes and cough are treated by using these plants (Table 1). Almost all of the species have more than one pharmaceutical properties.

3.3. Some medicinal plants and literature review

In the present study, *Urtica dioica* was mentioned to be used in treatment of kidney stones, fever-lowering, hypoglycemic, blood pressure. Other studies mention different diseases that treat by *Urtica dioica* such as analgesic and antimicrobial and anti-hyperglycemic activity (Bnouham *et al.*, 2003; Gülçin *et al.*, 2004), bronchitis, cardiovascular disease, cough, diabetes, respiratory disease and tonsillitis (Hayta *et al.*, 2014).

Teucrium polium is traditionally used in Hezar Jerib area to Antiseptic, analgesic and inflammation. There are many other uses for this species, antipyretic and intestinal motility activities (Autore *et al.*, 1984; Yaniv *et al.*, 1987; Gharaibeh *et al.*, 1988; Suleiman *et al.*, 1988; Hayta *et al.*, 2014).

There are many studies in other countries which they results are the same as the result of current study: *Achillea wilhelmsii* (Antihypertensive and hypolipidemic) (Asgary *et al*., 2000), *Allium sativum* (antibacterial activity) (Sokmen *et al.,* 1999), *Artemisia vulgaris* (hepatoprotective activity (Gilani *et al*., 2005), *Malva neglecta* (Antioxidant activity and anti-ulcer genic activity) (Gürbüz *et al*., 2005; Dalar *et al*., 2012), *Plantago lanceolate* (antioxidant activity) (Dalar *et al*., 2012).

3.4. IAR, RFC, CI calculations

Diseases that can be treated by plants sorted into 8 groups. The IAR values are presented in the Table2. It is clear that the ICF values range between 0.50 and 0.80. Nervous disease has the highest IAR value with the rate of 0.80. Diabetes and cardiovascular disease had rather high IAR value as 0.73 and 0.66, respectively, while cold, urinary disease and gastrointestinal disease had the same amount of IAR value as 0.62. Endocrine, nutritional and metabolic diseases were lowest IAR value as 0.50.

In some ethnobotanical survey, similar to this study, reported of ethnobotanical study in Kohghiluyeh and Boyer Ahmad Province in Iran, IAR of respiratory disease is 0.032 (Mosaddegh *et al.,* 2012) but in this study is 0.60 and its mean that the more frequent usage of herbal remedies by local people for Respiratory disease compared to other use categories.

Juárez-Vázquez *et al.,* (2013) result showed that diseases of the respiratory system had the highest 0.92 IAR but does not match with our study.

3.5. RFC and CI value

These indices will help better understanding of the traditional knowledge of plants used by local people in one area. As shown in Table 3, 32% (about 17 species) of the species studied have relative frequency of citation one (RFC = 1). It means these species are more popular plants in area. *Artemisia annua* and *Artemisia vulgaris* have the lowest number of citations and thus a few number of informants believed that these are useful species (Table 3).

A comparison between the RFC and the CI indices is shown in table 3. *Gallium verum* is placed in the first position by RFC and CI indices. Also, because of the highest values of CI index, this species has the most diverse uses. *Thymus kotschyanus* and *Achillea wilhelmsii* which were ranked first by RFC index, were ranked second and third by CI index, respectively. Based on Heinrich's view, the culturally important plants are those that are used by a large number of people for the same category of use (Heinrich *et al*., 1998).

4. Conclusion

Most commonly used plants are *Gallium verum*, *Thymus kotschyanus*, *Achillea wilhelmsii*, *Ziziphora sp*., *Mespilus germanica*, *Urtica diocia* and *Allium Akaka*. Most commonly used parts of the plants were the leaves (34%), fruits (12%) and flowers (9%). These results are similar to Hosseini *et al.,* (2009). They showed that leaves are the most commonly used parts in Golestan province. Differ from those of in Malatya, Turkey, Tetik *et al,* (2013) reported that most commonly used plants are *Anthemis* sp., *Armeniaca vulgaris*, *Crataegus* sp., *Juglans regia*, *Mentha* sp., *Malva neglecta*, *Plantago* sp., *Rosa canina*, *Rubus sanctus* and *Urtica dioica* and most commonly used parts of the plants were the leaves (42%), flowers (29%) and aerial parts (20%). But Naghibi *et al.,* (2012) concluded that aerial part is the used more.

Many plants are used for the treatment of asthma, diabetes, cardiovascular disorders, colds, expectorant, diabetes, gastric diseases, urinary diseases, respiratory, and throat diseases etc. Literature review showed that curative plants of Hezar Jerib are used in different countries in the treatment of similar diseases. Due to weather condition, most of plant became vanish in winter and fall so they have to collect medicinal plants in summer and spring, to use them during the year. Our interviews revealed that in the study area, plants are still commonly used for medicinal purposes by people in their daily lives.

Most of scientists believe that our ancestors used more medicinal plants than now but now days due to changes in the environment and life conditions and also expansion of modern care system, use of nature to treat diseases lost its position. For example, some youngsters didn't know that how use plants and or even name of indigenous plants.

Like other parts of Iran (Khajoei Nasab *et al.*, 2014; Mosaddegh *et al.*, 2012 and Gorbani, 2005), women information about medicinal plants are higher than men. In Kerman, Kohghiluyeh va Boyer Ahmad Province and Turkman sahra, the majority of informants were women. Studies regarding the medicinal plant used by current indigenous populations will upgrade traditional medicine and plant uses, as well as the integration of modern and traditional medicine. However, it is necessary to formulate policies for biodiversity conservation, sustainable management and community development.

5. References

Albuquerque, U.P., Lucena, R.F.P. 2005. Can appetency affect the use of plants by local people in tropical forests? Interciencia, 30: 506–511.

Asgary, S., Naderi, G.H., Sarrafzadegan, N., Mohammadifard, N., Mostafavi, S., Vakili, R. 2000. Antihypertensive and anti-hyperlipidemia effects of Achillea wilhelmsii. Drugs under Experimental and Clinical Research, 26: 89–93.

Autore, G., Capasso, F., De Fusco, R., Fasulo, M.P., Lembo, M., Mascolo, N., Menghini, A. 1984. Antipyretic and antibacterial actions of Teucrium polium (L.). Pharma-cological Research Communications, 16: 21–29.

Bnouham, M., Merhfour, F.M., Ziyyat, A., Mekhfi, H., Aziz, M., Legssyer, A. 2003. Antihyperglycemic activity of the aqueous extract of Urtica dioica. Fitoterapia, 74: 677–681.

Bulut, G., Tuzlaci, E. 2013. An ethnobotanical study of medicinal plants in Turgutlu (Manisa-Turkey). Journal of Ethnopharmacology. 149(3): 633-47.

Cakilcioglu, U., Turkoglu, I., 2010. An ethnobotanical survey of medicinal plants in Sivrice (Elazığ-Turkey). Journal of Ethnopharmacology. 132(1): 165–175.

Dalar, A., Türker, M., Konczak, I., 2012. Antioxidant capacity and phenolic consti-tuents of Malva neglecta Wallr. and Plantago lanceolata L. from Eastern Anatolia Region of Turkey. Journal of Herbal Medicine. 2: 42–51.

Dolatkhahi, M., Yousofi, M., Bagher nejad, J., 2010. Dolatkhahi A. Introductory study of the medicinal plants species of Kazeroon in Fars Province. Journal of Herbal Medicine. 3: 47-56.

Estrada, E., Villarreal, J.A., Cantú, C., Cabral, I., Scott, L., Yen, C., 2007. Ethnobotany in the Cumbres de Monterrey National Park, Nuevo León, México. Journal of Ethnobiology and Ethnomedicine. 3: 8–15.

Farooq, S., Barki, A., Yousaf Khan, M., Fazal, H. 2012. Ethnobotanical studies of the flora of Tehsil Birmal in South Wazirestan Agency, Pakistan. Pakistan journal of weed science research. 18: 277-291. (In Persian).

Gharaibeh, M.N., Elayan, H.H., Salhab, A.S., 1988. Hypoglycemic effects of Teucrium polium. Journal of Ethnopharmacology. Vol. 24: 93–99.

Ghollassimood, S. 2008. A contribution to some ethnobotanical aspects of Birjand flora (Iran). Pakistan Journal of Botany. Vol. 40: 1783–1791.

Ghorbani, A., 2005. Studies on pharmaceutical ethnobotany in the region of Turkmen Sahra, north of Iran (Part 1): general results. Journal of Ethnopharmacology. 102: 58–68. (In Persian).

Ghorbani, A., Longaberger, G., Feng, L., Sauerborn, J., 2011. Ethnobotanical study of medicinal plants utilized by Hani ethnicity in Naban River Watershed National Nature Reserve, Yunnan, China. Journal of Ethnopharmacology. 134: 651–667.

Gilani, A.H., Yaeesh, S., Jamal, Q., Ghayur, M., 2005. Hepatoprotective activity of aqueous-methanol extract of Artemisia vulgaris. Phytotherapy Research, 19: 170–172. (In Persian).

Gülçin, İ., Küfrevioğlu, O.I,, Oktay, M., Büyükokuroğlu, M.E., 2004. Antioxidant, antimicrobial, antiulcer and analgesic activities of nettle (Urtica dioica L.). Journal of Ethnopharmacology. 90: 205–215.

Gürbüz, I., Özkan, A.M., Yeşilada, E., Kutsal, O., 2005. Anti-ulcerogenic activity of some plants used in folk medicine of Pinarbasi (Kayseri, Turkey). Journal of Ethnopharmacology. 101: 313–318.

Gurdal, B., Kulturn, S., 2013. An ethnobotanical study of medicinal plants in Marmaris (Mugla, Turkey). Journal of Ethnopharmacology. 146; 113–126.

Hayta, S., Polat, R., Selvi, S., 2014. Traditional uses of medicinal plants in Elazığ (Turkey). Journal of Ethnopharmacology. 154: 613–623.

Heinrich, M., 2010. Ethno pharmacology in the 21st century – grand challenges. Frontiers in Pharmacology.1: 8-15.

Heinrich M, Ankli A, Frei B, Wiemann, C., Sticher, O., 1998. Medicinal plants in Mexico: healer's consensus and cultural importance. Social Science and Medicine, 47: 1859–1871.

Hosseini, S.A., Abarsaji, G.h., Hossaini, S.A., 2009. Medicinal plants of Golestan province. Iranian Journal of Medicinal Aromatic Plants. 24(4): 472-499.

Inta, A., Trisonthi, P., Trisonthi, C., 2013. Analysis of traditional knowledge in medicinal plants used by Yuanin Thailand. Journal of Ethnopharmacology. 149(1): 344–351.

Iranmanesh, M., Najafi, S.H., Yousofi, M., 2010. Ethnobotany survey of medicinal plant of Sistan region. Journal of Herbal Drugs. 2: 61-68.

Khajoei Nasab, F., Khosravi, A.R. 2014. Ethnobotanical study of medicinal plants of Sirjan in Kerman Province, Iran. Journal of Ethnopharmacology. 154(1): 190-197.

Mosaddegh, M., Naghibi, F., Moazzeni, H., Pirani, A., Esmaeili, S., 2012. Ethnobotanical survey of herbal remedies traditionally used in Kohghiluyeh va Boyer Ahmad province of Iran. Journal of Ethnopharmacology. 141(1): 80-95.

Mosaddegh, M., Esmaeili, S., Hassanpour, A., Malekmohammadi, M., Naghibi, F., 2016. Ethnobotanical study in the highland of Alvand and Tuyserkan, Iran. Iranian Journal of Pharmaceutical Research. 3(1): 7-17.

Naghibi, F., Mosaddegh, M., Mohammadi Motamed, S., Ghorbani, A., 2005, Labiatae family in folk medicine in Iran: from ethnobotany to pharmacology. Iranian Journal of Pharmaceutical Research. 2: 63-79.

Naghibi, F., Esmaeili, S., Malekmohammadi, M., Hassanpour, A., Mosaddegh, M., 2014. Ethnobotanical survey of medicinal plants used traditionally in two villages of Hamedan, Iran, Iranian Journal of Pharmaceutical Research. 1(3): 7-14.

Rates, S.M.K., 2001. Plants as source of drugs. Toxicon, 39: 603–613.

Rajaei, P., Mohamadi, N., 2012. Hezar Mountain allocated in south east of Iran. Journal of Ethnopharmacology. 11(4): 1153-1167.

Rehecho, S., Uriarte-Pueyo, I., Calvo, J., Vivas, L.A,, Calvo, M.I., 2011. Ethno pharmacological survey of medicinal plants in Nor-Yauyos, a part of the Landscape Reserve Nor-Yauyos-Cochas, Peru. Journal of Ethnopharmacology. 133: 75–85.

Sharififar, F., Moharam-Khani, M.R., Moattar, F., Babakhanloo, P., Khodami, M., 2014. Ethnobotanical study of medicinal plants of Joopar Mountains of Kerman province, Iran. Journal of Kerman University of Medical Sciences, 21(1): 37-51.

Sadeghi, Z., Kouhestani, K., Abdollahi, V., 2014. Mahmood A. Ethno pharmacological studies of Indigenous medicinal plants of Saravan region, Baluchistan, Iran. Journal of Ethnopharmacology.153(1): 111-118.

Safa, O., Soltanipoor, M.A., Rastegar, S., Kazemi, M., Nourbakhsh Dehkordi, K.H., Ghannadi, A. 2013. An Ethnobotanical survey on Hormozgan Province, Iran. *Avicenna Journal of Phytomedicine.* 3: 64-81.

Sharififar, F., Koohpayeh, A., Motaghi, M.M., Amirkhosravi, A., Puormohseni Nasab, E., Khodashenas, M., 2010. Study the ethnobotany of medicinal plants in Sirjan, Kerman Province, Iran. *Journal of Herbal Drugs*. 3: 19-28.

Sokmen, A., Jones, B.M., Erturk, M., 1999. The in vitro antibacterial activity of Turkish medicinal plants. Journal of Ethnopharmacology. 67: 79–86.

Suleiman, M.S., Abdul-Ghani, A.S., Al-Khalil, S., Amin, R., 1988. Effect of Teucrium polium boiled leaf extract on intestinal motility and blood pressure. Journal of Ethnopharmacology. 22: 111–116.

Tardio, J., Pardo-de Santayana, M., 2008. Cultural importance indices: a comparative analysis based on the useful wild plants of southern Cantabria (northern Spain).Economic Botany, 62: 24–39.

Tetik, F., Civelek, S., Cakilcioglu, U., 2013. Traditional uses of some medicinal plants in Malatya (Turkey). Journal of Ethnopharmacology. 146: 331–346.

Trotter, R.T., Logan, M.H.,1986. Informant consensus: a new approach for identifying potentially effective medicinal plants. In: Etkin, N.L. (Ed.), Plants in Indigenous Medicine and Diet, Behavioral Approaches. Redgrave Publishing Company, Bradford Hills, New York.

UICN, OMS, WWF. 1993. Directories Sobre Conservation de Plantas Medicinal Organization Mundial de la Salud (OMS). Union International para la Conservation de la Naturaleza (UICN) and World Wildlife Fund (WWF). Gland, Switzerland..

Uprety, Y., Asselin, H., Boon, E.K., Yadav, S., Shrestha, K.K., 2010. Indigenous use and bio-efficacy of medicinal plants in the Rasuwa District, Central Nepal. Journal of Ethnobiology and Ethnomedicine . 6:3-12.

WHO. WHO Traditional Medicine Strategy 2002–2005. World Health Organization, Geneva.

Yaniv, Z., Dafni, A., Friedman, J., Palevitch, D., 1987. Plants used for the treatment of diabetes in Israel. Journal of Ethnopharmacology. 19: 145–151.

Zargari, A., 1989–1992. Medicinal Plants. University Publication, Tehran, pp.5.

Juárez-Vázquez, M., Carranza-Álvarez, C., Alonso-Castro, A.J., González-Alcaraz, V., Bravo-Acevedo, E., 2013. Chamarro-Tinajero FJ, Solano E. Ethnobotany of medicinal plants used in Xalpatlahuac, Guerrero, México. Journal of Ethnopharmacology. 148: 521–527.

Chemical composition and antimicrobial activity of essential oil of *Salvia officinalis L. and Salvia virgata Jacq*

Ahmad Reza Golparvar[1,*], Amin Hadipanah[2], Mohammad Mehdi Gheisari[3], Davood Naderi[4], Shima Rahmaniyan[5], Mojtaba Khorrami[6]

[1]*Department of Agronomy and plant Breeding, Isfahan (Khorasgan) Branch, Islamic Azad University, Isfahan, Iran;*
***Email:** dragolparvar@gmail.com*
[2]*Department of Horticultural Sciences, Science and Research Branch, Islamic Azad University, Tehran, Iran;*
[3]*Toxicology Research Center, Isfahan (Khorasgan) Branch, Islamic Azad University, Isfahan, Iran;*
[4]*Department of Horticulture, Isfahan (Khorasgan) Branch, Islamic Azad University, Isfahan, Iran;*
[5]*Department of Horticultural Sciences, Yasouj Branch, Islamic Azad University, Yasouj, Iran;*
[6]*Department of Horticultural Sciences, Hormozgan University, Bandar Abbas, Iran;*

ARTICLE INFO

Topic: *Medicinal Plants*

Key words:
- ✓ *Salvia officinalis L*
- ✓ *Salvia virgata Jacq*
- ✓ *Chemical constitutes*
- ✓ *Antimicrobial activity*

ABSTRACT

Background & Aim: The genus *Salvia* (commonly known as sage) is a broad genus belonging to the family Lamiaceae. This study is aimed at assessing the essential oil composition and antimicrobial activities of two Salvia species.

Experimental: The chemical composition of the essential oils of *Salvia officinalis* L. and *Salvia virgata* Jacq, cultivated in Estahban (Fars, South Iran), was studied by means of GC-MS analyses. Antimicrobial activity was tested against a panel of microorganisms including one Gram-positive (*Staphylococcus epidermidis* PTCC NO. 1435) and one Gram-negative (*Escherichia coli*) and three fungal strain (*Alternaria alternata* PTCC NO. 5224, *Penicillium funiculosum* PTCC NO. 5301 and *P. funiculosum* PTCC NO. 5169) using the disk diffusion and agar-well diffusion methods and the Minimum Inhibitory Concentration (MIC) technique.

Results: In all, 57 compounds were identified, 42 for *S. officinalis*, accounting for 98.94% of the total oil, 29 for *S. virgata* (98.81%). The major components of *S. officinalis* essential oil were α-thujone (37.18%), 1,8-cineole (12.71%), β-thujone (9.10%) and the major components of *S. virgata* essential oil were caryophyllene oxide (30.23%), β-caryophyllene (22.63%), sabinene (11.82%). The antimicrobial activity of the total essential oil evaluated by the agar-well diffusion method, the results showed that the highest active against *S. epidermidis* and also the least active against *E. coli.* Inhibition of growth was tested by the disk diffusion method, the results showed that essential oil of *S. officinalis* and *S. virgata* were highest active against *E. coli* and *P. funiculosum* (PTCC NO. 5301), respectively. Also the least active against *A. alternata*.

Recommended applications/industries: The results showed that *S. officinalis* oil had higher antimicrobial activity compare to *S. virgata*.

1. Introduction

Throughout human history, medicinal and aromatic plants have been used for flavor enrichment in culinary and medicinal purpose in folk medicine. The family of Lamiaceae has been of great importance due to the unique aroma and nutritional value. One of the most important members of the Lamiaceae family is salvia (Naghibi *et al.,* 2010). Several species of Salvia are cultivated for their aromatic characteristics and reported to have wide range of biological activities, such as antibacterial, fungistatic, astringent, antiseptic, antifungal and digestive effects. Leaves are used in antiseptic and astringent herbal mixtures. Some compounds present in the essential oil are microbiologically active (Lu and Foo, 2002; Fellah *et al.,* 2006; Farhat *et al.,* 2009). The antimicrobial effects of essential oils derived from Medicinal and aromatic plants are the basis of copious applications, in various revenue generating sectors such as pharmaceutical, nutraceutical, cosmetic, perfume, agronomy, and sanitary industries (Raut and Karuppayil, 2014). Plants and their essential oils are potentially useful sources of antimicrobial compounds. Numerous studies have been published on the antimicrobial activities of plant compounds against many different types of microbes, including food-borne pathogens (Friedman *et al.,* 2002). The most antibacterial effects of the essences and their components refer to hydrophobia traits in the essential oils which are caused to infiltrate the lipidic walls of bacterial cells and can be changed its structures (Skaltsa *et al.,* 2003) and consequently many ions and cellular substrates percolate toward to outside of cells and be ultimately dying of bacteria (Carson *et al.,* 2002). The antifungal and antibacterial activity exhibited by the extracts and essential oils of medicinal plants has been demonstrated by several researchers (Ghasemi Pirbalouti *et al.,* 2009; Ghasemi Pirbalouti *et al.,* 2010). The antimicrobial activity of the essential oils is due to its major compounds. The minor compounds possess also an important role on anti-microbial activity (Ceylan and Fung, 2004). Velickovic *et al.* (2003) reported sage ethanol extract possesses antibacterial activity against standard strains of Gram positive bacteria (*Staphylococcus aureus*, *Bacillus subtilis*) and Gram negative bacteria (*Escherichia coli*, *Pseudomonas aeroginosa* and *Salmonella enteritidis*) and the result showed the inhibitory effect of sage ethanol extract with MIC= 10 mg/mL for *S. aureus*, MIC= 6 mg/mL for *B. subtilis*, MIC= 60 mg/mL for *E. coli*, MIC= 60 mg/mL for *P. aeroginosa* and MIC= 50 mg/mL for *S. enteritidis.* Investigation of Javidnia *et al.* (2008) on the antibacterial activity of the essential oil of *Salvia reuterana* and *Salvia multicaulis* districted that essential oil are more active against Gram-negative bacteria. The essential oil of *S. officinalis* is also effective against several bacteria, *e.g.*, *Listeria monocytogenes*, *Bacillus cereus*, *Bacillus subtilis*, *Escherichia coli* and *Staphylococcus aureus*, all recognized foodborne pathogens (Delamare, 2007; Klaus *et al.*, 2009). The aim of the present investigation was to study essential oil composition and antimicrobial activities of *Salvia officinalis* L. and *Salvia virgata* Jacq.

2. Materials and Methods

2.1. Plant material

The aerial parts of two *Salvia* species including *S. officinalis* and *S. virgata* were collected from Estahban (Fars province) in South Iran (29° 07′ N and 54° 02′ E) about 1700 m above sea level during 2014.

2.2. Essential oil extraction

Harvested fresh aerial parts of two *Salvia* species were dried at room temperature (25 ± 5 °C). Dried plant material was powered (100 gm, and subjected to hydro–distillation (1000 ml distilled water) for 3 hrs using a Clevenger-type apparatus according to the method recommended in BP (British Pharmacopoeia, 1988). Samples were dried with anhydrous sodium sulfate and kept in amber glass vials at 4°C ± 1°C until use.

2.3. Identification of the oil components

Compositions of the essential oils were determined by GC–MS. The GC/MS analysis was carried out with an Hewller-packard 6890 GC-MS system. HP-5MS column (30 m × 0.25 mm, 0.25 μm film thickness) was used with helium as carrier gas with flow rate of 1.0

mL/min. The injector temperature was set at 280°C. The oven temperature was kept at 50 °C for 4 min and programmed to 280 °C at a rate of 5 °C /min, and kept constant at 280 °C for 5 min. MS were taken at 70 eV. Mass range was from m/z 35 to 450. Identification of the essential oil components was accomplished based on comparison of retention times with those of authentic standards and by comparison of their mass spectral fragmentation patterns (WILLEY/ChemStation data system) (Adams, 2007).

2.4. Bacterial and fungal strains

Extracts were individually tested against a panel of microorganisms including one Gram-positive (*Staphylococcus epidermidis* PTCC NO. 1435) and one Gram-negative (*Escherichia coli*) and three fungal strain (*Alternaria alternata* PTCC NO. 5224, *Penicillium funiculosum* PTCC NO. 5301 and *P. funiculosum* PTCC NO. 5169) were all clinical isolates obtained from the Food Medicine Faculty, (I.A.U.) Islamic Azad University of Jahrom Branch, Iran. Stock cultures of the bacteria were kept in 10% glycerol PBS (phosphate buffered saline) at 37°C. The yeast was cultured overnight at 30°C in Sabouraud dextrose agar (SDB) (Merck, Germany).

2.5. *Antimicrobial test*

These experiments were performed by the disc diffusion method and agar-well diffusion method with some modification. The extracts were dissolved in dimethyl sulfoxide (DMSO, 20 μl) before testing for antimicrobial activity. Normal saline was used for the preparation of inoculants having turbidity equal to 0.5 McFarland standards.

Disc assay was applied on nutrient agar media with adjusting pH at 7.0. Bacteria were spread on the media and the plates were allowed to dry for 5 minutes. The fungus was maintained on Potato Dextrose Agar (PDA) at 25 ± 1°C. Molten PDA (20 ml) was poured into sterilized petri dishes and seven concentrations of oil including (0.312, 0.625, 1.25, 2.5, 5, 10 and 20 μl/disc) were added into the medium. Bacterial plates were incubated at 30°C for 24 hours while fungal was incubated at 28°C for 48 hours. Diameter of inhibition zones was measured to the nearest millimeter for five replicates and the average diameter were calculated.

3. Results and discussion

3.1 Composition of the essential oils

Table 1 shows the chemical composition of the two essential oils; a total of 42 and 29 compounds were identified in the essential oil from the aerial parts of *S. officinalis* and *S. virgata*, respectively. The yield of *S. officinalis* oil is 2.4% (v/w), and its main components were α-thujone (37.18%), 1,8-cineole (12.71%), β-thujone (9.10%), camphene (5.54%) and viridiflorol (5.33%) (Fig. 1). The yield of *S. virgata* oil is 1.6% (v/w), and the main components were caryophyllene oxide (30.23%), β-caryophyllene (22.63%), sabinene (11.82%), 1-octan-3-ol (6.64%) and thujene (6.28%) (Fig. 2).

3.2 Antimicrobial activity

The results of antimicrobial activity of the essential oils obtained from *S. officinalis* and *S. virgata* are shown in (Table 2-5). The results showed that the essential oil of *S. officinalis* and *S. virgata* were most active against *S. epidermidis* and also the least active against *E. coli* (Table 2 and 3). Correlation coefficient between essential oil concentration of *S. officinalis* and diameter of inhibition zones by the agar-well diffusion method in *S. epidermidis*, *A. alternata*, *P. funiculosum* (PTCC NO. 5301), *P. funiculosum* (PTCC NO. 5169) and *E. coli* were 90%, 76%, 15%, 76% and 90%, respectively. Correlation coefficient between essential oil concentration of *S. virgata* and diameter of inhibition zones by the agar-well diffusion method in *S. epidermidis*, *A. alternata*, *P. funiculosum* (PTCC NO. 5301), *P. funiculosum* (PTCC NO. 5169) and *E. coli* were 72%, 75%, 82%, 92% and 92%, respectively.

The results showed that the essential oil of *S. officinalis* and *S. virgata* were most active against *E. coli* and *P. funiculosum* (PTCC NO. 5301), respectively. Also the least activity was observed against *A. alternata* (Table 4 and 5).

Table 1. Chemical composition of the essential oils of *S. officinalis* and *S. virgata*

No	Compound	RI	*S. officinalis*(%)	*S. virgata* (%)
1	Cis-Salvene	852	0.43	-
2	Trans-Salvene	859	0.06	-
3	Tricyclene	915	0.19	-
4	Thujene	928	0.11	6.28
5	α-Pinene	937	5.20	1.14
6	Camphene	955	5.54	-
7	Sabinene	974	0.05	11.82
8	β-Pinene	978	2.03	-
9	1-Octan-3-ol	985	0.15	6.64
10	Myrcene	992	0.74	-
11	3-Octanol	995	0.03	-
12	α -Phellandrene	999	0.08	-
13	Cyclotetrasiloxane	1003	-	1.76
14	α-Terpinene	1008	0.20	1.04
15	*p*-Cymene	1021	1.07	-
16	Limonene	1025	1.75	1.45
17	1,8-Cineole	1029	12.71	2.09
18	Cis -Ocimene	1030	0.01	-
19	γ-Terpinene	1044	0.30	1.12
20	Cis- Sabinene hydrate	1050	0.11	0.23
21	Linalool oxide	1076	0.12	-
22	α-Terpinolene	1083	0.13	-
23	Trans-Sabinene hydrate	1093	0.09	0.32
24	Linalool	1101	0.42	-
25	α-Thujone	1112	37.18	-
26	β-Thujone	1115	9.10	-
27	trans-p-Menth-2-en-1-ol	1117	-	0.75
28	α-Campholene aldehyde	1119	0.07	-
29	Camphore	1126	0.15	-
30	trans-Pinocarveol	1136	-	0.34
31	Borneol	1155	6.47	-
32	Terpinene-4-ol	1177	0.64	5.25
33	α-Terpineol	1184	0.24	-
34	Thymol	1290	-	0.75
35	Trans-Sabinyl acetate	1291	0.28	-
36	Carvacrol	1300	0.11	-
37	Carvacryl acetate	1352	0.07	-
38	*β*-Caryophyllene	1418	1.69	22.63
39	α-Humulene	1454	1.72	0.95
40	Naphthalene	1480	0.05	-
41	γ-Curcumene	1483	-	1.08
42	Ledene	1499	0.05	-
43	γ-Elemene	1524	-	0.24
44	Bicyclogermacrene	1565	-	0.53
45	Spathulenol	1577	-	0.17
46	Caryophyllene oxide	1581	0.71	30.23
47	Viridiflorol	1590	5.33	-
48	β-Selinene	1604	0.18	-
49	Humullene epoxide Π	1606	0.93	-
50	α–Cadinol	1626	-	0.23
51	Heptadecane	1700	-	0.19

52	Octadecane	1800	-	0.46
53	Manool	2056	2.45	-
54	Heneicosane	2100	-	0.34
55	Docosane	2200	-	0.23
56	Octacosane	2800	-	0.36
57	Nonacosane	2900	-	0.23
	Total		98.94	98.81
	Essential oil yield (%)		2.4	1.6

RI = Retention indices in elution order from DB-5 column

Table 2. Antimicrobial activity of the essential oil of *S. officinalis* determined by the agar-well diffusion method.

	Essential oil concentration (µl/disc)						
Microorganisms	**0.312**	**0.625**	**1.25**	**2.5**	**5**	**10**	**20**
Staphylococcus epidermidis (PTCC NO. 1435)	0	0.7	1	1.2	1.4	1.8	2.2
Alternaria alternata (PTCC NO. 5224)	0.1	0.2	0.4	1	0.7	1	1.5
Penicillium funiculosum (PTCC NO. 5301)	0	0.4	1	1	1.1	1.4	1
Penicillium funiculosum (PTCC NO. 5169)	0	0.3	0.8	1	1	1.2	1.6
Escherichia coli	0	0	0	0.4	0.6	0.8	1

Table 3. Antimicrobial activity of the essential oil of *S. virgata* determined by the agar-well diffusion method.

	Essential oil concentration (µl/disc)						
Microorganisms	**0.312**	**0.625**	**1.25**	**2.5**	**5**	**10**	**20**
Staphylococcus epidermidis (PTCC NO. 1435)	0	0	0.4	1	1.5	1.7	2
Alternaria alternata (PTCC NO. 5224)	0	0	0.2	0.5	1	1.2	1.4
Penicillium funiculosum (PTCC NO. 5301)	0	0	0.3	0.8	1.2	1.7	2
Penicillium funiculosum (PTCC NO. 5169)	0	0	0.3	0.6	1	1.4	1.9
Escherichia coli	0	0	0	0.4	0.6	0.8	1

Table 4. Antimicrobial activity of the essential oil of *S. officinalis* determined by disc diffusion method.

	Essential oil concentration (µl/disc)						
Microorganisms	**0.312**	**0.625**	**1.25**	**2.5**	**5**	**10**	**20**
Staphylococcus epidermidis (PTCC NO. 1435)	0	0.2	0.5	0.8	1.2	1.5	2
Alternaria alternata (PTCC NO. 5224)	0	0.1	0.1	0.5	0.6	0.7	1
Penicillium funiculosum (PTCC NO. 5301)	0	0.5	0.8	0.8	1	1	1.2
Penicillium funiculosum (PTCC NO. 5169)	0	0.2	0.4	0.7	1	1.3	2
Escherichia coli	0	0.7	0.7	1	1	1.2	3.1

Table 5. Antimicrobial activity of the essential oil of *S. virgata* determined by disc diffusion method.

	Essential oil concentration (µl/disc)						
Microorganisms	**0.312**	**0.625**	**1.25**	**2.5**	**5**	**10**	**20**
Staphylococcus epidermidis (PTCC NO. 1435)	0	0	0.3	0.8	1.2	1.4	1.7
Alternaria alternata (PTCC NO. 5224)	0	0	0.3	0.4	0.7	1	1.2
Penicillium funiculosum (PTCC NO. 5301)	0	0	0.2	0.7	1	1.2	1.8
Penicillium funiculosum (PTCC NO. 5169)	0	0	0.5	0.8	0.1	1.1	1.6
Escherichia coli	0	0	0.3	0.8	1.2	1.4	1.7

Correlation coefficient between essential oil concentration of *S. officinalis* and diameter of inhibition zones by the disk diffusion method in *S. epidermidis*, *A. alternata*, *P. funiculosum* (PTCC NO.

5301), *P. funiculosum* (PTCC NO. 5169) and *E. coli* were 84%, 81%, 71%, 94% and 91%, respectively. Correlation coefficient between essential oil concentration of *S. virgata* and diameter of inhibition zones by the disk diffusion method in *S. epidermidis, A. alternata, P. funiculosum* (PTCC NO. 5301), *P. funiculosum* (PTCC NO. 5169) and *E. coli* were 76%, 88%, 88%, 90% and 77%, respectively.

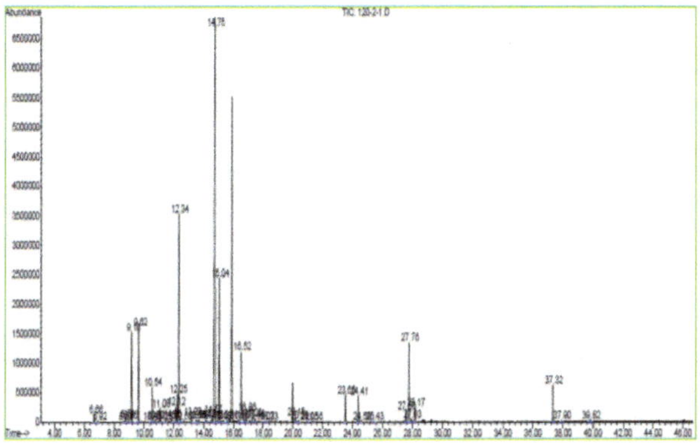

Fig. 1. The chromatogram of *S. officinalis* essential oil.

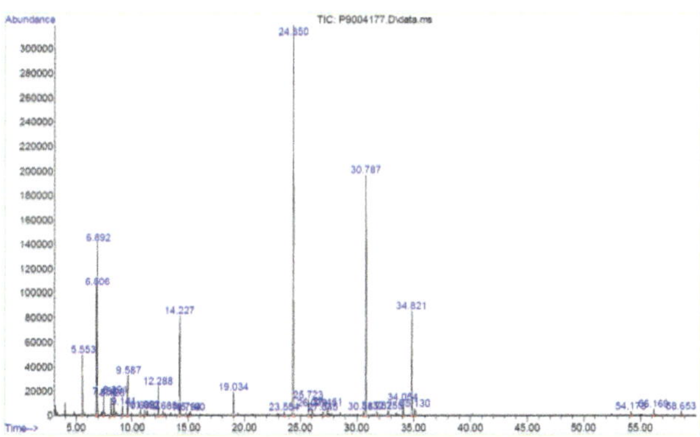

Fig. 2. The chromatogram of *S. virgata* essential oil

Many studies showed that herbs from the Lamiaceae family have a potent antioxidant and antibacterial activities. Among these, eugenol, carvacrol and thymol which are the major components of essential oils, are primarily responsible for their bactericidal/bacteriostatic properties. It was also observed, that the antimicrobial effect of plant extracts varies from one herb to another in different regions of the world. This may be due to many factors such as: the effect of climate, soil composition, the type of solvent used` in the extraction process, and also on the volume of inoculum used and culture medium or the type of strains within the same species of bacteria (Kozlowska *et al.,* 2015; Hadipanah and Khorrami, 2016). *Salvia officinalis* produces monoterpenes with a broad range of carbon skeletons, including acyclic, monocyclic, and bicyclic compounds. Three distinct monoterpene synthases are responsible for the first steps in the formation of the most characteristic monoterpenes of *S. officinalis* essential oil. The (+)-sabinene synthase catalyzes the production of sabinene, which undergoes further rearrangements leading to the two major monoterpenes, α- and β-thujone. The 1,8-cineole synthase produces in one-step 1,8-cineole. Finally, (+)-bornyldiphosphate synthase produces bornyl diphosphate, which is subsequently hydrolyzed to borneol and then oxidized to camphor (Wise *et al.,* 1998; Said-Al Ahl *et al.,* 2015). Golparvar and Hadipanah (2013) reported the major components *S. officinalis* cultivated in Isfahan (Iran) were camphor (17.75%), thujone (13.25%) and 1,8-cineole (13.03%). Sefidkon and Mirza (1999) reported the major components *Salvia virgata* cultivated in Tabriz (north of Iran) were β-caryophyllene (46.6%), germacrene-B (13.9%) and β-caryophyllene epoxide (13.2%).

Antimicrobial activity of essential oil is one of the most examined features, important for both food preservation and control of human and animal diseases of microbial origin. Some studies claim that the phenolic compounds present in spices and herbs might also play a major role in their antimicrobial effects (Hara-Kudo *et al.,* 2004). There has been no large scale, systematic investigation of the relationship between bacterial inhibition and the total phenolic content of spices and herbs. That oxygenated monoterpenes, exhibit strong antimicrobial activity, especially pronounced on whole cells, while hydrocarbon derivatives possess lower antimicrobial properties, as their low water solubility limits their diffusion through the medium. Hydrocarbons tend to be relatively inactive regardless of their structural type, and this inactivity is closely related to their limited hydrogen bound capacity and water solubility (Sokovic *et al.,* 2010). Compounds from *S. officinalis* essential oil have been shown to exhibit high antibacterial activity against *Staphyloccocus aureus, Escherichia coli, Pseudomonas aeruginosa* and *Bacillus subtilis* (Valero and Salmeron, 2003).

Khalil and Li (2011) during their study on the essential oil of *S. officinalis* against *E. coli, P. aeruoginosa, S. typhi, S. aureus, Streptococcus group D* and *C. albicans*, showed that *S. aureus, Streptococcus* and *C. albicans* were most susceptible than *E. coli, S. typhi* and *P. aeruoginosa*.

In most of the studies, the antimicrobial activity of *Salvia* species was considered to be related to 1,8-cineole, β-caryophyllene, thujone, camphor, borneol in their contents (Akin *et al.*, 2010; Tenore *et al.*, 2010). However, the role of other minor compounds should not be neglected. Some studies have concluded that whole essential oils have a greater antibacterial activity than the major components mixed. Chemical compounds have direct activity against many species of bacteria such as terpenes and a variety of aliphatic hydrocarbon (alcohols, aldehydes and ketones) (Bachir Raho *et al.*, 2016).

4. Conclusion

The composition of the essential oil of *S. officinalis* and *S. virgata* growing in Iran has been analyzed and its antimicrobial activity investigated. The results indicate that the oil may be used in the treatment of diseases caused by the microorganisms tested. Antimicrobial activity of essential oil is one of the most examined features, important for both food preservation and control of human and animal diseases of microbial origin.

5. Acknowledgements

This research project has been supported by Islamic Azad University, Jahrom branch, Iran.

6. References

Adams, R.P. 2007. Identification of Essential Oil Components by Gas Chromatography/Mass Spectrometery, 4th edition (Allured Publishing Corporation, Carol Stream, IL) 456.

Akin, M., Demirci, B., Bagci, Y. and Baser, K.H.C. 2010. Antibacterial activity and composition of the essential oils of two endemic *Salvia* sp. from Turkey. *African Journal of Biotechnology*, 9: 2322-2327.

Bachir Raho, G., Benattouche, Z., Bevilacqua, A., Corbo, M.R., Sinigaglia, M. and Pignatiello, S. 2016. Antimicrobial Activity of Extracts from *Salvia officinalis* L on some Bacteria and Yeast. *Journal of Biotechnology Research*, 2(5): 31-35.

British Pharmacopoeia. 1988. British pharmacopoeia, vol. 2. HMSO, London, pp. 137–138.

Carson, C.F., Mee, B.J. and Riley, T.V. 2002. Mechanism of action of *Melaleuca alternifolia* (tea tree) oil on *Staphylococcus aureus* determined by time-kill, lysis, leakage and salt tolerance assays and electron microscopy. *Antimicrobial Agents and Chemotherapy*, 46: 1914-1920.

Ceylan, E. and Fung, D.Y.C. 2004. Antimicrobial Activity of Spices. *Journal of Rapid Methods and Automation in Microbiology*, 12: 1-55.

Delamare, A.P.L. 2007. Antibacterial activity of the essential oils of *Salvia officinalis* L. and *Salvia triloba* L. cultivated in South Brazil. *Food Chemistry*, 100. 603-608.

Farhat, M.B., Jordan, M.J. and Chaouech-Hamada, R. 2009. Variations in essential oil, phenolic compounds, and antioxidant activity of Tunisian cultivated *Salvia officinalis* L. *Journal of Agricultural and Food Chemistry*, 57: 10349-10356.

Fellah, S., Diouf, P.N. and Petrissans, M. 2006. Chemical composition and antioxidant properties of *Salvia officinalis* L. oil from two culture sites in Tunisia. *Journal of Essential Oil Research*, 18(5): 553-556.

Friedman, M., Henika, R.P. and Mandrell, E.R. 2002. Bactericidal activities of plant essential oils and some of their isolated constituents against *Campylobacter jejuni*, *Escherichia coli*, *Listeria monocytogenes*, and *Salmonella enterica*. *Journal of Food Protection*, 65: 1545-1560.

Ghasemi Pirbalouti, A., Jahanbazi, P., Enteshari, S., Malekpoor, F. and Hamedi, B. 2010. Antimicrobial activity of some Iranian medicinal plants. *Archives of Biological Science Belgrade*, 62(3): 633-642.

Ghasemi Pirbalouti, A., Taheri, M., Raisee, M., Bahrami, H.R. and Abdizadeh, R. 2009. In vitro antifungal activity of plant extracts on *Saprolegnia parasitica* from cutaneous lesions of rainbow trout (*Oncorhynchus mykiss*) eggs. *The Journal of Food, Agriculture & Environment,* 7: 94-96.

Golparvar A.R. and Hadipanah, A. 2013. Identification of the components of sage (*Salvia officinalis* L.) and thyme (*Thymus vulgaris* L.) cultivated in Isfahan climatic conditions. *Electronic Journal of Biology*, 9(2): 42-45.

Hadipanah, A. and Khorrami, M. 2016. Chemical composition and antibacterial activity of essential oil from two Thymus species. *Journal of Herbal Drugs,* 6(4): 211-217.

Hara-Kudo, Y., Kobayashi, A., Sugita-Konishi, Y. and Kondo, K. 2004. Antibacterial activity of plants used in cooking for aroma and taste. *Journal of Food Protection,* 67: 2820–2824.

Javidnia, K., Miri, R., Soltani, M., Gholami, M. and Khosravi, A. 2008. Antimicrobial activity and chemical composition of the essential oils of six Iranian *Salvia* species. *Chemistry of Natural Compounds*, 44(5): 654–658.

Klaus, A., Beatovic, D., Niksic, M. Jelacic, S. and Petrovic, T. 2009. Antibacterial activity of aromatic plants essential oils from Serbia against the *Listeria monocytogenes. Journal of Agricultural Sciences,* 54(2): 95-104.

Kozlowska, M., Laudy A.E., Przybyl, J., Ziarno, M. and Majewska, E. 2015. Chmical composition and antibacterial activity of some medicinal plants from Lamiaceae family. *Acta Poloniae Pharmaceutica-Drug Research,* 72(4): 757-767.

Lu, Y. and Foo, L.Y. 2002. Polyphenolics of *Salvia.* A review. *Phytochemistry*, 59: 114-140.

Naghibi, F., Mosaddegh, M., Mohammadi Motamed, M. and Ghorbani, A. 2010. Labiatae family in folk medicine in Iran: From ethnobotany to pharmacology. *Iranian Journal of Pharmaceutical Research*, 4: 63-79.

Raut, J.S. and Karuppayil, S.M. 2014. A status review on the medicinal properties of essential oils, *Industrial Crops and Products*, 62: 250–264.

Said-Al Ahl, H., Hussein, M.S., Gendy, A.S.H. and Tkachenko, K. 2015. Quality of sage (*Salvia officinalis* L.) Essential Oil Grown in Egypt. *International Journal of Plant Science and Ecology,* 1(4): 119-123.

Sefidkon, F. and Mirza, M. 1999. Chemical composition of the essential oils of two Salvia species from Iran, *Salvia virgata* Jacq. and *Salvia syriaca* L. *Flavour and Fragrance Journal,* 14(1): 45-46.

Skaltsa, H.D., Demetzos, C., Lazari, D. and Sokovic, M. 2003. Essential oil analysis and antimicrobial activity of eight *Stachys* species from Greece. *Phytochemistry,* 64(3): 743-752.

Sokovic, M., Glamoclija, J., Marin, P.D., Brkic, D. and Van Griensven, L.J.L. 2010. Antibacterial effects of the essential oils of commonly consumed medicinal herbs using an *In Vitro* model. *Molecules*, 15: 7532-7546.

Tenore, G.C., Ciampaglia, R., Arnold, N.A., Piozzi, F., Napolitano, F., Rigano, D. and Senatore, F. 2010. Antimicrobial and antioxidant properties of the essential oil of *Salvia lanigera* from Cyprus. *Food and Chemical Toxicology,* 49(1): 238-243.

Velickovic, D., Randjelovic, N. and Ristic, M. 2003. Chemical constituents and antimicrobial activity of the ethanol extracts obtained from the flower, leaf and stem of *Salvia officinalis* L. *Journal of the Serbian Chemical Society,* 68(1): 17-24.

Wise, M.L., Savage, T.J., Katahira, E. and Croteau, R. 1998. Monoterpene synthases from common sage (*Salvia officinalis*). cDNA isolation, characterization, and functional expression of (+)-sabinene synthase, 1,8-cineole synthase, and (+)-bornyl diphosphate synthase. *Journal of Biological Chemistry,* 273(24): 14891-14899.

24

Effect of Different Drying Methods on Some Biochemical Properties of Iranian Ox-tongue (*Echium amoenum* Fisch. & Mey.)

Arash Saeedi, Hossein Ali Asadi-Gharneh*
Department of Horticulture, Islamic Azad University, Isfahan (Khorasgan) Branch. Isfahan, Iran;
***Email:** h.asadi@khuisf.ac.ir

ARTICLE INFO

***Topic:** Medicinal Plants*

Key words:
- ✓ *Drying methods*
- ✓ *Iranian ox-tongue*
- ✓ *Pigment content*
- ✓ *Traditional drying*

ABSTRACT

Background & Aim: Iranian ox-tongue (*Echium amoenum* Fisch. & Mey.) is an endemic Iranian medicinal plant belongs to Boraginaceae family. The violet-blue petals of this plant have been used in traditional medicine. Drying is one of the most critical and fundamental operations in the post-harvest processing of medicinal plants.

Experimental: This research was carried out in Islamic Azad University, Isfahan (Khorasgan) branch in 2015. The experiment was arranged based on completely randomized design with three repetitions. Drying methods are including sun and shade drying, oven-drying (45, 65 and 85°C) and microwave drying (200, 300 and 400 W). Drying time of Iranian Ox-tongue petals and some biochemical properties such as total chlorophyll, the amount of carotenoids, anthocyanin content and total flavonoids were measured.

Results: The results showed that different drying methods had significant effects on drying time, chlorophyll, carotenoids, total flavonoid and anthocyanin contents of Iranian ox-tongue petals. The maximum and minimum drying times were measured in shade drying and microwave 400 W, respectively. The anthocyanin content gradually decreased with the increase of oven temperatures and microwave powers. Also shade drying method had the highest amount of total chlorophyll and carotenoids. Generally, regarding the biochemical composition, traditional shade drying is the optimum method for dying of Iranian ox-tongue petals.

Recommended applications/industries: According to this study, shade drying could be recommended in terms of qualitative characteristics of mentioned medicinal plant.

1. Introduction

Iranian ox-tongue (*Echium amoenum* Fisch. & Mey.) belongs to Boraginaceae family and is an herbaceous and perennial endemic Iranian medicinal plant and naturally is grown in mountainous regions of North of Iran (Babakhanzadeh-Sajirani *et al.,* 2014) at an altitude ranging from 60-2200 meters (Soltani, 2005; Mozaffarian, 1998).

Flowers and leaves are the main medicinal parts of the Iranian ox-tongue (Abed *et al.,* 2014). Dried violet–blue petals of ox-tongue in Iranian traditional medicine have been used as diaphoretic, tranquillizer, cough suppressant, tonic and as a remedy for sore throat (Amin, 1991; Mehrabani *et al.,* 2005). The major components of Iranian ox-tongue petals including anthocyanin, flavonoids, saponins, unsaturated terpenoids, sterols and essential oils (Shafaghi *et al.,* 2002).

The most fundamental and common method for post-harvest preservation of medicinal plants is drying. The reduction of the water content of freshly harvested medicinal plants is imperative for handling and storage purpose and less susceptible to microorganisms (Tanko *et al.,* 2005: Ghasemi-Pirbalouti *et al.,* 2013). Drying reduces the enzymatic activity inhibiting chemical reaction as hydrolysis, oxidation, and fermentation (Santana et *al.,* 2014). Drying of medicinal plants must be carefully performed in order to preserve the aroma, appearance, and nutritional values (Crivelli *et al.,* 2002). According to basis of heat source of energy utilization, the methods for drying medicinal plants could be categorized into natural and mechanical (Cai *et al.,* 2004).

Sun drying is the cheapest and is traditionally practiced for medicinal plants; however, the long drying time, contamination and spoilage of product exposed to the open environment are undesirable in terms of economic reasons (Kostaropoulos and Saravacos, 1995).

Due to the advantages such as a lower impact on product quality, reduction in drying time, and less energy use, microwave drying is becoming surprisingly popular as an alternative conventional drying technique (Zhang *et al.,* 2006; Vadivambal and Jayas, 2007).

There is little information about the influence of the different drying methods on the quality characteristics of Iranian ox-tongue; therefore the aim of present study is to evaluate the effect of different drying methods on some biochemical properties of Iranian ox-tongue petals.

2. Materials and Methods

2.1. Plant materials

The fresh flowers of Iranian ox-tongue (*Echinum amoenum* Fisch & Mey.) were collected in April 2015 from natural habitat at the Sajiran region in Gilan province. This area located to the north region of Iran (Latitude: 36° 52′97′′N, Longitude: 50° 14′ 31′′E, elevation 770 m). Plants were kept in cooled bags for transport to the laboratory. In this experiment the fresh petals at eight different methods of drying were evaluated as sun-drying of plant material under open air sunny conditions, shade-drying under conventional open air conditions, oven-drying (Memmert 660, Germany) at 45, 65 and 85°C and microwave drying (Panasonic NN-1000W) at 200, 300 and 400 W.

A 300 gr samples was used in each experiment and the drying process was continued until the mass of the samples reduced to a moisture content of about 10% on a wet weight basis.

2.2. Determination of Biochemical properties

The total chlorophyll and carotenoid content was determined according to a method introduced by Arnon (1967). The content of chlorophyll was obtained by summarizing chlorophyll a and b content and results were expressed in mg/g of FW (equations 1, 2 and 3). Also the amount of carotenoid content was calculated by the equations 4, and results **were** reported in mg/g of FW.

(1) $Chl_a = [12.25A_{663} - 2.79A_{645}] \times V/W \times 1000$

(2) $Chl_b = [12.12A_{645} - 5.10A_{663}] \times V/W \times 1000$

(3) $Chl_{total} = Chl_a + Chl_b$

(4) Carotenoid= $[(1000\ A_{470}) - 1.82\ Chl_a - 85.02\ Chl_b) / 198$

Where Chl_a= (chlorophyll a), Chl_b= (chlorophyll b), V= (volume of used acetone) and W= (used leaf fresh weight).

The total anthocyanin content was measured by Wagner (1979) methods. Briefly, a mass of 0.1 g of sample was soaked in 10 ml of acidified methanol. The tissue was crushed and kept at 25 °C for 24 h in dark. The extracts were then centrifuged at 4000×g for 5 min at room temperature. The absorption rate of the supernatant was read by spectrophotometer at 550 nm. In order to measure the amount of anthocyanin's the molar absorption coefficient of 33000 mol^{-1} cm^{-1} was used and anthocyanin content was reported in mmol per g of fresh mass.

Total flavonoids content was determined by aluminum chloride colorimetric method (Pourmorad *et al.,* 2006). Plant extracts (0.5 ml) were separately mixed with 1.5 ml of methanol, 0.1 ml of 10% aluminum chloride, 0.1 ml of 1 M potassium acetate and 2.8 ml of distilled water. They were kept at room temperature for 30 min; the absorbance of the reaction mixture was measured at 415 nm with a spectrophotometer and results were reported as mg dry weight equivalents per gram quercetin.

2.3. Statistical analysis

The experiment was arranged based on completely randomized design (CRD) with three repetitions. Statistical analyses were performed using SAS 9.1 software. Mean were separated using Duncan's multiple test at 5% significance.

3. Results and discussion

The results indicated that the dying time and some biochemical characteristics such as total chlorophyll, carotenoids, anthocyanin content and total flavonoids were varied in different drying methods and significant difference (P <0.01) was observed between them.

The mean value of drying time in different drying methods showed significant difference (P <0.01). The maximum drying time (2280 min) was measured at the shade drying method. Although, the minimum drying time (57 min) was spent in the microwave 400 W, the longest drying period was 40 times higher compared with the shortest drying period. Sun drying methods and oven drying at 45 °C has not significant differences in terms of drying time. Among the oven dying methods, oven 85 °C has the lowest drying time (Fig 1). The higher energy power of microwave and oven drying made the drying process faster but contributed more significantly to the loss of the active compounds than a smaller energy input (Dermelj *et al.,* 1995). In over all, Water content and temperature has effect on drying time of medicinal plants and the ideal temperatures can vary greatly among species. In terms of drying time, our results in high temperatures and high microwave watts were agreement with Ebadi *et al.* (2011) on drying of Savory (*Satureja hortensis* L.).

The sun drying is the most common and the cheapest drying method of agricultural products in several countries. This method is successfully employed in various agricultural products (Doymaz, 2009), but for medicinal plants this method is not recommended, because solar drying as commonly leads to photodecomposition reactions (Santana *et al.*, 2014) and the long drying time is undesirable for economic reasons.

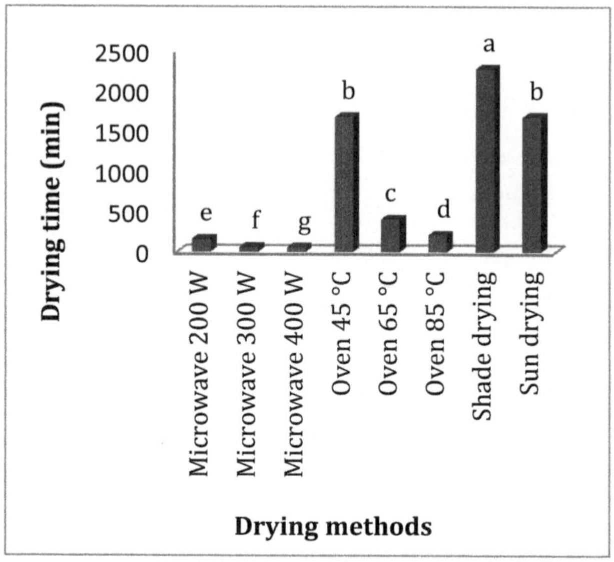

Fig 1. Drying time of Iranian ox-tongue dried petals in different drying methods. (Significant difference at 5% probability level has been indicated with different letters).

Chlorophyll is a group of compounds responsible for color intensity of plants. Mean comparison results showed significant differences in total chlorophyll content among drying methods. The highest amounts of total chlorophyll were observed in shade dying and oven drying at 45 °C. also microwave 400 W and oven 85 °C have the lowest amounts of total chlorophyll content (Fig 2). These results are agreement with flinging of Diaz-Moroto *et al.* (2002) on parsley leaves drying. It is generally accepted that the different drying techniques affect different pigments in a variety of ways and that the dehydration process results in the qualitative and quantitative changes in dried plants (Drostinova *et al.,* 2015). In tumor or cancer therapy chlorophyll or chlorophyll derivatives can be utilized as a photodynamic agent (Brandis *et al.*, 2006).

The amount of carotenoid content varied from 0.026 mg/g in microwave 200 W to 0.048 mg/g in shade drying methods (Fig 3). These finding are agreement with previous study by Komes *et al.* (2011) of dehydrated lemon balm leaves (*Mellisa officinalis*

L.), marigold flowers (*Calendula officinalis* L.) and borage petals (*Borago officinalis* L.). The results obtained by Kamel *et al.* (2013) have shown that all methods of drying used (air drying, oven drying, microwave drying) significantly decreased the yield of carotenoids in the edible parts of leafy vegetables and the greatest reduction was observed using microwave drying method and less effect was observed using air drying. Susceptibility of these beneficial compounds to degradation at high temperatures was reported by Komes *et al.* (2013).

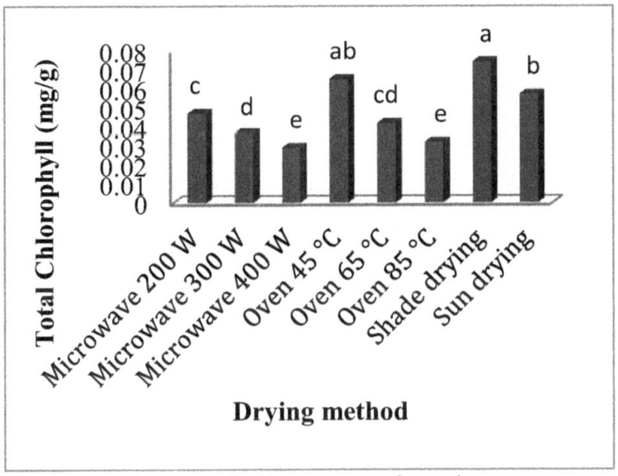

Fig 2. Total chlorophyll content of Iranian ox-tongue dried petals in different drying methods (Significant difference at 5% probability level has been indicated with different letters).

Also Diaz-Moroto *et al.* (2002) reported that increasing the temperature, usually results in a decrease of the quality of dried herbs. The biological importance of carotenoids is related to antioxidants properties. Carotenoids can fact as antioxidant and may possess some anti-carcinogenic properties (Krinsky, 1989).

In terms of total anthocyanin content the highest and lowest amounts were measured by using shade drying (1.051 mmol/g) and oven drying at 85 °C (0.442 mmol/g) respectively (Fig 4). The anthocyanin content gradually decreased with the increasing of temperature. Anthocyanins are sensitive to pH, temperature, light, oxygen, enzyme and sulfur dioxide (Nadi, 2016). Anthocyanins have been reported to be destroyed by high heat during processing and storage of food (Morales-Delgo*et al.,* 2014). Anthocyanins were responsible for biological membrane stability and protect against free radical produced by radiation (Handley *et al.,* 2011).

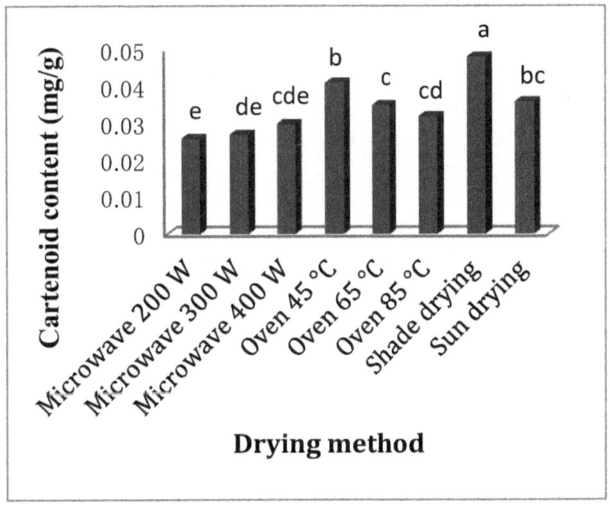

Fig 3. Carotenoid content of Iranian ox-tongue dried petals in different drying methods (Significant difference at 5% probability level has been indicated with different letters).

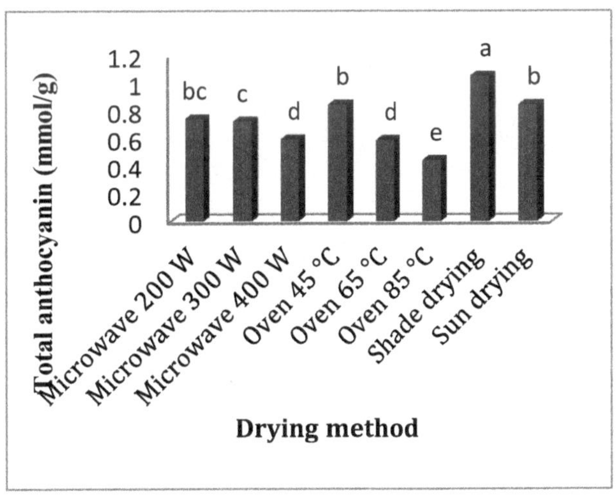

Fig 4. Total anthocyanin content of Iranian ox-tongue dried petals in different drying methods (Significant difference at 5% probability level has been indicated with different letters).

In terms of total anthocyanin content the highest and lowest amounts were measured by using shade drying (1.051 mmol/g) and oven drying at 85 °C (0.442 mmol/g) respectively (Fig 4). The anthocyanin content gradually decreased with the increasing of temperature. Anthocyanins are sensitive to pH, temperature, light, oxygen, enzyme and sulfur dioxide (Nadi, 2016). Anthocyanins have been reported to be destroyed by high heat during processing and storage of food (Morales-Delgo*et al.,* 2014). Anthocyanins were responsible for biological membrane stability and protect against free radical produced by radiation (Handley *et al.,* 2011).

Different drying methods have significant effects on total flavonoids content of dried petals. As you can see in Fig 5, with the increase of microwave power and oven temperature, the flavonoids content were increased. On the other hand, the natural drying methods have not significant differences in total flavonoids. These components might be formed in high temperatures. The differences in flavonoids content in dried petals of ox-tongue might be due to the duration of samples to high temperatures exposure. The concluded results were agreement with Ben Haj Saeid *et al.* (2013) on drying leaves of *Allium roseum* L. Flavonoids are the group of plant metabolites which provide health benefits through cellsignaling pathways and antioxidant effects.

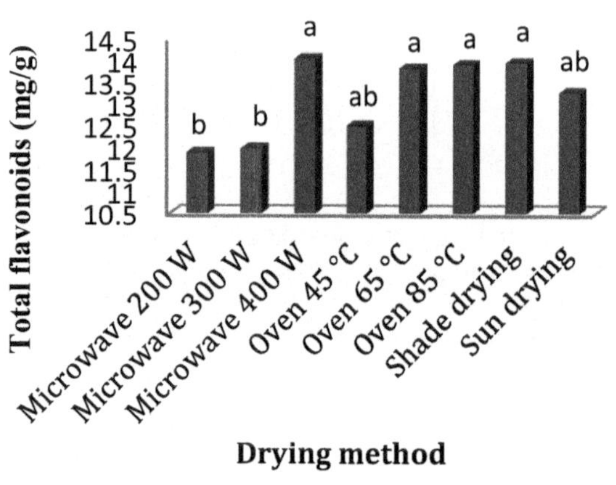

Fig 5. Total flavonoids content of Iranian ox-tongue dried petals in different drying methods (Significant difference at 5% probability level has been indicated with different letters).

4. Conclusion

Drying is one of the basic process of medicinal plants that is affected on quantitative and qualitative characteristics. As the bioactive components of medicinal plants may be very sensitive to drying procedures, for obtaining the highest quality of medicinal plants, it is necessary to investigate the influence of drying methods on quality parameters. According to our results, shade drying was the most favorable among the different drying methods which preserves the higher amount of all biochemical compounds.

5. References

Abed, A., Vaseghi, G., Jafari, E., Fattahian, E., Babhadiashar, N., Abed, M. (2014). *Echium Amoenum* Fisch. Et Mey: A Review on its Pharmacological and Medicinal Properties. *Asian Journal of Medicinal Pharmaceutical Researches*, 4(1): 21-23.

Amin, Gh.R. (1991). *Popular Medicinal Plants of Iran*. Iranian Research Institute of Medicinal Plants. Tehran, Iran. 230 pp.

Arnon, A. N. (1967). Method of extraction of chlorophyll in the plants. *Agronomy Journal,* 23:12-121.

Babakhanzadeh, E., Hadian, J., Abdosi, V., Larijani, K. (2014). Evaluation content of flavonoids and anthocyanin's in Iranian borage subject in Eshkevari accessions affected by different habitats in North of Iran. *Journal of Biodiversity and Environmental Science,*4 (2): 364-368.

Ben Haj Said, L., Neffati, H.N.M., Bellagha, S. (2013). Color, Phenolic and antioxidant characteristic changes of *Allium roseum* leaves during drying. Journal of *Food Quality*, 36: 403-410.

Brandis, A. S., Y. Salomon, Scherz, A. (2006). Chlorophyll snsitizers in photodynamic therapy advances in photosynthesis and respiration, 25: 461– 483.

Cai, T., Chen, F. and Qi, J. (2004). Dehydrated oriental mushrooms, leafy vegetables, and food preparation herbs and condiments. p.373–393. In: Y.H. Hui, S.

Ghazala, D.M. Graham, K.D. Murrell and W. Nip (eds.), Handbook of Vegetable Preservation and Processing, Marcel Dekker, New York.

Crivelli, G., Nani, R.C. Di Cesare, L.F. (2002). Influence of processing on the quality of dried herbs. Atti VI Giornatescientifiche SOI. Spoleto 23-25 April, 2002, vol. II, p. 463-464.

Dermelj, M., Bogenrieder, C., Hidvegi, M., Lasztitit, R. (1995). Effect of microwave vacuum drying on protein and chlorophyll contents of blind nettle (*Urtica urens* L.).*Periodica Polytechnica Chemical Engineering*, 39(1):77-84.

Diaz-Maroto M.C., Perez-Coello M.S., Cabezudo, M.D. (2002). Effect of different drying methods on the volatile components of parsley (*Patroselinum crispum* L.). *European Food Research and Technology*, 215: 227-230.

Doymaz, I. (2009). An experimental study on drying of green apples. *Drying Technology*, 27: 478–485.

Droštinová,L., Braniša, J., Bončíková,D., Jomová, K. (2015). Effect of Drying methods in content of some natural pigment in *Urtica dioica* L. and *Mellissa officinalis* L. *Journal of Microbial Biotechnology and Food Science*, 5 (2):182-185.

Ebadi, M.T., Rahmati, M., Azizi, M., Hassanzadeh Khayyat, M. (2011). Effects of different drying methods (natural method, oven and microwave) on drying time, essential oil content and composition of Savory (*Satureja hortensis* L.). *Iranian Journal of Medicinal and Aromatic Plants*, 26 (4): 476-489.

GhasemiPirbalouti, A., Mahdad, E. and Craker, L. (2013). Effects of drying methods on qualitative and quantitative properties of essential oil of two basil landraces. *Food Chemistry*, 141(3): 2440-2449.

Handley S.A., Raja K.B., Sharpe C., Flanagan R.J. (2011). Measurement of serum lanthanum in patients treated with lanthanum carbonate by inductively coupled plasma-mass spectrometry. *Annals of Clinical Biochemistry*, 48(2): 178-182.

Kamel, M.S., Thabet, A.H., Algada, A. E. (2013). Influence of drying process on the functional properties of some plants. *Chemistry and Materials Research*, 3(7): 1-8.

Komes, D., Cvitanovic, A.B., Horzic, D., Markovic, K., Ganic, K.K. (2011). Characterization of pigments and antioxidant properties of three medicinal plants dried under different drying conditions. *Proceedings of the 11th International Congress on Engineering and Food.*

Kostaropoulos, A.E.; Saravacos, G.D. (1995). Microwave pre-treatment for sun-dried raisins. *Journal of Food Science*, 60: 344–347.

Krinsky, N. I. (1989). Antioxidant functions of carotenoids. *Free Radical Biology and Medicine*, 7(6): 617-635.

Mehrabani M., Ghassemi N., Sajjadi, E., Ghannadi, A., Shams-Ardakani, M. (2005). Main phenolic compound of petals of *Echium amoenum* Fisch and Meya famous medicinal plant of Iran. *Daru*, 13 (2): 65-69.

Morales-Delgado, D.Y.; Tellez-Medina, D.I.; Rivero-Ram′Irez, N.L.; Arellano- Maz′On, M. (2014). Effect of convective drying on total anthocyanin content, antioxidant activity and cell morphometric parameters of strawberry parenchymal tissue.*Revista Mexicana De Ingeniería Química Journal*, (13):179-187.

Mozaffarian, V. (1998). *A dictionary of Iranian plants names*. Tehran: Farhang Moaser Publishers. pp. 547-548.

Nadi, F. (2016). Bioactive compound retention in *Echium amoenum* Fisch. &C. A. Mey. Petals: Effect of fluidized bed drying conditions. *International Journal of Food Properties*, 1-12.

Pourmorad, F., Hosseinimehr, S.J., Shahabimajd, N. (2006). Antioxidant activity, phenol and flavonoid contents of some selected Iranian medicinal plants. *African Journal of Biotechnology*, 5 (11): 1142-1145.

Santana, A.M., Pereira, G.S., Boaventura, C.M., Uetenabaro, A.T., Costa, L.C., Oliveria, R.A. (2014). Rupture of glandular trichomes in *Ocimum gratissimum* leaves influences the content of essential oil during the drying method. *Revista Brasileria de Farmacognosia*, 24: 524-530.

Shafaghi, B., Naderi, N., Tahmasb, L., Kamalinejad, M. (2002). Anxiolytic effect of *Echium amoenum*

L. in mice. *Iranian Journal of Pharmaceutical Research*, 1: 37-41.

Soltani , A . (2005). *Encyclopedia of medicinal plants in traditional medicine*, Arjmand Publications, Tehran. Iran.

Tanko, H., Carrier, D.J., Duan, L., Clausen E. (2005). Pre- and post-harvest processing of medicinal plants. *Plant Genetic Resources*, 3: 304-313.

Vadivambal, R., Jayas, D. (2007). Changes in quality of microwave-treated agricultural products—a review. *Biosystematics Engineer*, 98:1–16.

Wagner, G.J. (1979). Content and vacuole extra vacuoles distribution of neutral sugars, free amino acid, and anthocyanins in protoplast. *Plant Physiology*, 64: 88-93.

Zhang, M., Tang, J., Mujumdar, A. S., Wang, S. (2006). Trends in microwave-related drying of fruits and vegetables. *Food Science and Technology*, 17: 524–534.

Study of phytohormones effects on UV-B stress seeds of thyme species

Mehrab Yadegari

Department of Agronomy and Medicinal Plants, Faculty of Agriculture, Shahrekord Branch, Islamic Azad University, Po.Box:166. Shahrekord, Iran;

***Email: mehrabyadegari@gmail.com**

ARTICLE INFO

Topic: *Medicinal Plants*

Key words:

- ✓ *Phytohormones*
- ✓ *Thyme species*
- ✓ *UV-B Stress*

ABSTRACT

Background & Aim: *Thymus vulgaris* L. and *Thymus daenensis* Celak (Thyme), members of the family Lamiaceae, are widely used in Iranian folk medicine. The aim of this research was to study how salicylic acid (SA), gibberellin (GA), and indole acetic acid (IAA)-seed priming affect UV-B radiation in seeds of Thyme (*T. vulgaris, T. daenensis* Celak) under both laboratory and outdoor conditions.

Experimental: The effects of phytohormones (200, 400, 600 ppm) and irradiation performed in a 60 Co Gamma cell 220 source at a dose of 3 kGy (10, 20 and 30 min) on seeds of Thyme species were studied. Seeds were tested under *in vitro* and outdoor conditions in a complete randomized factorial layout with 4 and 3 replications, respectively. The characters measured under *in vitro* condition were seed germination percentage, mean time of germination, root and stem length. On the field, the characters evaluated were number of leaf, length of plant, root and shoot dry matter and essential oil.

Results: SA treatment was better under *in vitro* conditions. No significant effects were obtained from GA and IAA. The most destructive effects and the best beneficial phytohormones were UV 30 min and SA (200 and 400 ppm), respectively. The effects of foliar application of hormones were determined on growth and essential oil production in medicinal plants in two consecutive years. Shoot dry matter increased in both years with SA applications but IAA and GA had no beneficial effects on germination characters after UV radiation.

Recommended applications/industries: SA-priming of seeds protects thyme seedlings against UV-B radiation. The results of this study also showed that elevation of free SA levels in plants, either by exogenous feeding or genetically may enhance their tolerance to abiotic stress.

1. Introduction

Thymus species are commonly used as flavoring agents and medicinal plants. Seeds of this plant do not exhibit dormancy and the best time for harvesting this plant is at the beginning of its flowering period (Yadegari, 2015).

During the past decades, the thinning of the stratospheric ozone has led to enhanced ultraviolet-B (UV-B) radiation on the earthsurface. UV-B radiation (280-320 nm) represents only 0.3% of the radiation reaching the Earth, but it is significant since it is absorbed by important macromolecules, including proteins and nucleic acids (Caldwell *et al.,* 2007). Increases in solar UV-B have raised concerns about the damaging impact of UV-B radiation on crop plants (Taipina *et al.,* 2011). Numerous studies have shown that enhanced UV-B radiation can affect the physiological and biochemical processes of many plant species, including altered plant photosynthesis (Sunita and Guruprasad, 2012), changes in carbon partitioning from growth pools to secondary metabolic pathways (Liu *et al.*, 2013), and thus changes in crop morphology, crop reproductive organ abortion and yield reduction (Choudhary and Agrawal, 2014), plant growth and development, photosynthesis and biomass production (Lavola *et al.,* 2013; Nawkar *et al.,* 2013). UV stress might influence the ratio of seed materials such as total anthocyanin (Eguchi and Sato, 2009), phenolic compounds (Kondo and Kawashima, 2000), as well as malondialdehyde, superoxide dismutase, catalase and peroxidase (Chen, 2008). Enhanced UV decreased the leaf area per unit plant biomass but increased biomass productivity (Weih *et al.,* 1998), had no significant effects on height growth, shoot and root biomass of birch seedlings (Kostina *et al.,* 2001), increased superoxide dismutase (SOD) activity (Li *et al.,* 2014), number of seeds per fruit as well as mean individual seed mass but the germination rates of produced seeds were unaffected (Stephanou and Manetas, 1998). In wheat, the combination of drought and UV-B caused more severe damage to wheat seedlings than stress factors applied separately (Tian and Lei, 2007). UV induces fluorescence of cotton foreign matter (Mustafic *et al.,* 2014). Responses to high energy UV-B cause noticeably different effects in different varieties of plants. If plant experience higher energy UV in the early stages of growth, the effects can cause heritable changes, which will in turn affect yield and impact the viability of the next generation of seed (Brown and Jenkins, 2008). Application of UV-B light can be used as a strategy to improve antioxidant phenolic compounds of plants (Lee *et al.,* 2013).

Plant hormones play important roles in plant growth and yield formation (Xu and Li, 2006). Salicylic acid (SA) is considered to be an important signaling molecule, which plays an important role in regulating a number of physiological processes and plant resistances to stresses (Saruhan *et al.,* 2012). Many reports have illustrated that SA can ameliorate the injurious effects of UV on plants (Moussaand El-Gamal, 2010; Liu *et al.*, 2012). SA seed priming reduced UV-B radiation on growth (Singh *et al.*, 2015), concentrations of several polyphenols and produced more total phenolic, flavonoids, and antioxidants (Lee *et al.*, 2013). Plants accumulate large amounts of SA when exposed to UV radiation (Bandurska and Cieślak, 2013). Furthermore, SA stimulates the photosynthetic machinery by increasing the content and accumulation of chlorophyll in UV-stressed plants (Mahdavian *et al.,* 2008) in response to oxidative stress. Although UV induced oxidative stress and increased lipid peroxidation that was significantly decreased by SA pre-treatment (Saruhan *et al.,* 2012). The application of SA to plants improved shoot growth and photosynthesis (Fattahi *et al.,* 2011). Depending on the plant species, the application of Gibberellin (GA), a phytohormone, can improve plant growth, ion uptake and transport, nutrient utilization and is responsible for seed germination, stem elongation, leaf expansion and flowering, and prevents chlorophyll breakdown (Rashad and Hussien, 2014).

Auxin is another phytohormone and was first isolated and characterized for plant growth. Indole-3-acetic acid (IAA) is a type of auxin (Nakamura *et al.,* 2006; Bilkay *et al.,* 2010). The application of Indole Acetic Acid (IAA) resulted in more starch accumulation and is thus an essential compound required for the growth and development of roots and shoots (Yang *et al.,* 2014).

The aim of this study was to investigate the effect of phytohormones and irradiation on measured characters such as speed of germination, mean time of germination, root and stem length under *in vitro* and outdoor conditions. Number of leaf, length of plant, root and shoot dry matter and essential oil were measured.

2. Materials and Methods

2.1. Plant material and treatments

The seeds of *T. vulgaris* and *T. daenensis* Celak were collected from the fields. The treatments were salicylic acid (SA), Gibberellin (GA), Indole Acetic Acid (IAA) and regulation of UV-B toxicity in seeds under both laboratory and outdoor conditions at the Islamic Azad University, Shahrekord Branch. In this research, seeds of thyme were studied to determine the effects of phytohormones (200, 400, 600 ppm) and irradiation was performed in a 60 Co Gamma cell 220 source at a dose of 3 kGy (10, 20 and 30 min). Under *in vitro* and outdoor conditions a complete randomized block design in factorial layout with 4 and 3 replications, respectively was used. Before medicinal plants culture, each petri was washed with alcohol, disinfected by fire and placed on a stain paper. After disinfection, seeds were treated with 2000 ppm Carboxin thiram at 25°C temperature, under light. When water in the petri dish was relatively evaporated, irrigation was conducted in the field. The number of seedling produced by each plant was counted every day. Measured characters under *in vitro* condition were seed germination percentage, mean time of germination, root and stem length. Number of leaf, length of plant, root and shoot dry matter and essential oil were measured. The germination ratio was measured with the following formula (Fattahi *et al.*, 2011):

Speed of Germination (SP) = X1 /Y1 + (X2-X1)/Y2 + ... + (Xn-Xn-1)/Yn

Mean Time of Germination (MTG) = N1T1+N2T2+N3T3+ … (NnTn)/ N

Where N1, N2 are the number of seeds germinated on the first and second days, respectively; T1=N1, T2=N1+N2, N is the total seed germinated, Y_n number of days to final germination period.

Three replicates of the control and treated plants (three plants of each) were harvested and the shoot of each plant was collected separately for estimation of shoot fresh weight and height which were expressed as g/plant and cm/shoot, respectively. Irradiation was performed in a ^{60}Co Gamma cell 220 (AECL) source with a dose rate of about 3.5 kGy/h at doses of 3 kGy having a dose uniformity factor of 1.13. Dosimetry mapping was previously performed by Fricke dosimetry.

2.2. Essential oil extraction

Fresh aerial parts of *T. vulgaris* L. and *T. daenensis* Celak were dried at room temperature (25±3°C). Plant material was powdered (100 g) and subjected to hydro–distillation with 1000 ml distilled water for 3 h using a Clevenger-type apparatus.

2.3. Statistical analysis

All data were subjected to ANOVA using the statistical computer package SAS ver. 8. When the treatment effects were significant ($p<0.05$) in relation to the control, treatment means were separated using Least Significant Difference test at the significance level ($P<0.05$).

3. Results and discussion

IAA and GA hormones had no significant effects on seeds treated with UV. Results from the field showed that there was a significant difference between concentrations of SA. Although in some single treatments, there were no significant differences, but in combined treatments, there were differences in most characters as the SA400×UV10 treatment was the best (Tables 1 to 4). It seems that by increasing UV radiation, most of the measured characters were diminished. The application of SA treatment significantly improved growth characters including stem and root length, number of lateral stem/ leaf, fresh weight of root and shoot, dry weight of root and shoot and essential oil percentage in two species of thyme. The destructive effects of UV on seeds under laboratory conditions of the two species were in appearance; only SA could repair morphological measured characters.

Table 1. L.S.D comparisons of measured characters of *Thymus vulgaris* L. that affected by SA and UV in first year under field condition.

Treat	SL[†] (cm)	RL (cm)	MTG	SP (%)	FWR (g/plant)	FWS (g/plant)	DWR (g/plant)	DWS (g/plant)	EO (%)	NLS	NL
M1[¥]	6.7±0.1^{a}	5.9±0.1^{a}	8.1±1.1^{a}	0.18±0.01^{a}	95.4±5.1^{a}	111.1±8.1^{a}	35.2±3.1^{a}	41.1±5.3^{a}	0.8±0.01^{a}	11.1±1.1^{a}	99.2±3.3^{a}
M2	7.2±0.1^{a}	6.1±0.06^{a}	8.2±0.9^{a}	0.19±0.02^{a}	96.3±4.2^{a}	117.5±7.1^{a}	36.3±4.2^{a}	45.2±4.3^{a}	0.8±0.01^{a}	11.4±2.2^{a}	99.4±4.2^{a}
M3	4.3±0.09^{b}	4.4±0.1^{b}	7.4±0.8^{a}	0.17±0.01^{a}	92.1±3.1^{a}	98.9±6.7^{ab}	33.1±3.2^{a}	39.4±2.1^{a}	0.8±0.01^{a}	10.7±1.3^{a}	90.4±6.1^{a}
M4	5.5±0.08^{ab}	5.5±0.05^{ab}	6.6±0.7^{b}	0.15±0.01^{b}	85.4±5.2^{a}	94.2±4.1^{b}	27.2±4.2^{ab}	34.3±3.2^{ab}	0.6±0.01^{b}	9.5±1.4^{a}	73.2±5.2^{b}
M5	5.3±0.08^{ab}	5.2±0.1^{ab}	6.7±0.6^{b}	0.16±0.01^{b}	86.1±3.3^{a}	97.1±5.7^{ab}	28.2±3.2^{ab}	35.7±2.7^{ab}	0.6±0.02^{b}	9.6±2.2^{a}	74.2±6.3^{b}
M6	3.3±0.09^{c}	3.2±0.05^{b}	5.9±1.1^{b}	0.12±0.01^{b}	72.1±4.1^{b}	88.1±4.1^{b}	25.6±2.2^{ab}	8.2±4.5^{b}	0.5±0.01^{b}	8.8±1.1^{a}	65.1±5.3^{b}
M7	1.3±0.1^{d}	1.2±0.04^{c}	4.8±1.1^{c}	0.09±0.01^{c}	61.1±5.5^{b}	72.2±3.3^{c}	22.3±2.1^{ab}	25.2±4.3^{b}	0.2±0.01^{c}	4.5±1.7^{b}	26.4±1.2^{c}
M8	1.4±0.09^{d}	1.4±0.1^{c}	4.9±0.5^{c}	0.1±0.06^{c}	62.2±5.5^{b}	75.2±4.2^{c}	23.3±3.1^{ab}	25.5±6.1^{b}	0.2±0.01^{c}	4.4±0.9^{b}	27.2±1.2^{c}
M9	1.1±0.08^{d}	1±0.07^{c}	3.9±0.8^{c}	0.07±0.05^{c}	48.2±3.1^{c}	61.1±5.1^{c}	18.2±1.1^{b}	19.1±3.3^{c}	0.2±0.01^{c}	3.1±0.9^{b}	19.1±1.1^{c}

Means in each column followed by the same letters are not significantly different ($P<0.05$).

[†]SL: Stem length, RL: Root length, NLS: Number of lateral stem, NL: Number of leaf, FWR: Fresh weight of root, FWS: Fresh weight of shoot, DWR: Dry weight of root, DWS: Dry weight of shoot, EO: Essential oil, MTG: Mean Time of Germination, SP: SP: Speed of Germination.

[¥]M1: UV10×SA200, M2: UV10×SA400, M3: UV10×SA600, M4: UV20×SA200, M5: UV20×SA400, M6: UV20×SA600, M7: UV30×SA200, M8: UV30×SA400, M9: UV30×SA600.

Table 2. L.S.D comparisons of measured characters of *Thymus vulgaris* L. that affected by SA and UV in second year under field condition.

Treat	SL[†] (cm)	RL (cm)	MTG	SP (%)	FWR (g/plant)	FWS (g/plant)	DWR (g/plant)	DWS (g/plant)	EO (%)	NLS	NL
M1[¥]	7.7±0.1^{a}	5.8±0.05^{a}	8.5±1.1^{a}	0.17±0.01^{a}	88.2±2.1^{a}	114.4±2.1^{a}	30.2±3.2^{a}	39.2±1.1^{a}	0.72±0.01^{a}	12.4 ±1.1^{a}	93.2 ±5.5^{a}
M2	7.4±0.2^{a}	6.2±0.04^{a}	8.5±1.2^{a}	0.18±0.01^{a}	89.3±3.2^{a}	121.5±3.4^{a}	32.1±2.1^{a}	41.1±2.3^{a}	0.81±0.01^{a}	14.2 ±1.8^{a}	96.7 ±3.1^{a}
M3	5.3±0.2^{b}	4.7±0.03^{b}	7.2±1.3^{a}	0.11±0.01^{b}	72.1±2.1^{a}	98.2±4.4^{ab}	28.2±2.2^{a}	35.3±1.1^{ab}	0.74±0.01^{a}	11.7 ±2.1^{a}	96.4 ±3.3^{a}
M4	5.7±0.3^{ab}	5.7±0.04^{ab}	6.4±0.5^{b}	0.1±0.01^{b}	82.2±3.2^{a}	92.2±3.5^{b}	29.1±1.1^{a}	34.3±2.4^{ab}	0.49±0.01^{b}	9.7± 1.1^{b}	75.4 ±2.1^{b}
M5	4.8±0.1^{ab}	5.5±0.1^{ab}	6.4±0.6^{b}	0.1±0.01^{b}	71.1±4.1^{a}	90.3±2.2^{b}	32.2±2.1^{a}	35.7±3.1^{ab}	0.51±0.01^{b}	9.4± 0.2^{b}	75.2 ±2.1^{b}
M6	3.7±0.2^{c}	3.1±0.02^{b}	5.8±0.7^{b}	0.09±0.01^{b}	72.1±5.5^{a}	70.2±3.3^{c}	28.6±1.2^{a}	27.1±2.6^{b}	0.47±0.01^{b}	8.6± 0.2^{b}	65.6 ±2.2^{b}
M7	0.99±0.3^{d}	1.3±0.01^{c}	4.9±0.1^{c}	0.09±0.01^{b}	59.1±3.1^{b}	67.7±2.4^{c}	15.4±2.1^{b}	24.2±2.1^{b}	0.26±0.02^{c}	4.3± 0.31^{c}	25.3 ±2.1^{c}
M8	0.95±0.2^{d}	1.4±0.01^{c}	4.9±0.8^{c}	0.08±0.01^{b}	54.2±2.2^{b}	55.2±3.2^{d}	15.5±2.2^{b}	25.2±1.2^{b}	0.25±0.02^{c}	4.9± 0.2^{c}	22.4 ±2.3^{c}
M9	0.87±0.3^{d}	0.99±0.01^{c}	3.6±0.1^{c}	0.05±0.01^{c}	44.9±2.4^{b}	45.1±2.3^{d}	11.1±2.3^{b}	18.2±1.1^{c}	0.19±0.02^{c}	3.7± 0.1^{c}	16.5 ±2.7^{c}

Means in each column followed by the same letters are not significantly different ($P<0.05$).

[†]SL: Stem length, RL: Root length, NLS: Number of lateral stem, NL: Number of leaf, FWR: Fresh weight of root, FWS: Fresh weight of shoot, DWR: Dry weight of root, DWS: Dry weight of shoot, EO: Essential oil, MTG: Mean Time of Germination, SP: SP: Speed of Germination.

[¥]M1: UV10×SA200, M2: UV10×SA400, M3: UV10×SA600, M4: UV20×SA200, M5: UV20×SA400, M6: UV20×SA600, M7: UV30×SA200, M8: UV30×SA400, M9: UV30×SA600.

Table 3. L.S.D comparisons of measured characters of *Thymus daenensis* L. that affected by SA and UV in first year under field condition.

Treat	SL† (cm)	RL (cm)	MTG	SP (%)	FWR (g/plant)	FWS (g/plant)	DWR (g/plant)	DWS (g/plant)	EO (%)	NLS	NL
M1	10.2±0.7^{a}	7.6±0.5^{a}	10.1±1.2^{a}	0.21±0.02^{a}	81.2±3.2^{a}	99.4±3.2^{a}	22.2±0.6^{a}	29.3±1.2^{a}	0.62±0.02^{a}	11.4±1.1^{a}	83.2±0.6^{a}
M2	10.7±0.8^{a}	8.7±0.2^{a}	10.5±0.9^{a}	0.22±0.01^{a}	82.3±2.4^{a}	111.1±4.2^{a}	21.1±0.6^{a}	31.1±1.4^{a}	0.7±0.03^{a}	12.2±1.3^{a}	86.7±0.4^{a}
M3	8.4±0.7^{b}	6.3±0.1^{b}	9.2±0.8^{a}	0.17±0.01^{b}	73.1±2.2^{a}	98.6±3.2^{a}	20.2±0.5^{a}	25.3±2.1^{a}	0.66±0.01^{a}	10.7±1.2^{a}	86.4±0.4^{a}
M4	6.8±0.5^{b}	5.4±0.1^{b}	7.4±0.7^{b}	0.15±0.01^{b}	62.2±2.2^{b}	82.2±2.1^{b}	19.1±0.5^{a}	24.3±1.1^{a}	0.44±0.01^{b}	8.7±0.9^{b}	75.4±0.1^{b}
M5	7.3±0.4^{b}	5.7±0.2^{b}	7.7±0.6^{b}	0.14±0.02^{b}	66.1±3.1^{b}	88.3±3.2^{b}	18.2±0.1^{a}	25.7±0.8^{a}	0.51±0.01^{b}	8.4±0.8^{b}	75.2±0.1^{b}
M6	5.4±0.3^{c}	5.1±0.2^{b}	5.8±0.7^{b}	0.11±0.01^{c}	58.1±1.1^{b}	81.2±1.1^{b}	16.6±0.1^{b}	22.1±0.9^{b}	0.43±0.02^{b}	7.6±0.6^{b}	55.6±0.1^{c}
M7	3.6±0.1^{c}	2.3±0.2^{c}	4.9±0.1^{c}	0.09±0.01^{c}	49.1±3.2^{c}	57.7±2.1^{c}	14.4±0.6^{b}	19.2±0.7^{b}	0.22±0.02^{c}	4.2±0.5^{c}	15.3±0.5^{d}
M8	3.9±0.1^{c}	3.4±0.1^{c}	4.9±0.1^{c}	0.07±0.01^{c}	44.2±2.2^{c}	54.2±2.2^{c}	14.5±0.5^{b}	18.2±0.4^{b}	0.21±0.01^{c}	4.5±0.4^{c}	12.4±0.8^{d}
M9	2.8±0.2^{c}	2.9±0.1^{c}	4.6±0.3^{c}	0.04±0.01^{d}	34.9±2.1^{c}	44.1±2.7^{c}	13.1±1.1^{c}	15.2±0.1^{b}	0.17±0.01^{c}	3.7±0.6^{c}	11.5±0.9^{d}

Means in each column followed by the same letters are not significantly different (P<0.05).

†SL: Stem length, RL: Root length, NLS: Number of lateral stem, NL: Number of leaf, FWR: Fresh weight of root, FWS: Fresh weight of shoot, DWR: Dry weight of root, DWS: Dry weight of shoot, EO: Essential oil, MTG: Mean Time of Germination, SP: SP: Speed of Germination.

¥M1: UV10×SA200, M2: UV10×SA400, M3: UV10×SA600, M4: UV20×SA200, M5: UV20×SA400, M6: UV20×SA600, M7: UV30×SA200, M8: UV30×SA400, M9: UV30×SA600.

Table 4. L.S.D comparisons of measured characters of *Thymus daenensis* L. that affected by SA and UV in second year under field condition.

Treat	SL† (cm)	RL (cm)	MTG	SP (%)	FWR (g/plant)	FWS (g/plant)	DWR (g/plant)	DWS (g/plant)	EO (%)	NLS	NL
M1$^{¥}$	11.7±1.2^{a}	7.8±0.4^{a}	9.5±0.5^{a}	0.22±0.01^{a}	78.2±2.2^{a}	99.4±1.6^{a}	22.2±1.3^{a}	35.2±0.9^{a}	0.65±0.02^{a}	12.7±0.3^{a}	85.2±2.5^{a}
M2	12.4±1.1^{a}	7.2±0.5^{a}	9.9±0.6^{a}	0.23±0.01^{a}	79.3±3.2^{a}	111.5±1.1^{a}	23.1±1.1^{a}	40.1±0.8^{a}	0.66±0.01^{a}	14.6±0.2^{a}	86.7±3.6^{a}
M3	10.3±0.9^{a}	6.7±0.6^{a}	8.2±0.3^{a}	0.2±0.01^{a}	76.1±3.3^{a}	88.2±1.1^{ab}	21.2±1.2^{a}	32.3±0.7^{ab}	0.59±0.01^{a}	11.5±0.1^{a}	81.4±4.1^{a}
M4	7.7±0.8^{b}	5.2±0.4^{b}	6.4±0.2^{b}	0.17±0.02^{b}	62.2±1.1^{ab}	72.2±1.1^{b}	19.1±1.4^{ab}	29.3±0.8^{ab}	0.47±0.01^{b}	8.7±0.1^{b}	65.4±2.1^{b}
M5	7.8±0.7^{b}	4.6±0.1^{b}	6.4±0.4^{b}	0.16±0.02^{b}	66.1±1.2^{ab}	75.3±1.1^{b}	18.2±1.1^{ab}	31.7±0.9^{ab}	0.48±0.01^{b}	8.8±0.1^{b}	66.2±2.1^{b}
M6	6.7±0.1^{b}	4.3±0.1^{b}	5.8±0.4^{b}	0.15±0.03^{b}	59.1±2.6^{ab}	66.2±2.3^{c}	15.6±1.3^{ab}	28.1±0.9^{b}	0.39±0.01^{b}	7.8±0.1^{b}	67.6±2.7^{b}
M7	3.9±0.6^{c}	4.9±0.3^{b}	5.9±0.1^{b}	0.14±0.01^{b}	44.1±2.9^{c}	52.7±2.5^{c}	11.4±1.6^{b}	19.2±0.9^{b}	0.17±0.03^{c}	4.7±0.3^{c}	17.3±3.1^{c}
M8	3.6±0.5^{c}	4.4±0.3^{b}	5.9±0.1^{b}	0.12±0.01^{c}	412±1.1^{c}	55.2±2.1^{c}	11.5±1.1^{b}	19.2±1.2^{b}	0.18±0.04^{c}	4.9±0.3^{c}	18.4±1.1^{c}
M9	2.8±0.1^{c}	3.1±0.4^{c}	3.6±0.5^{c}	0.11±0.01^{c}	34.9±1.5^{c}	44.1±2.7^{c}	9.1±1.2^{b}	17.2±1.3^{c}	0.15±0.05^{c}	3.5±0.2^{c}	16.5±1.9^{c}

Means in each column followed by the same letters are not significantly different (P<0.05).

†SL: Stem length, RL: Root length, MTG: MTG: Mean Time of Germination, SP: SP: Speed of Germination, FWR: Fresh weight of root, FWS: Fresh weight of shoot, DWR: Dry weight of root, DWS: Dry weight of shoot, EO: Essential oil, NLS: Number of lateral stem, NL: Number of leaf.
¥M1: UV10×SA200, M2: UV10×SA400, M3: UV10×SA600, M4: UV20×SA200, M5: UV20×SA400, M6: UV20×SA600, M7: UV30×SA200, M8: UV30×SA400, M9: UV30×SA600.

Table 5. Results of correlation between characters in *Thymus vulgaris* L. that affected by SA and UV in first year under field condition.

Characters	SL† (1)	RL (2)	NLS (3)	NL (4)	FWR (5)	FWS (6)	DWR (7)	DWS (8)	EO (9)	MTG (10)	SP (11)
1	1										
2	0.49*	1									
3	0.68**	0.57**	1								
4	0.78**	0.48*	0.5**	1							
5	0.6**	0.78**	0.45*	0.5**	1						
6	0.65**	0.76**	0.65**	0.59*	0.6**	1					
7	0.79**	0.65**	0.65**	0.65**	0.6**	0.65**	1				
8	0.68**	0.74**	0.69**	0.69**	0.72**	0.69**	0.66**	1			
9	0.88**	0.78**	0.73**	0.66**	0.77**	0.73**	0.71**	0.73**	1		
10	0.82**	0.71**	0.78**	0.75**	0.72**	0.74**	0.67**	0.55**	0.73**	1	
11	0.81**	0.73**	0.66**	0.71**	0.73**	0.67**	0.66**	0.8**	0.57**	0.66**	1

ns,* and ** : Non significant, significant at the 5% and 1% levels of probability, respectively.
†SL: Stem length, RL: Root length, NLS: Number of lateral stem, NL: Number of leaf, FWR: Fresh weight of root, FWS: Fresh weight of shoot, DWR: Dry weight of root, DWS: Dry weight of shoot, EO: Essential oil, MTG: Mean Time of Germination, SP: SP: Speed of Germination.

Table 6. Results of correlation between characters in *Thymus vulgaris* L. that affected by SA and UV in second year under field condition

Characters	SL† (1)	RL (2)	NLS (3)	NL (4)	FWR (5)	FWS (6)	DWR (7)	DWS (8)	EO (9)	MTG (10)	SP (11)
1	1										
2	0.49*	1									
3	0.68**	0.37ns	1								
4	0.78**	0.2 ns	0.55**	1							
5	0.6**	0.68**	0.48*	0.3 ns	1						
6	0.65**	0.66**	0.61**	0.51*	0.55**	1					
7	0.79**	0.61**	0.65**	0.55**	0.34 ns	0.61**	1				
8	0.68**	0.74**	0.65**	0.62**	0.65**	0.62**	0.62**	1			
9	0.88**	0.75**	0.81**	0.77**	0.71**	0.76**	0.66**	0.55**	1		
10	0.77**	0.7**	0.71**	0.55**	0.66**	0.71**	0.6**	0.5**	0.8**	1	
11	0.61**	0.66**	0.55**	0.66**	0.7**	0.62**	0.55**	0.72**	0.5**	0.6**	1

ns,* and ** : Non significant, significant at the 5% and 1% levels of probability, respectively.
†SL: Stem length, RL: Root length, NLS: Number of lateral stem, NL: Number of leaf, FWR: Fresh weight of root, FWS: Fresh weight of shoot, DWR: Dry weight of root, DWS: Dry weight of shoot, EO: Essential oil, MTG: Mean Time of Germination, SP: SP: Speed of Germination.

Table 7. Results of correlation between characters in *Thymus daenensis* L. that affected by SA and UV in first year under field condition.

Characters	SL† (1)	RL (2)	NLS (3)	NL (4)	FWR (5)	FWS (6)	DWR (7)	DWS (8)	EO (9)	MTG (10)	SP (11)
1	1										
2	0.33^{ns}	1									
3	0.62^{**}	0.33^{ns}	1								
4	0.71^{**}	0.38^{ns}	0.35^{ns}	1							
5	0.62^{**}	0.58^{**}	0.33^{ns}	0.44^{ns}	1						
6	0.55^{**}	0.56^{**}	0.56^{**}	0.59^{*}	0.6^{**}	1					
7	0.65^{**}	0.35^{ns}	0.61^{**}	0.65^{**}	0.6^{**}	0.65^{**}	1				
8	0.6^{**}	0.54^{**}	0.6^{**}	0.65^{**}	0.7^{**}	0.63^{**}	0.61^{**}	1			
9	0.66^{**}	0.5^{**}	0.7^{**}	0.8^{**}	0.66^{**}	0.53^{**}	0.55^{**}	0.8^{**}	1		
10	0.55^{**}	0.66^{**}	0.45^{**}	0.58^{**}	0.44^{*}	0.35^{ns}	0.45^{**}	0.48^{**}	0.8^{**}	1	
11	0.34^{ns}	0.65^{**}	0.37^{ns}	0.68^{**}	0.35^{ns}	0.55^{**}	0.3^{ns}	0.4^{ns}	0.88^{**}	0.8^{**}	1

ns,* and ** : Non significant, significant at the 5% and 1% levels of probability, respectively.

†SL: Stem length, RL: Root length, NLS: Number of lateral stem, NL: Number of leaf, FWR: Fresh weight of root, FWS: Fresh weight of shoot, DWR: Dry weight of root, DWS: Dry weight of shoot, EO: Essential oil, MTG: Mean Time of Germination, SP: SP: Speed of Germination.

Table 8. Results of correlation between characters in *Thymus daenensis* L. that affected by SA and UV in second year under field condition.

Characters	SL† (1)	RL (2)	NLS (3)	NL (4)	FWR (5)	FWS (6)	DWR (7)	DWS (8)	EO (9)	MTG (10)	SP (11)
1	1										
2	0.49^{*}	1									
3	0.68^{**}	0.57^{**}	1								
4	0.78^{**}	0.48^{*}	0.5^{**}	1							
5	0.6^{**}	0.78^{**}	0.45^{*}	0.3^{ns}	1						
6	0.65^{**}	0.76^{**}	0.65^{**}	0.3^{ns}	0.56^{**}	1					
7	0.79^{**}	0.65^{**}	0.65^{**}	0.55^{**}	0.62^{**}	0.65^{**}	1				
8	0.68^{**}	0.74^{**}	0.69^{**}	0.61^{**}	0.62^{**}	0.59^{**}	0.62^{**}	1			
9	0.88^{**}	0.78^{**}	0.83^{**}	0.72^{**}	0.73^{**}	0.55^{**}	0.66^{**}	0.71^{**}	1		
10	0.81^{**}	0.7^{**}	0.73^{**}	0.7^{**}	0.6^{**}	0.5^{**}	0.6^{**}	0.7^{**}	0.57^{**}	1	
11	0.82^{**}	0.7^{**}	0.7^{**}	0.66^{**}	0.61^{**}	0.75^{**}	0.76^{**}	0.55^{**}	0.59^{**}	0.59^{**}	1

ns,* and ** : Non significant, significant at the 5% and 1% levels of probability, respectively.

†SL: Stem length, RL: Root length, NLS: Number of lateral stem, NL: Number of leaf, FWR: Fresh weight of root, FWS: Fresh weight of shoot, DWR: Dry weight of root, DWS: Dry weight of shoot, EO: Essential oil, MTG: Mean Time of Germination, SP: SP: Speed of Germination.

Thus, the foliar application of SA in 400 ppm concentration resulted in an increase which when compared with other treatments.

SA was found to be the most effective resisting the severe UV effects on its seeds. In almost the same order, the destructive effects of UV on the seeds could be reduced. UV radiation may be controlled but to a limited extent by SA. MTG as well as the SP ratio of the seeds, significantly increased as affected by SA and decreased upon non-application of SA. Stem length, root length, number of lateral stem/ leaf, fresh weight of root and shoot, dry weight of root and shoot, essential oil percentage were measured on the two species of thyme in control. Most of the measured characters decreased upon application of more than 10 minutes of UV. Control treatment in many places produced the same yield components with SA400×UV10 treatment. It was clear from the presented data that the higher levels of UV were more effective than the lower levels, and SA hormone was superior to other hormones. However, the highest essential oil percentage was found with the SA400×UV10 treatment. Essential oil percentage positively correlated with the weight of shoot/root dry and fresh matter in the two species (tables 5-8). The results of this study showed just only the beneficial effects of SA hormone application on thyme plants. Increasing UV can result in lesser yield of essential oil content from thyme. In the present study, the effects of hormones applications were determined on the growth and yield of medicinal plants in two consecutive years. Shoot dry matter increased in both years with SA applications but IAA and GA had no beneficial effects on seeds after UV radiation.

Enhanced UV radiation has been found to suppress plant growth, decrease germination and growth (Ervin *et al.,* 2004). The highest germination rate was observed with SA (Fattahi *et al.,* 2011). SA can ameliorate oxidative stressed plants and the application of 400 ppm SA was beneficial and after this dosage, the expression of characters decreased. Under UV conditions in the laboratory, essential oil, yield and phytochemical materials in plant decreased (Eguchi and Sato, 2009; Weih *et al.,* 1998; Kondo and Kawashima 2000; Chen, 2008), or increased total phenolic, flavonoids, antioxidants (Lee et al., 2013), number of seeds per fruit (Stephanou and Manetas, 1998). Enhanced UV-B reduced plant height, dry weight of individual stem, yield per plant, pod number per plant and seed number per pod (Liu *et al*., 2013), concentrations of several polyphenols and had positive impacts on germination. Increasing UV-B radiation may have had no significant effects on the height growth, shoot and root biomass of birch seedlings (Kostina *et al*., 2001) or might alter biosynthesis of SA as indicated by a decreased level of SA (Singh *et al.,* 2015; Tian and Lei, 2007; Mustafic *et al.,* 2014). Plant responses to high energy UV-B cause noticeably different effects in different varieties of plants (Brown and Jenkins, 2008). SA pre-treatment significantly decreased UV induced oxidative stress and also acts as a stabilizer of membrane integrity to improve plant resistance to UV (Li *et al.,* 2014; Taipina *et al*., 2011).

This is the first report in which the effects of phytohormones applications on certain physiological characteristics were determined for seeds of thyme plants and also their relationship with yield and essential oil content. It is obvious that weight and number of stem can be used as a tool for selecting new cultivars with high yield under UV-B radiation. It seems the weight of shoot dry matter was the best character correlated by most characters. From the present data, it is thus concluded that the application of SA is beneficial to thyme plants at concentrations of 400 ppm or lower, and can result in an increase in dry matter yield of up to 40%. There are still many unanswered questions about how SA acts in increasing yield and essential oil content. One possibility is that the foliar applied SA can affect dry matter accumulation and increase shoot/root dry matter; also, SA affected the absorption and transition of essential nutrients which changes metabolism, growth and development and thus increased upper phytochemicals. It seems that control plants (no foliar application) performed better than plants subjected to upper UV radiation. These results reflect the role of applying SA in improving the total essential oils in thyme plants. Plants treated with 400 ppm of SA resulted in more fresh and dry weight of shoots and roots and essential oil percentage. Many researchers have stated that SA is an important signaling molecule which plays an important role in regulating plant resistance to stresses (Saruhan *et al.,* 2012; Moussa and El-Gamal, 2010; Liu *et al.,* 2012; Bandurska and Cieślak, 2013; Mahdavian *et al.,* 2008). SA pre-treatment enhanced seed germination percentage, mean time of germination, root and stem length; and in outdoor conditions, number of leaf, length of plant, root and shoot dry matter and essential oil percentage in the two species of thyme plant (Fariduddin *et al.,* 2003; Li *et al.,* 2014).

4. Conclusion

In this research, the SA-priming of seeds protects thyme seedlings against UV-B radiation. The results of this study also point out that the elevation of free SA levels in plants, either by exogenous feeding or genetically may enhance their tolerance against abiotic stress. Furthermore, the findings are also significant as it has been shown that UV stress occurs in natural fields where one stressor may modify the effects of others and SA may play a positive role in regulating toxicity in plants. It could be concluded from the results that SA hormone had significant effects on measured characters as well as the chemical component of the essential oil of thyme plants. The most suitable amount of SA supply for the production of thyme plants to obtain the highest weight of dry/fresh root and shoot in Shahrekord, Iran is 400 ppm foliar application. The effects of the combined application of UV10 × SA400 is suggested in comparison with their individual use. This study provides some useful information about the efficacy of foliar application of phytohormones under *in vitro* and *in vivo* conditions. These methods are relatively new and need further improvement with regard to rates, timing, and technique.

5. References

Bandurska, H. and Cieślak, M. 2013. The interactive effect of water deficit and UV-B radiation on salicylic acid accumulation in barley roots and leaves. *Environmental of experimental and Botanical*, volume 94: 9-18.

Bilkay, I.S., Karakoç, S. and Aksöz, N. 2010. Indole-3-acetic acid and gibberellic acid production in *Aspergillus niger*. *Turkish Journal of Biology*, volume 34: 313-318.

Brown, B.A. and Jenkins, G.I. 2008. UV-B signaling pathways with different flounce-rate response profiles are distinguished in mature Arabidopsis leaf tissue by requirement for UVR8, HY5, and HYH. *Plant Physiology,* volume 146: 576- 588.

Caldwell, M.M., Bornman, J.F., Ballare, C.L. and Kulandaivelu, G. 2007. Terrestrial ecosystems, increased solar ultraviolet radiation and interactions with other climatic factors. *Photochemistry Photobiology Science*, volume 6: 252-266.

Chen, Y.P. 2008. *Isatis indigotica* seedlings derived from laser stimulated seeds showed improved resistance to elevated UV-B. *Plant Growth Regulators*, volume 55: 73–79.

Choudhary. K.K. and Agrawal, S.B. 2014. Ultraviolet-B induced changes in morphological, physiological and biochemical parameters of two cultivars of pea (*Pisum sativum* L.). *Ecotoxicology Environment Safety,* volume 100:178–187.

Eguchi, K. and Sato, T. 2009. Differences in the Ratios of Cyanidin-3-O-glucoside and Cyanidin-3-O-rutinocide to Total Anthocyanin under UV and Non-UV Conditions in Tartary Buckwheat (*Fagopyrum tataricum* Garten). *Plant Production Science*, volume 12 issue 2: 150—155.

Ervin, E.H., Zhang, X. andFike, J.H. 2004. Ultraviolet-B radiation damage on Kentucky bluegrass. II. Hormone supplement effects. *Horticultural Science*, volume 39: 1471-1474.

Fattahi, M., Nazeri, V., Sefidkon, F., Zamani, Z. and Palazon, J. 2011. The Effect of Pre-sowing Treatments and Light on Seed Germination of *Dracocephalum kotschyi* Boiss: An Endangered Medicinal Plant in Iran. *Horticultural Environmental Biotechnology*, volume 52 issue 6: 559-566.

Kostina, E., Wulff, A. andTiitto, R.J. 2001. Growth, structure, stomatal responses and secondary metabolites of birch seedlings (*Betula pendula*) under elevated UV-B radiation in the field. *Trees*, volume 15: 483–491.

Lavola, A., Nybakken, L., Rousi, M., Pusenius, J. and Petrelius, M. 2013. Combination treatment of elevated UVB radiation, CO2 and temperature has little effect on silver birch (*Betula pendula*) growth and phytochemistry. *Physiology Plant*, volume 149: 499–514.

Liu, B., Liu, X.B., Li, Y.S. and Herbert, S.J. 2013. Effects of enhanced UV-B radiation on seed growth characteristics and yield components in soybean. *Field Crop Research*, volume 154: 158-163.

Lee, M.J., Son, J.E. and Oh, M.M. 2013. Growth and phenolic content of Sowthistle grown in a closed-type plant production system with a UV-A or UV-B

Lamp. *Horticultural EnvironmentalBiotechnology,* volume 54 issue 6: 492-500.

Li, X.M., Ma, L.J., Bu, N., Li, Y.Y. and Zhang, L.H.2014. Effects of salicylic acid pre-treatment on cadmium and/or UV-B stress in soybean seedlings. *Biologia Plantarum*, volume 58 issue 1: 195-199.

Mahdavian, K., Kalantari, K.M., Ghorbanli, M. and Torkzade, M. 2008. The effects of salicylic acid on pigment contents in ultraviolet radiation stressed pepper plants. *Biology of Plant,* volume 52:170-172.

Moussa, H.R. and El-Gamal, S.M. 2010. Effect of salicylic acid pretreatment on cadmium toxicity in wheat. *Biology of Plant*, volume 54: 315-320.

Mustafic, A., Li, Ch. and Haidekker, M. 2014. Blue and UV LED-induced fluorescence in cotton foreign matter. *Journal of Biology Engineering,* volume 8 issue 29: 2-11.

Rashad, R.T. andHussien, R.A. 2014. A comparison study on the effect of some growth regulators on the nutrients content of maize plant under salinity conditions. *Annals of Agricultural Science*, volume 59 issue 1: 89-94.

Saruhan, N., Saglam, A. and Kadioglu, A. 2012. Salicylic acid pretreatment induces drought tolerance and delays leaf rolling by inducing antioxidant systems in maize genotypes. *Acta Physiology Planetarium,* volume 34: 97-106.

Singh, V.P., Kumar, J., Singh, M., Singh, S., Prasad, S.M. and Dwivedi, R. 2015. Role of salicylic acid-seed priming in the regulation of chromium (VI) and UV-B toxicity in maize seedlings. *Plant Growth Regulators*, DOI 10.1007/s10725-015-0076-4.

Sunita, K., and Guruprasad, K.N. 2012. Solar UV-B and UV-A/B exclusion effects onintra specific variations in crop growth and yield of wheat varieties. *Field Crop Research,* volume 125: 8–13.

Taipina, M.S., Garbelottib, M.L., Leda, C.A. and Rodas, A.B. 2011. The effect of gamma irradiation on the nutrional properties of sunflower whole grain cookies. *Procedia Food Science,* volume 1:1992-1996.

Tian, X.R. and Lei, Y.B. 2007. Physiological Responses of Wheat Seedlings to Drought and UV-B Radiation. Effect of Exogenous Sodium Nitroprusside Application. *Russian Journal of Plant Physiology*, volume 54 issue 5: 676–682.

Xu, Z.H. and Li, J.Y. 2006. Plant hormones research in China: past, present and future. *Chaining Bulletin of Botany*, volume 23: 433–442.

Yadegari, M. 2015. Foliar application of micronutrients on essential oils of borago, thyme and marigold. *Journal of Soil Science and Plant Nutrition*, volume 15 issue 4: 949-964.

Yang, D., Luo, Y., Ni, Y., Yin, Y., Yang, W., Peng, D., Cui, Z. and Wang, Z. 2014. Effects of exogenous ABA application on post-anthesis dry matter redistribution and grain starch accumulation of winter wheat with different stay green characteristics. *Crop Journal*, volume 2: 144-153.

26

Effects of cell phone radiation on estrogen and progesterone levels and ovarian changes in rats treated with garlic (*Allium sativum* L.) hydro-alcoholic extract

Behnaz Hajiuon[*]

[1]*Department of Physiology, Islamic Azad University, Kazeroon Branch, Kazeroon, Iran;*
Email:** ***behnazhajiuon@gmail.com

ARTICLE INFO

Topic: *Physiology-Pharmacology*

Key words:
- ✓ *Electromagnetic wave*
- ✓ *Estrogen*
- ✓ *Garlic*
- ✓ *Ovary*
- ✓ *Progesterone*

ABSTRACT

Background & Aim: Electromagnetic waves can damage sex organs and cause hormonal disorders, whereas garlic is known as reducing risk factors for various diseases. The aim of this study was to investigate the probable effects of mobile phone radiation and consumption of garlic on estrogen and progesterone levels and ovarian changes.
Experimental: Five groups of rats (n = 8) were used which groups included control, sham (exposed to 900 MHz wavelength), receiving garlic extract, and receiving both extract and microwaves. After a month, rats were weighed and serum levels of estrogen and progesterone were measured. Ovaries were also removed, weighed and their probable histological changes were studied.
Results & Discussion: The mean body weights in different groups showed no significant changes, whereas a significant increase was seen in serum level of progesterone in experimental groups-II and III. Also, there were no observable histological changes in the ovaries of different groups.
Recommended applications/industries: Although microwaves can cause weight lost in mails and presence of allicin and vitamins A and B in garlic can compensate some of this weight lost, this isn't the case in females. In addition, both microwaves and garlic extract have less effect on female reproductive system, reflected only in the serum progesterone concentration.

1. Introduction

As the use of cell phone technology has grown throughout the world in recent years, the tendency for determining its potential harmful impacts on human health has also increased significantly (Ferreri *et al.*, 2006). The spectrum of electromagnetic (EM) waves is very wide, but microwave frequency and wave length range from 300 MHz to 300 GHz and 1 mm to 1 m, respectively (Verschaeve & Maes, 1998; Banik *et al.*, 2003; Baharara *et al.*, 2004; Hemayatkhah Jahromi *et al.*, 2012). Microwave spectrum is used in mobile phones and mean frequency they emit is about 900 MHz to 1 GHz (Verschaeve & Maes, 1998; Hyland, 2000; Baharara *et al.*, 2004; Hemayatkhah Jahromi *et al.*, 2012).

Skull exposure to microwave may damage central nervous system, including the hypothalamus- pituitary axis, while direct exposure of abdomen, pelvis or spine might affect the gonads, leading to interference in the function of sex hormones and infertility. Gonads are very sensitive to electromagnetic waves, and depending on the amount of radiation, they can affect the reproductive activities temporarily or permanently (Rowley *et al.*, 1974; Shalet *et al.*, 1976; Amanda & Stephen, 1993).

The evidence for the harmful effects of mobile phone on fertility are still equivocal and biological effects of electromagnetic field (EMF) emitted from these devices are controversial as well (Sarookhani *et al.*, 2011). Results a study of female rat gonads by Baharara et al. (2004) indicated that long-term cell phone radiation changes reproductive endocrine system, alters the ultra-structure of oocytes and reduces the rate of successful mating (Baharara *et al.*, 2004). Moreover, in a study by Ozguner et al. (2005) on histopathology of testes exposed to RF field, reported a decrease in testosterone level. In contrast, the effects of GSM (Global system for mobile communications, originally Group Special Mobile) 1800 MHz radiation on serum testosterone level, steroidogenic capacity of Leydig cells and histology of reproductive organs have been investigated and results showed a higher level of testosterone with no histological changes in the organs examined (Forgacs *et al.*, 2006). Similarly, results a research on the effects of 950 MHz electromagnetic field on the adrenal and sex organs of mail rabbits in 2010, it was found that there were abnormalities in the levels of testosterone and FSH, likely to affect reproductive functions (Sarookhani et al., 2011).

On the other hand, recent scientific studies have been focusing on the use of plant products as therapeutic agents (Sarkar *et al.*, 2006). Garlic is one of these plant products, traditionally used for its cytotoxic, antitumor, antifungal, antibacterial, antiviral and anti protozoal properties (Sarkar *et al.*, 2006).

As a member of the Aliaceae family, *Allium sativum* or garlic (Ulbricht *et al.*, 2010), contains various substances including minerals, carbohydrates, proteins, fats and vitamins (Kemper Kathi., 2000; Haciseferogullari *et al.*, 2005; Cobas *et al.*, 2010). Vitamins found in garlic include vitamin A, various kinds of vitamin B, such as riboflavin, thiamine, nicotinic acid, and vitamins C and E. Among many different compounds found in garlic, studies suggest that biological and pharmacological effects of this plant are mainly due to its sulfur compounds (Kemper Kathi, 2000; Khalid & Gordon, 2006; Lanzotti, 2006; Cobas *et al.*, 2010). Some of these sulfur compounds are aliin, allicin, ajoene, allylpropyl disulfide, diallyltrisulfide, sallylcysteine, vinyldithiines, S-allylmercaptocystein, etc (Kemper Kathi., 2000; Khalid & Gordon, 2006; Sarkar *et al.*, 2006).

Because of their high costs, their potential side effects and restrictions of their use, in recent years, there has been a tendency among researchers in attempting to treat disorders by replacing chemical drugs with some natural plant components (Mahmoodi *et al.*, 2011). Although, cell phone use is wide spread and some of their inevitable deleterious effects on the body have been documented, there has been little attempt to reduce these effects through diet or use of herbs. Since garlic has some health benefits and microwaves have some adverse effects on the same area of human health, in this study we tried to investigate the effects of cell phone radiation along with the consumption of hydro alcoholic extract of garlic on female reproductive system in particular, ovaries. The importance of fertility and vital roles of ovaries in reproduction as well as, the ubiquity of cell phone use is sufficient enough to urge detailed studies of the physiology, cell biology, and molecular effects of microwaves. These studies offer the potential to enhance our understanding of garlic and the optimal use of cell phones. Therefore, the goal of present research was to investigate the probable effects of mobile phone radiation and consumption of the extract of garlic on estrogen and progesterone levels and ovarian changes.

2. Material and methods

2.1. Plant material

Soaking method (Maceration) was used to prepare garlic extract (Lachance, 1997; Tatara Marcin et al., 2005).

2.2. Animals

40 Wistar rats with average body weight of 200 ±10 g and 80 to 90 days old were used in this study. In order to adapt to new environmental condition all animals were kept in the Animal House of Kazeroon Islamic Azad University for one week before entering into the trial. They were placed in special cages under standard

conditions of 23-25 °C and 12 h of light and 12 h of dark cycle. They had unlimited access to food and water, and all moral principles on using and treating animals were taken into consideration.

2.3. Treatments

Animals were randomly divided into five groups of eight, including control (left untreated), sham group (exposed to wavelength of 900 MHz), the experimental group-I (receiving 400mg/kg garlic extract), Experimental group-II (receiving 200mg/kg extract plus 900 MHz waves), and experimental group-III (receiving 400mg/kg extract plus 900 MHz waves). Groups receiving radiation were exposed 12 times a day, each time 10 min. Nokia 1200 cell phone was used to make EMF and cages were surrounded by aluminum foil to focus waves and limit the electromagnetic field to the interior of the cages. During wave exposure, the cell phone was sat in different modes, including call, missed call and turn on mode (without real talk). After the first round of irradiation, animals of experimental groups II and III received the extract followed by 11 rounds of daily exposure.

2.3. Measurements

At the end of the experiment (lasting a month), animals were weighed, blood samples were collected and serum levels of estrogen and progesterone were measured using ELISA kits (Made by Biosouece Europe). Ovaries were also removed, prepared using classical method of hematoxylin and eosin staining and studied by light microscope.

2.4. Statistical analysis

The results were examined by SPSS software and ANOVA/Tukey tests and the significant difference was sat at $P < 0.05$.

3. Results and discussion

Results of body weight and serum estrogen and progesterone levels are shown in Table 1. As seen, there are no significant differences in the mean body weights of various groups (Fig. 1 and Table 1). In addition, mean serum levels of estrogen in the experimental groups showed a decrease compared to control, but this decrease wasn't significant (Fig. 2 and Table 1). Conversely, the levels of progesterone elevated significantly in experimental groups II and III (Figu3 and Table 1). Finally, microscopic examination of ovarian sections revealed no visible morphological changes among different groups (Fig. 4). As seen, there are no adverse effects on corpus luteum groups receiving extract and exposed to microwaves (Fig. 4).Since mobile phones are wide spread and generally kept close to the body, they are considered as the main source of EM radiation that an average person is exposed to. Indeed, the whole body can act as an efficient antenna for absorption of EM radiation. Therefore, radiation emitted from a cell phone can reach all parts of the body and penetrate into the living tissues, and influence the body at the cellular level (Sarookhani *et al.*, 2011).

In fact, magnetic fields (MFs) can enhance fat breakdown and glycogenesis (Aghdam shahryar *et al.*, 2009). It also increases body metabolism, body temperature and activity of the sweat glands (Russelreiter, 2007). In addition, the results by Atilla Ilhan et al. (2004) indicated that exposure of rats to microwave frequencies at 900 MHz (used in cell phones) can cause weight loss. According to their findings, exposure to microwave frequencies can cause oxidative stress in animals and decrease their antioxidant activities, leading to weight lost (Ilhan *et al.*, 2004). In contrast, our studies indicated that male and female rats respond differently to EM waves, and that mails appear more sensitive than females. According to our results, exposure of female rats to cell phone radiation has no significant effect on body weight (Table 1 and Fig. 1), while this treatment can cause weight loss in mail rats and administration of garlic extract, especially high dose, can prevent weight loss caused by radiation (in the press). The study by Lotfi et al. (2009) indicates that plasma cholesterol and triglyceride levels decline in mail rodents following exposure to900 MHz radiation emitted from cell phones leading to weight lost (Lotfi & Aghdam shahryar, 2009). The observed weight loss in mails might be related to the decline in testosterone level. This hormone is involved in weight gain, especially in the production of muscle (Srinivas-Shankar & Frederick, 2009). Indeed, testosterone and/or its derivatives are used in body building by athletes (Te-Chi *et al.*, 2009). As a probable site for deleterious effects of microwaves, hormone testosterone is almost absent in females.

In addition, the effects of low frequency electromagnetic waves on gonads and fertility have been studied by many researchers. Some of these reports are indicative of reduced fertility, impaired spermiogenesis and reduction in the number of live fetuses in rats (Soeradi & Tadjudin, 1989; Mevissen &. Buntenkotten, 1994; Fernie & Bird, 2000; Baharara *et al.*, 2004). Most of these studies, however, are related to mail reproductive functions, and show that microwave radiation can harm testes, reflected in their structures and testosterone level.

In his report, Sultan (2010) stated that mobile phone radiation can cause a decrease in serum testosterone concentration (Sultan *et al.*, 2010). Similarly, in their study, Jelodar et al. (2008) reported that the mean testosterone level is reduced in mice exposed to radiation leaked from microwave ovens (Jelodar & Zare, 2008). They stated that the decrease in testosterone concentration could be due to the effects of radiation on Leydig cells, pituitary or hypothalamus and alteration of gonadotropin secretion (Jelodar & Zare, 2008). Moreover, the physiological and morphological impacts of cell phones on testis lead to disorders in seminiferous epithelium, and decrease in germinal epithelium and testosterone level (Ozguner *et al.*, 2005). Conversely, Ozguner (2002) found that EMF causes Leydig cell proliferation, increase in testosterone level and testicular weight, and lowering of testicular germ cells (Ozguner *et al.*, 2002). On the other hand, the effects of microwaves on female reproductive system are less clear.

According to the results of this study, cell phone radiation can elevate progesterone level, while estrogen concentration remains unaffected (Fig. 2 and 3 and Table 1). This is partly in agreement with the study of Baharara (2004) who investigated the levels of estrogen and progesterone in female rats exposed to radiation, and showed reduction in the serum concentration of progesterone and no change in estrogen level (Baharara *et al.*, 2004). Jahromi et al. (2012) also reported that FSH, Estrogen and progesterone levels rise after exposure to radiation (Hemayatkhah Jahromi *et al.*, 2012). These differences are probably due to the differences in the radiation dose, conditions and the way in which waves are administered. It seems that radiation emitted from mobile phones can alter levels of FSH, LH and progesterone through influencing CNS (especially hypothalamus) and changes in the secretion of gonadotropin-releasing hormone (GnRH) (Baharara *et al.*, 2004; Hemayatkhah Jahromi *et al.*, 2012).

Huuskonen (2001) noticed no significant changes in the levels of estrogen and progesterone after the initial exposure to microwaves (Huuskonen & Saastamoinen, 2001; Baharara *et al.*, 2004). However, they reported reduction in the levels of LH and FSH. This decrease in the levels of FSH and LH can be regarded as the effects of electromagnetic fields on brain and GnRH release (Hyland, 2000).

In 2010, the effect of garlic oil on the thickness of zygote wall was measured and indicated that garlic oil plays a direct or in direct role in ovarian activity and Increases secretion of sex hormones, including estrogen (Kadhim *et al.*, 2012). Apparently, garlic extract stimulates the secretion of gonadotropins and ovarian hormones through activation of pituitary gland, promotion of exit from the Golgi cells, cell cycle, and increased ability of binding to estrogen receptors (Obochi *et al.*, 2009). This might be one reason for the observed increase in progesterone level (Fig. 3).

Based on our results, both garlic and cell phone radiation have no observable effects on ovarian tissues, and primary follicles and corpus luteum appear unchanged in various groups (Fig. 4). These results support the study of Jahromi et al. (2012) who stated that the number of primary follicles and corpus luteum show no significant changes after exposure to radiation (Hemayatkhah Jahromi *et al.*, 2012). Conversely, microwaves can damage testes, particularly Leydig cells, which are responsible for secretion of testosterone (Carmela, 2004; Jelodar & Zare, 2008). While garlic extract is known as a lowering factor in blood cholesterol levels (in both human and animal) and inhibits cholesterol biosynthesis (Campbell *et al.*, 2001), presence of compounds, such as thiamine and organic sulfur in garlic affect male and female differently. It seems that the production of testosterone and progesterone are not related to cholesterol metabolism (Hammami *et al.*, 2008), rather their levels are dependent on the modulation of steroidogenic enzymes. It has been shown that green garlic can damage Leydig cells, which are responsible for secretion of testosterone (Chakrabarti & Bhattacharyya, 2003; Ebomoyi & Ahumibe, 2010). Likewise, garlic causes a dose-dependent decrease in plasma and intra testicular testosterone concentrations in rats and Leydig cells are known as its target (Hammami *et al.*, 2008). In contrast, garlic extract has no observable pathological effects on ovaries and their secretion (Fig 2, 3, and 4).

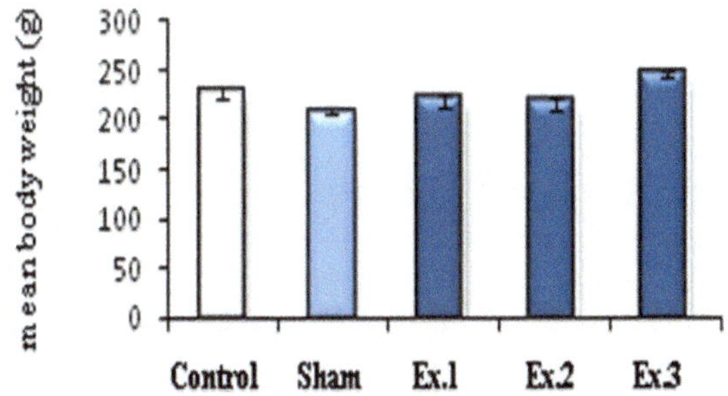

Fig 1. Mean body weight differences among various groups exposed to cell phone radiation and/or received garlic extract.
* indicates a significant difference.

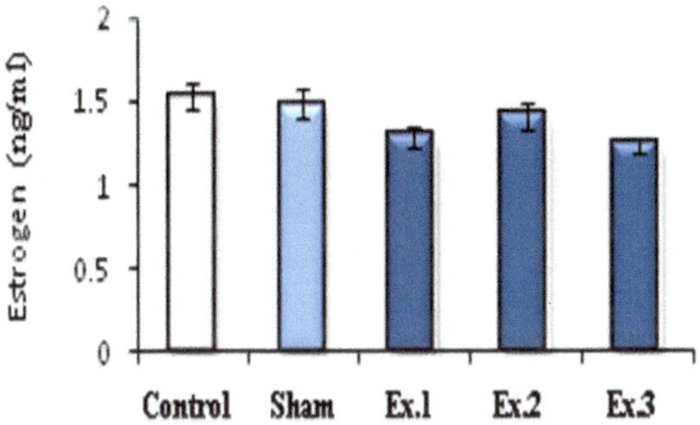

Fig 2. Mean estrogen levels in various groups exposed to cell phone radiation and/or received garlic extract.

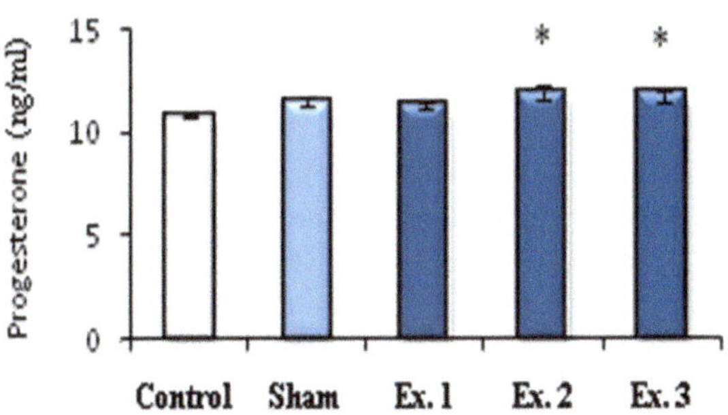

Fig 3. Mean serum levels of progesterone hormone in various groups exposed to cell phone radiation and/or received garlic extract.
* indicates a significant difference.

The apparent difference in the sensitivity of male and female reproductive systems, particularly gonads to microwaves is probably related to the position of testes and ovaries in the body. While testes are located out of the body within the testicular sac (Scrotum), ovaries are positioned deep in the body within the coelom, protected from the environmental factors (John & Guyton, 2011). On the other hand, microwaves have long wave lengths and cannot penetrate deep in the body (Vaessen, 2009). Hence, ovaries are less accessible to cell phone radiation than testes, and cannot be directly affected by their microwaves.

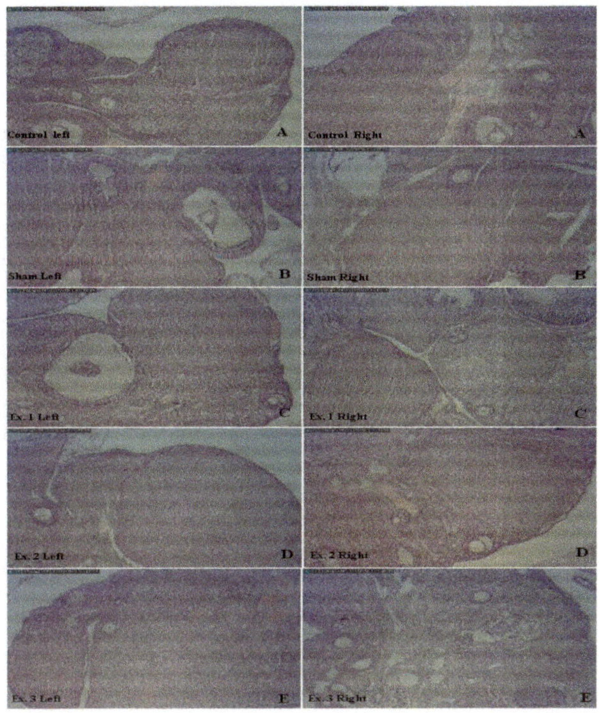

Fig 4. Cross sections of ovarian tissues in different groups exposed to cell phone radiation and/or received garlic extract. A: control, B: sham, C: experimental I, D: experimental II and E: experimental III. (Magnification=70X)

Table 1. Mean body weight and serum levels of estrogen and progesterone in different groups.

Groups	Weight (g)	Estrogen (ng/ml)	Progesterone (ng/ml)
	Female	Female	Female
Control	227.3 ±5.23	1.53 ±0.08	10.8 ±0.1
Sham	228.5± 3.33	1.48± 0.09	11.5± 0.2
Experimental-I	219± 6.32	1.28± 0.06	11.3± 0.14
Experimental –II	215.6± 6.79	1.4± 0.08	11.9± 0.37 *
Experimental _III	244.8±3.56	1.23±0.04	11.8±0.28 *

Mean ± SEM Difference with control : *
($p \leq 0.05$) Difference with sham : **
* indicates a significant difference.

Nevertheless, the observed differences in the sensitivities of testes and ovaries to garlic extract are not clear. Considerable attention should be given to the molecular functioning of the compounds present in garlic, particularly organic sulfur, as new insights on deleterious effects of cell phones will emerge. Such studies shed further light on the molecular functioning of the reproductive system and factors (including microwaves and various food products) effecting it, and provide insight for additional experimentation.

4. Conclusion

We showed that cell phone radiation can differently affect male and female reproductive systems, and garlic extract can only partially protect males against microwaves. These differences are probably due to the location of gonads in the body, because testes are placed out of the body within the testicular sac, and ovaries are positioned within coelom and thus less exposed to cell phone radiation. Thus, it appears that men are more sensitive to microwave irradiation than women, and they should be more cautious in using cell phones and perhaps, should stay away from mobile relaying ground antenna.

5. Acknowledgment

This article is based on the results of master thesis of Behnaz Hajioun, Physiology Student of Islamic Azad University-Kazeroon Branch. We sincerely appreciate all people who supported her in this project, especially lab staff of KAU. We also thank Mr. Esfandiar Sharifi for his help in translation and editing of this article.

6. References

Aghdam shahryar, H., Lotfi, A.R., Bahojb, M., and karamibonary, A.R. 2009. Effects of 900 MHz electromagnetic fields emitted from a cellular phone on T3, T4, and cortisol levels in Syrian hamsters. *Bulletin of Veterinary Institute in Pulawy.*, 53: 233-236.

Baharara, J., Parivar, K., Oryan, SH. and Ashraf, A. 2004. The effects of long-term exposure with simulating cell phone waves on gonads of female Balb/C mouse. *Journal of Reproduction and Infertility.*, 5(3): 217-226.

Banik, S., Bandyopadhyay, S. and Ganguly, S. 2003. Bioeffects of microwave – a brief review. *Bioresource Technology.*, 87: 155–159.

Campbell, J.H., Efendy, J.L., Smith, N.J. and Campbell, G.R. 2001. Molecular basis by which garlic suppresses atherosclerosis. *Journal of Nutrition.*, 131: 1006-1009.

Carmela, M. 2004. EMF-NET: effects of the exposure to electromagnetic fields: from science to public health and safer workplace, *SSPE-CT.,* 34: 502-173.

Chakrabarti, K., Pal, S. and Bhattacharyya, A.K. 2003. Sperm immobilization activity of *Allium sativum* L. and other plant extracts. *Asian Journal of Andrology.,* 5(2), 131-136.

Cobas, AC., Soria, AC., Martinez, M.C. and Villamiel, M. 2010. A comprehensive survey of garlic functionality. *Nova Science Publishers.,* 5: 1-60.

Ebomoyi, M. I. and Ahumibe, K. C. 2010. Serum testosterone and morphology of the testes in wistar rats following chronic garlic feeding. *Journal of Physiology and Pathophysiology.* 1(3): 39-43.

Fernie, K.J. and Bird, D.M. 2000. Effects of electromagnetic fields on the reproductive success of American Kestres. *Physiological and Biochemical Zoology.*, 73(1): 60-5.

Ferreri, F., Curcio, G., Pasqualetti, P., De Gennaro, L., Fini, R. and Rossini, P. M. 2006. Mobile phone emissions and human brain excitability. *American Neurological Association.*, 60: 188–196.

Forgacs, Z., Somosy, Z., Kubinyi, G., Bakos, J., Hudak, A., Surjan, A. and Thuroczy, G. 2006. Effect of whole-body 1800 GSM-like microwave exposure on testicular steroidogenesis and histology in mice. *Reproductive Toxicology.*, 22: 111-117.

Haciseferogullari, H., Ozcan, M., Demir, F. and Calisir, S. 2005. Some nutritional and technological properties of garlic (*Allium sativum*). *Journal of Food Engineering.*, 68: 463-469.

Hammami, I., Nahdi, A., Mauduit, C., Benahmed, M., Amri, M., Ben Amar, A., Zekri, S., May, A. and May, M.V. 2008. The inhibitory effects on adult male reproductive functions of crude garlic (Allium sativum) feeding. *Asian Journal of Andrology.,* 10: 593-601.

Hemayatkhah Jahromi, V., Dehghani, Kh., Fatahi, E., Nazari, M. and Farzam, M. 2012. The effects of mobile phone waves on the reproductive physiology in adult female rats. *Advances in Environmental Biology.*, 6(10): 2735-2741.

Huuskonen, H. and Saastamoinen, V. 2001. Effects of low-frequency magnetic fields on implantation in rats. *Reproductive Toxicology*., 15(1), 49-59.

Hyland, G. 2000. Physics and biology of mobile telephony .*The Lancet*., 356(9244): 1833-6.

Hyland, G. 2000. Physics and biology of mobile telephony. *Lancet*., 356(9244): 1833-1836.

Ilhan, A., Gurel, A., Armutcu, F., Kamisli, S., Iraz, M., Akyol, O. and Ozen, S. 2004. *Ginkgo biloba* prevents mobile phone-induced oxidative stress in rat brain, *Clinica Chimica Acta*., 1-2: 153-16.

Jelodar, G. and Zare, Y. 2008. Effect of radiation leakage of microwave oven on rat serum testosterone at pre and post pubertal stage. *Journal of Shahid Sadoughi University of Medical Sciences and Health Services*., 15 (4) :64-68.

John, E. and Guyton, C. 2011. Guyton & Hall Physiology Review. Illustrated. The University of California. *Elsevier Saunders*., 978:4160-4574.

Kemper Kathi, J. 2000. Garlic (*Allium sativum*). *Longwood Heral Task Force and the Center for Holistic Pediatric Education and Research.,* 1-49.

Lachance, P.A. 1997. Designer Foods III: Garlic, Soy, and Licorice. *Nutrition Press Trumbull*, CT., 52-58.

Lanzotti, V. 2006. The analysis of onion and garlic. *Journal of Chromatography A*., 1112: 3–22.

Lotfi, A.R. and Aghdam Shahryar, H. 2009. Effects of 900 MHz electromagnetic fields emitted by cellular phone on total cholesterol and trglyceride levels of plasma in Syrian hamsters (mesocricetusauratus). *Journal of Applied Biology Science.*, 2(3): 85-88.

Mahmoodi, M., Hosseini Zijoud, S.M., Hassanshahi, G.H., Toghroli, M.A., Khaksari, M., Hajizadeh, M.R., and Mirzajani, E. 2011. The effects of consumption of raw garlic on serum lipid level, blood sugar and a number of effective hormones on lipid and sugar metabolism in hyperglycemic and/or hyperlipidemic individuals. *Advances in Biological Chemistry*., 1: 29-33.

Mevissen, M. and Buntenkotten, S. 1994. Effects of static and time-varing magnetic fields on Reproduction and fetal development in Rats. *Teratology*., 50(3): 229-37.

Murad Kadhim Mohammed, A., Ahmed Thamir, W., Haider Kadhim, S. and Mohammed jabbar, A. 2012. Effect of garlic oil in some qualitative characteristics of laying hens eggs .*International Journal of Advanced Biological Research.,* 2 (4): 653 656.

Obochi, G.O., Malu, S.P., Obi-Abang, M., Alozie, Y. and Iyam, M.A. 2009. Effect of Garlic Extracts on Monosodium Glutamate (MSG) Induced Fibroid in Wistar Rats. *Pakistan Journal of Nutrition*., 8 (7): 970-976.

Ogilvy-Stuart, A.L. and Shalet, S.M. 1993. Effect of radiation on the human reproductive system. *Environmental Health Perspectives Supplements*., 101 (Suppl.2): 109-116.

Ozguner, I.F., Dindar, H., Yagmurlu, A., Savas, C., Gokcora, I.H. and Yucesan, S. 2002. The effect of electromagnetic field on undescended testis after orchiopexy. *International Urology and Nephrology*, *33*(1), 87-93.

Ozguner, M., Koyu, A., Cesur, G., Ural, M., Ozguner, F., Gokcimen, A. and Delibas, N. 2005. Biological and morphological effects on the reproductive organ of rats after exposure to electromagnetic field. *Saudi Medical Journal*., 26:(3): 405-410.

Rahman K. and Gordon, M. Lowe. 2006. Significance of garlic and its constituents in cancer and cardiovascular disease. *American Society for Nutrition*., 136: 736S–740S.

Rowley, M.J., Leach, D.R., Warnei, G.A. and Heller C.G. 1974. Effect of graded doses of ionising irradiation on the human testis. *Radiation Research*., 59: 665-678.

Russel, J.T. Reiter. 2007. A Review of neuroendocrine and neurochemical changes associated with static and extremely low frequency electromagnetic field exposure. *Integrative Psychological and Behavioral Science*., 28(1): 57-75.

Sarkar, P., Kumar, H., Rawat, M., Varshney, V.P., Goswami, T.K., Yadav, M.C. and Srivastava, S.K. 2006. Effect of administration of garlic extract and PGF2α on hormonal changes and recovery in endometritis cows. *Asian - Australasian Journal of Animal Sciences.,* 19: 964 – 969.

Sarookhani, M.R., Asiabanha Rezaei, M., Safari, A., Zaroushani, V. and Ziaeiha, M. 2011. The influence of 950 MHz magnetic field (mobile phone radiation) on sex organ and adrenal functions of male rabbits. *African Journal of Biochemistry Research*., 5(2): 65-68.

Shalet, S. M., Beardwell, C. G., Jones, P. H., Pearson, D. and Orrell, D. H. 1976. Ovarian failure following abdominal irradiation in childhood. *British Journal of Cancer*, 33(6), 655.

Soeradi, O. and Tadjudin, M.K. 1989. Congenital Anomalies in the offspring of rats after exposure of the testis to an electrostatic field. *International Journal of Andrology.*, 9(2): 152-60.

Srinivas-Shankar, U. and Frederick, C.W. 2009. Frailty and Muscle Function: Role for Testosterone. Advances in the Management of Testosterone Deficiency. *Front Horm Res. Basel,* Karger., 37: 133–149.

Sultan, A.M., Abdul, M.A.D., Sufia, H., Mubammad, M.K. and Mubammad, B.I. 2010. Effects of mobile phone radiation on serum testosterone in Wistar rats. *Saudi Medial Journal.*, 31(8): 869 – 873.

Tatara Marcin, R., Śliwa, E., Dudek, K., Mosiewicz, J. and Studziński, T. 2005. Effect of aged garlic extract and allicin administration to sows during pregnancy and lactation on body weight gain and gastrointestinal tract development of piglets. PART I. *Bulletin of the Veterinary Institute in Pulawy.*, 49: 349-355.

Te-Chi, L., Chia-Hua, K. and Paulus, S.W. 2009. Exercise and Testosterone. *Adaptive Medicine.*, 1(1): 26-31.

Ulbricht, C., Basch, E., Basch, S., Kathryn Bryan, J., Conquer, J., Grimes Serrano, J.M., Hammerness, P. and et al. 2010. An evidence-based review of garlic and its hypolipidemic properties by the natural standard research collaboration. *Natural Medicine Journal.*, 2 (4): 1-7.

Vaessen, P. 2009. Wireless Power Transmission. *Briefing Paper.*, 1-13.

Verschaeve, L. and Maes, A. 1998. Genetic carcinogenic and teratogenic effects of radiofrequency fields. *Mutation Research.*, 410: 141-165.

Isolation of borneol and bornyl acetate from *Ferulago macrocarpa* by microwave irradiation

Jila Asghari*, Mohammad Salehi, Mohsen Mazaheri Tehrani

Department of Chemistry, Faculty of Science, Golestan University, PO. Box: 49138-15739, Gorgan, Iran;
***Email:** *jasghari@gu.ac.ir*

ARTICLE INFO **ABSTRACT**

Topic: *Phytochemistry*

Key words:
- ✓ Ferulago macrocarpa
- ✓ *Microwave irradiation*
- ✓ *Borneol*
- ✓ *Bornyl acetate*

Abbreviations:
Microwave- assisted extraction (MAE), Solvent-free microwave extraction (SFME), Microwave-assisted hydro-distillation (MAHD), Hydro-distillation (HD), Microwave irradiation (MW).

Background & Aim: A simple and rapid microwave- assisted extraction (MAE) procedure was developed and optimized for the isolation of borneol and bornyl acetate from *Ferulago macrocarpa*. *Ferulago macrocarpa* (Apiaceae) is an endemic plant in Iran.
Experimental: Dried powdered aerial parts of plants were soaked in water and irradiated with microwave in a Clevenger extraction approach under optimum conditions (520 W and 0.5 h).
Results & Discussion: Compared to traditional heating methods by Clevenger, the present method is more efficiency and proceeds in a short time. The isolation rates of borneol and bornyl acetate increased by about 2 and 1.3, respectively, as compared to the conventional thermal methods. Low cost, easy extraction, high purity of the extracted products and high efficiency are the advantages of this method. Furthermore, solvent free extraction of the essential oils is a good method for the development of green chemistry.
Recommended applications/industries: The essential oil of this plant obtained by MAHD and HD methods, contained bornyl acetate as the most abundant component. The extracted essential oil by MAHD was qualitatively similar to that obtained by HD however; it was achieved in a much short time. Therefore pilot microwave reactor might be proven suitable for large scale extraction with potential industrial applications.

1. Introduction

Natural products have been served as a major source of drugs; the latter contribute to human health. Essential oils and plant extracts are the most promising groups of natural compounds for the development of safer new drugs. Many efforts have been scientifically increased to discover new compounds from various kinds of plants for treatment of some diseases (Clark, 1996). One resource in the discovery of novel effective compounds may result from the traditional uses of natural compounds.

The genus *Ferulago* comprises of 35 species worldwide which seven species are found in Iran (Mozaffrian, 1996). *F. macrocarpa* belongs to the family Apiaceae (Mozaffarian, 2008). *F. macrocarpa* is a medicinal herb. A number of bioactive constituents have been reported from the essential oil of *F. macrocarpa*, with anti-anopheles and anti-malaria mosquito activities (Hadji-akhoondi *et al.*, 1992). The essential oil from *F. macrocarpa* contains borneol (Fig. 1a) and bornyl acetate (Fig. 2b). These components have sedative effects, especially on the nervous system (Buchbauer *et al.*, 1992). A research on bovine brain neurotransmitters indicated that the anesthesia effect of borneol is more than a standard drug such as Lidocaine. In addition, it makes preventing stroke in mice (Xiao-Jing *et al.*, 2006) and the life of rats suffered from stroke has increased significantly (Meirong *et al.*, 1993; Chun-Jie *et al.*, 2006). Results of several studies have also recommended the use of borneol in the eye drops, because borneol selectively increases the penetration of eye drop into the cornea (Li *et al.*, 2006; Chun-Jie *et al.*, 2006). Modern sample preparation techniques have been described for the extraction of components from the medicinal plants (Hao *et al.*, 2002); these include ultrasound extraction, super-hot water extraction and microwave-assisted extraction process (Kaufmann *et al.*, 2002). In recent years, the microwave-assisted hydro-distillation (Mohamad *et al.*, 2006), solvent-free microwave extraction (Wang *et al.*, 2006; Lucchesi *et al.*, 2004, 2007), and a combination of microwave heating and dry distillation are developed as new techniques for the production of the essential oils. Development and application of modern sample-preparation techniques for extraction process toward gave a much cleaner analytical extract profile was increased.

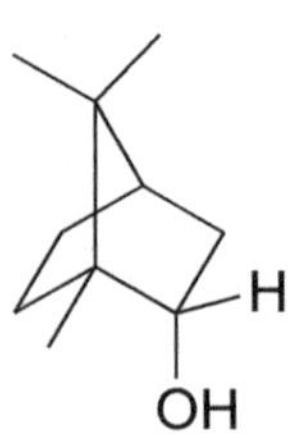

(1)

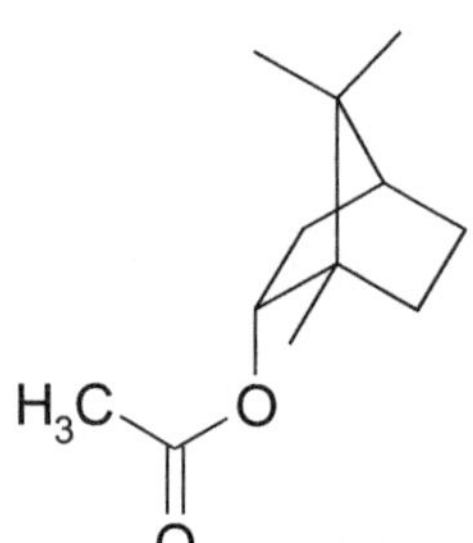

(2)

Fig 1. Structure of borneol andbornyl acetate

Extraction of essential oils through microwaves achieved by the following mechanisms, with irradiation of the plant surfaces, the essential oils are heated and ripple to the plant cells and then it get dissolved in the solvent (Ganzler *et al.*, 1990), and microwave irradiation can decay the cell walls from the oil containing glands and with their disintegration, oil is dissolved in the solvent (Kaufmann *et al.*, 2002).

In the present research, much effort has been focused on the isolation of potentially useful products from the plant by using MAE method without solvent. The samples, getting soaked in water, were irradiated with microwave in a Clevenger extraction approach under optimum conditions. The extracted components of the essential oils from this method were compared with those obtained by the conventional solvent extraction method.

2. Materials and Methods

2.1. Plant material

The aerial portions of *F. macrocarpa* were collected from Sanandaj in Kurdistan province, western Iran on April 2009. Voucher herbarium specimen (No. 4097) of the plant was identified and deposited at the Agricultural Research Center of Sanandaj, Iran. The aerial parts of plant were dried at room temperature for seven days.

2.2. Essential oil isolation

2.2.1. Extraction of essential oil by MAHD. The dried flower of *F. macrocarpa* were powdered using a blender into powdered pieces, whereby 50 g of dried powdered sample getting soaked in 750 mL water in the round-bottomed flask for 1h. The filtrated samples put in the microwave extractor were equipped with the Clevenger type apparatus, temperature and time controller. The essential oil was extracted from the collected material at 400, 500, and 600 W irradiation powers for 34 min. The essential oil was collected in a flask which was then dried over anhydrous sodium sulfate and evaporated the solvent using a vacuum rotary evaporator.

2.2.2. Extraction of essential oil by HD. In the traditional heating method, 50 g of the aerial part of *F. macrocarpa* was subjected to hydro-distillation for 3:30 h using a Clevenger type apparatus and the resulting oil was subsequently dried over anhydrous Na_2SO_4. The extracted oil from the two above described methods were kept in air-tight sealed glass vials and covered with aluminum foil at 4 °C for further analysis.

2.3. Essential oil analysis

2.3.1. Gas Chromatography (GC) analysis. The analysis of the essential oil was done by a GC (Agilent Technologies 6890 N) equipped with a FID detector, and HB-5 fused capillary silica columns (30 m x 0.25 mm, 0.25 μm film thickness). The samples, dissolved in ethanol were injected (20 μL) in the split less mode into Helium carrier gas with a constant flow rate of 2 mL/min. The injector and detector temperature was 280 °C. The column temperature was set at 40 °C for 3 min, and then programmed until 160 °C at a rate of 5 °C/min isothermal at this temperature for 2 min, and the finally increased at the rate of 10 °C/min to 280 °C.

2.3.2. Preparation of standard and sample solution. Quantitative data of the compounds (borneol and bornyl acetate) were determined from the appropriate calibration curve (Fig. 1 and Fig. 2). Standard solution was prepared by dissolving of borneol and bornyl acetate (4 mmol) in 25 mL ethanol separately. Calibration standard solutions were prepared by the dilution of stock standard solution with ethanol in concentration range of 0.1 to 2.0 mmol/L for borneol and 0.25 to1.5 mmol/L for bornyl acetate. All standard solutions were filtered through 0.45 μm pore-size membrane filter before injection. The sample solution was prepared by transferring the sample with equivalent of 2.2 mg in 5 mL ethanol, and then a portion of it was filtered before injection into GC. The linear regression analysis of the data for the calibration plots of borneol and bornyl acetate showed linear relationship with $r^2 = 0.9992$ and 0.9959, respectively.

Figures 3 and 4 were shown the yields of extracted essential oil and the content of borneol and bornyl acetate in the oil by thermal heating and microwave-assisted methods. The yield of extracted oil by MW (0.04% w/w) compared to HD method (0.03 w/w) was increased. The content of borneol and bornyl acetate by traditional heating method is 3.1% and 42.82% of the total oil, respectively. MW effect in the content of borneol and bornyl acetate showed the yields of these compounds as7.86%, 57.72%, at 400w, 9.6% and 49% at 520w and 5.04% and 33.5% at 620w power irradiation, respectively.

3. Results and Discussion

Using MAHD and HD apparatus, the essential oils from *F. macrocarpa* was appeared as clear, light yellow colored and oily layer on the top of aqueous distillate which was trapped with 10 mL $CHCl_3$ as an organic collecting solvent. Using MAHD, the contents of essential oil obtained after 34 min were 20, 35, and 40μL with yields of 0.4, 0.7 and 0.8 μL/mg at 400, 500 and 600 W, respectively. Extraction by HD methods resulted in 30 μL essential oil with yield of 0.6 μL/mg, however it took a much longer time of 3:30 h.

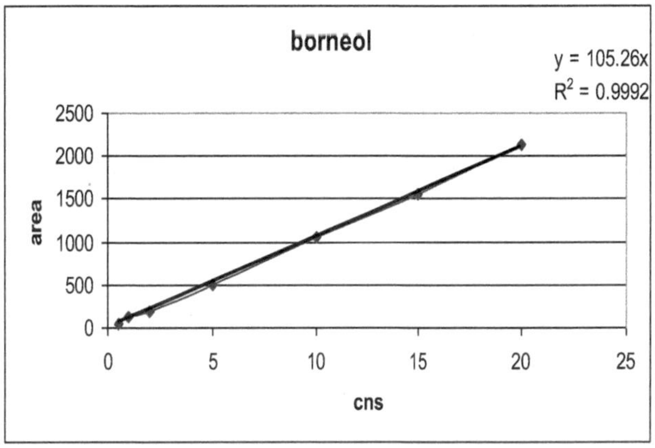

Fig 1. Calibration curve of standard solution of borneol at concentrations 0.1 to 2 mmol/L in ethanol

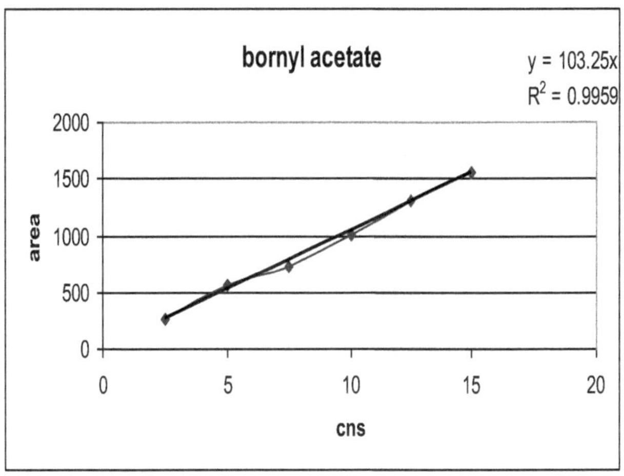

Fig 2. Calibration curve of standard solution of bornyl acetate concentrations 0.25 to1.5 mmol/L in Ethanol

The essential oil was subjected to detailed GC analysis in order to investigate borneol and bornyl acetate components. The signal at R_f = 15.2 and 17.1 min was identified borneol and bornyl acetate respectively with help of the chromatograms of their individual standard compounds (Fig. 6 and Fig. 7).

In order to evaluate the microwave power effect on the essential oil yields extraction was done under different power. As depicted in Fig. 3, with increasing the irradiation power from 400 to 620 W, the extraction of the essential oil increased and reached its maximum at 620 W. Although the essential oil yield increased to 0.04%, with increasing the irradiation power, from 400 to 620 W but, the applied high power irradiation decreased the yield of borneol and bornyl acetate (Fig. 4). This may be due to different materials having different appropriate microwave irradiation power and molecular interaction structure which can affect their yields of extraction. (Djouahri *et al.*, 2013). Hence, 400 W was chosen as the appropriate microwave irradiation power. The extraction of borneol and bornyl acetate in MW method was enhanced by 2 to2.5 and 1.5 folds, respectively as compared to the thermal heating method. It is due to the better interaction of MW with polar compounds. Since the polarity of borneol is more than bornylacetat, therefore, the quantity of borneol in the essential oil increased.

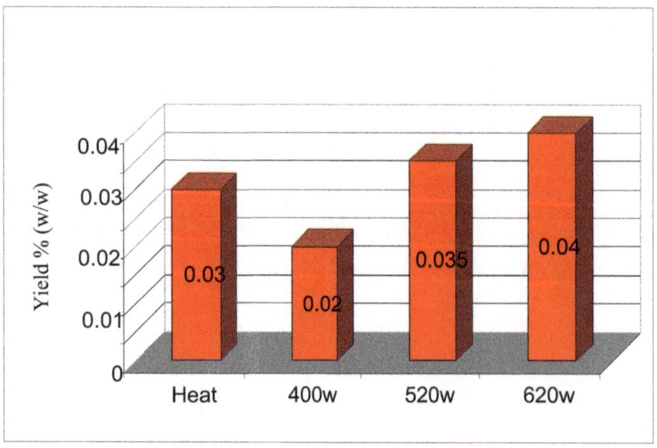

Fig 3. Compared the effect of microwave power and traditional heating method on the extraction of essential of *Ferulago macrocarpa*

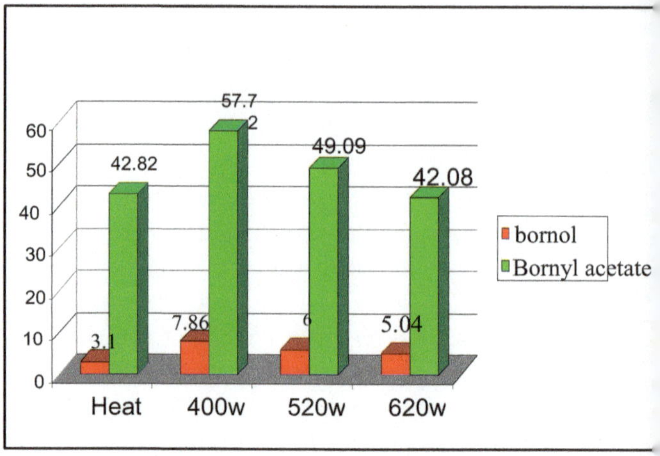

Fig 4. Compared the effect of microwave power with traditional heating method on the extraction yield of borneol and bornyl acetate

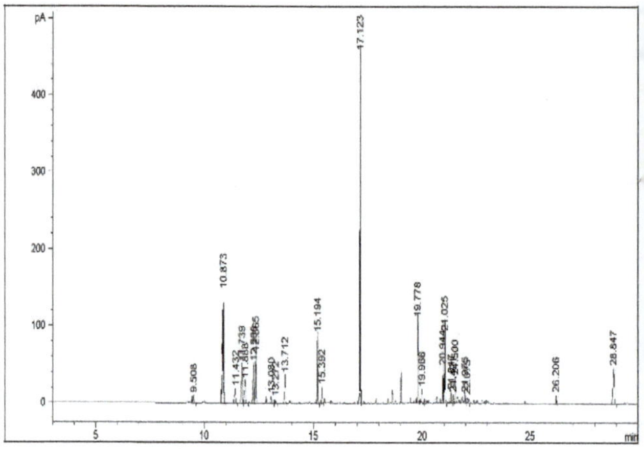

Fig 5. Chromatogram of the essential oil from *Ferulago macrocarpa* extracted by MAHD

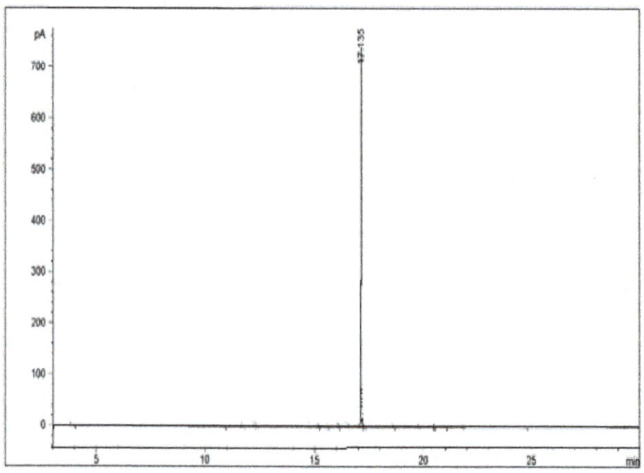

Fig 6. Chromatogram of standard solution of bornyl acetate

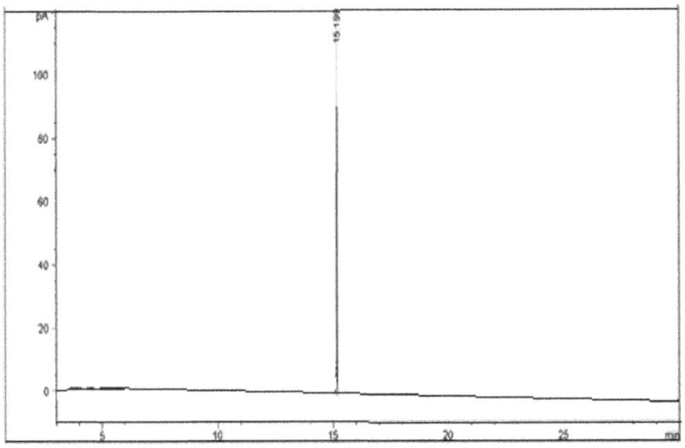

Fig 7. Chromatogram of standard solution of borneol

4. Conclusion

A simple and rapid microwave-assisted hydro-distillation (MAHD) protocol has been established for the isolation of borneol and bornyl acetate from *F. macrocarpa* at optimal condition. To evaluate the MAHD efficiency, we compared our results with those of hydro-distillation (HD) using the conventional Clevenger in terms of extraction time, extraction yield and efficiency. The yields of borneol and bornyl acetate were increased by 2 and 1.3 folds respectively, compared to HD.

5. Acknowledgements

The authors are grateful to Golestan University for financial support.

6. References

Buchbauer, G., Jäger, W., Jirovetz, L., Meyer, F. and Dietrich, H. 1992. Effects of valerian root oil, borneol, isoborneol, bornyl acetate and Isobornyl acetate on the motility of laboratory animals (mice) after inhalation. *Pharmazie.*, 47: 620-622.

Chun-Jie W., Qin-wan H., Hong-yI Q., Ping G. and Shi-xiang, H. 2006. Promoting effect of borneol on the permeability of puerarin eye drops and timolol maleate eye drops through the cornea in vitro. *Pharmazie.*, 61: 783-788.

Clark, A.M. 1996. Natural products as a resource for new drugs. *Pharmaceutical Research.*, 13: 1133-1144.

Djouahri, A., Boudarene, L. and Meklati, E.Y., 2013. Effect of extraction method on chemical composition, antioxidant and anti-inflammatory activities of essential oil from the leaves of Algerian *Tetraclinis articulata* (Vahl) Masters. *Industrial Crops and Products.*, 44: 32-36.

Ganzler K., Bati J. and Valko K., 1990.Effective sample preparation method for extracting biologically active compounds from different matrices by a microwave technique. *Journal of Chromatography A.*, 520: 257-262.

Hadjiakhoondi A., Aghe L.N. and Etemadi R.. 1992. Chemical and biological study of essential oil of *Ferulago macrocarpa* (Fenzi) Boiss, Effects of valerian root oil, borneol, isoborneol, bornyl acetate and isobornyl acetate on the motility of laboratory animals (mice) after inhalation, Publisher: Bait al-Hikmah., 620-622.

Heywood, V.H. 1985. *Flowering Plants of the Word*, Croom Helm. London 219-221.

Hao, J., Han, W., Huang, S., Xue, B. and Deng, X. 2002. Microwave- assisted extraction of artemisinin from *Artemisia annua* L. *Separation and Purification Technology.,.*, 28: 191-196.

Kaufmann, B. and Christen, P. 2002. Recent extraction techniques for natural products: microwave-assisted extraction and pressurised solvent extraction. *Phytochemistry Analysis.*, 13: 105–113.

Lucchesi, M.E., Chemat, F. and Smadja, J. 2004. Solvent- free microwave extraction of essential oil from aromatic herbs: comparison with conventional hydro-distillation. *Journal of Chromatography A.*, 1043: 323- 327.

Lucchesi, M.E., Smadja, J., Bradshaw, S. Louw, W. and Chemat, F. 2007. Solvent free microwave extraction of *Elletaria cardamomum* L.: A multivariate study of a new technique for the extraction of essential oil. *Journal of Food Engineering.*, 79: 1079-1086.

Meirong, L., Shaomei, Y., Yingqing, Z., Weiping, Q. and Meirong, F. 1993. The effect of borneol on evan's blue staining of rabbit and rat brain tissue. Institute of Clinical Pharmacology. 4.

Mohamed, A., Ferhat, A., Brahim, Y., Meklati, A., Jacqueline, Smadja B. and Farid Hemat, C. 2006. An improved microwave Clevenger apparatus for distillation of essential oils from orange peel. *Journal of Chromatography A.*, 1112: 121–12.

Mozaffarian, V.1994.*Plant Systematics*, Vol. 2, Nashr Danesh Emrouz, Tehran 372.

Mozaffarian, V. 1996. *A Dictionary of Iranian Plant* Names, Farhang Moaser, Tehran 194-195.

Mozaffarian, V. 1983. *The family of Umbelliferae in Iran, Key and distribution*, Research Institute of Forests and Rangelands, Tehran, Iran, 35, 387.

Wang, Z., Ding, L., Li, T., Zhoua, X., Wanga, L. and Zhang, H. 2006 Improved solvent-free microwave extraction of essential oil from dried *Cuminum cyminum* L. and *Zanthoxylum bungeanum* Maxim. *Journal of Chromatography A.*, 1102: 11–17.

Xiao-Jing, H., Qing-jie, L. and Yu-lan, L. 2006. Effects of Borneol injection on inflammation in focal cerebral ischemia reperfusion rats. *West China Journal of Pharmaceutical Sciences*, 21:523-526.

Xue, L., Chen, X.W., Fan, H.X., Fan, Sh., Liang, Y., Xia, J.X., Zhou, H. and Hu, Zh. 2006. Effect of borneol on levels of monoamine neurotransmitters in prefrontal cortex of rat after long-term continuous operations, *Acta Academiae Medicinae Militaris Tertia*e, 18.

Chemical compositions of the essential oil from peppermint (*Mentha piperita* L.) cultivated in Isfahan conditions

Ahmad Reza Golparvar[1*], **Amin Hadipanah**[2]
Department of Agronomy and plant Breeding, Isfahan (Khorasgan) Branch, Islamic Azad University, Isfahan, Iran;
Email: *dragolparvar@gmail.com

[2]*Department of Horticultural, Science and Research Branch, Islamic Azad University, Tehran, Iran;*

ARTICLE INFO

Topic: *Agronomy*

Key words:
- ✓ Mentha piperita L.
- ✓ *Chemical constitutes*
- ✓ *GC/MS*

ABSTRACT

Background & Aim: Peppermint (*Mentha piperita* L.) oil is one of the most popular and widely used as an essential oil. The aim of this study was to identify of the chemical components of peppermint cultivated in Isfahan climatic conditions.
Experimental: The aerial parts of the plants were collected from a filed in Meymeh, Isfahan province in 2012. The essential oil was extracted by a Clevenger approach and analyzed using GC/MS.
Results & Discussion: In total, 29 compounds were identified in the essential oil from the aerial parts peppermint. The results obtained in our study indicated that the major components in the oil were camphane (14.01%), menthone (13.89%), menthol (12.37%) β-pinene (7.62%), pulegone (6.41%), β-cubebene (4.95%), α-pinene (4.743%), γ-terpinene (4.08%), delta-carane (3.81%) and piperiton (3.04%).
Recommended applications/industries: The oil contents of peppermint varied slightly from year to year mostly due to variations in yearly growing weather conditions.

1. Introduction

Peppermint (*Mentha piperita* L.) belongs the family Lamiaceae, is one of the most important medicinal plants which used in food, sanitary and cosmetic industries. The leaves of peppermint are strongly scented due to the presence of essential oils. Peppermint is widely used for its medicinal properties such as anti-spasmodic, anti-sickness, anti-helminthic, carminative, and stomachic, etc.

Peppermint cultivated in the temperate, Mediterranean and subtropical regions of the world (Nostro *et al.*, 2000 ; Ormancey *et al.*, 2001). Peppermint (*Mentha piperita* L.) which is tetraploid (2n=72), is a sterile natural hybrid of *M. aquatica* L. (2n=96) and *M. spicata* L. (2n = 48) (Tucker, 1992).The plant is a perennial with 50-60 cm tall. The square stems are usually reddish-purple and smooth. The leaves are short, oblong-ovate and serrate. The flowers are purple-pinkish and appear in the summer months. The plant has runners above and below ground (Mozaffarian, 1996; Yazdani *et al.*, 2003). The essential oil of peppermint is between 1 to 2.5% in the leaves dried which is mostly made up from menthol (50%), menthone (10 to 30%), menthyl esters (up to 10%) and further monoterpene derivatives (pulegone, piperitone, and menthofurane) (Murrray, 1995). Derwich et al. (2010) reported 29 compounds identified in the leaves oil. In addition they reported the yield of essential oil of *Mentha piperita* was 1.02% and the major compound in were menthone (29.01%), followed by menthol (5.58%), menthyl acetate (3.34%), menthofuran (3.01%), 1,8-cineole (2.40%), isomenthone (2.12%), limonene (2.10%), α-pinene (1.56%), germacrene-D (1.50%), β-pinene (1.25%), sabinene (1.13%), and pulegone (1.12%). A report by Ka et al. (2005) on the chemical composition of *M. piperita* essential oil indicated that the major constitutes were menthol (18 mg/g) and neo-menthol (0.72 mg/g) (), as well as menthol (28-42 %), menthone (19-27 %), and 1,8-cineole (4-5 %) (Iscan *et al.,* 2002). The aim of this study was to identify of chemical components in the essential oil from peppermint (*Mentha piperita* L.) cultivated in Isfahan province.

2. Materials and Methods

2.1. Plants materials

The aerial parts of the plant samples of *Mentha piperita* L. were collected from a field of the center of Iran, Meymeh is a city in and the capital of Meymeh district, in Shahin Shahr and Meymeh county, Isfahan province, (latitude. 33˚, 26′ N, longitude. 51˚, 10′ E, altitude 1965 m above sea level), during summer 2012. Climate in this province varies from semi-dry. The soil of the field was clay loam with pH 7.45, contains total N (0.81%), total P_2O_5 (39 ppm) and total K_2O (465 ppm) with an EC of 4.74(dS/m).

2.2. Essential oil extraction

The fresh aerial of *M. piperita* were dried inside for six days at room temperature (25 ± 5 °C), and the ground to fine a powder using Moulinex food processor. The essential oil was extracted from 50 g of ground tissue in 1 L of water contained in a 2 L flask and heated by heating jacket at 100 °C for 3 h in a Clevenger–type apparatus, according to producers outlined British Pharmacopoeia. The collected essential oil was dried over anhydrous sodium sulphate and stored at 4 °C until analyzed.

2.3. GC/MS analysis

GC/MS analysis was carried out with an Agilent 5975 GC-MSD system. HP-5MS column (30 m x 0.25 mm, 0.25 μm film thickness) was used with helium as carrier gas with flow rate of 1.0 mL/min. The oven temperature was kept 20 °C at 50 °C for 4 min and programmed to 280 °C at a rate of 5 °C /min, and kept 20 °C constant at 280 °C for 5 min, at split mode. The injector temperature was at 20°C at 280 °C. Transfer 20 line temperatures 280 °C. MS were taken at 70 eV. Mass range was from *m/z* 35 to 450.

3. Results and discussion

Results of GC/MS indicated that 29 compounds were identified in the essential oil from the aerial parts of peppermint. The results indicated that the major components were camphane (14.01%), menthone (13.89%), menthol (12.37%) β-pinene (7.62%), pulegone (6.41%), β-cubebene (4.95%), α-pinene (4.743%), γ-terpinene (4.08%), *delta*-carane (3.81%), and piperiton (3.04%) (Table 1 & Fig. 1). The components of peppermint oil vary slightly from year to year. This may be mostly due to changes in climate conditions and the effect of climate on chemotypes of mints. Yazdani et al. (2003) reported the highest of menthol content in essential oil of *Mentha piperita* L. in different origin cultivated in Iran, was (56.4%) from Sari province. The highest of menthol content from the dried leaves was (1.49%) from Kerend-e Gharb, Kermanshah province.

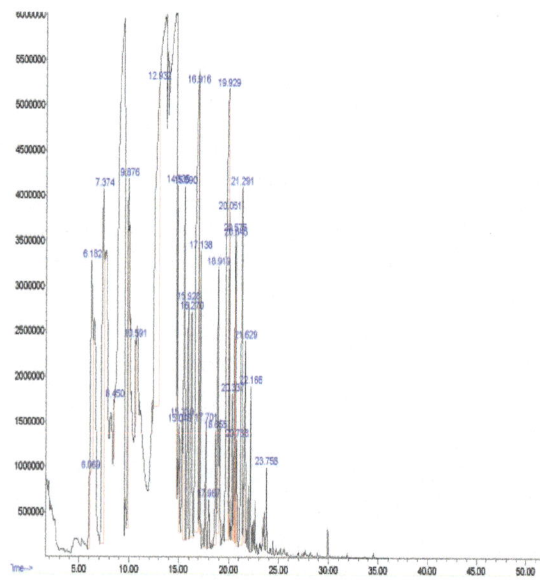

Fig 1. TIC of the essential oil from *Mentha piperita* L.

Jaimand et al. (2001) reported the main compinents of the oils from two cultivars of *M. piperita* were neo-menthol (42.62%), 1,8–cineole (16.51%), and piperitone (12.25%) in sample-1, and L-menthol (37.55%), L-menthone (19.13%), 1,8-Cineole (11.48%), and menthofuran (4.45%) in sample-2. Soltani et al. (2009) reported the main constituents of the oil were menthone, menthol, menthofuran, pulegone, 1,8-cineole, and menthyl acetate for first harvested and whereas the main constituents of the oil at second harvest were menthol, menthone, neo-menthone, 1,8-cineole and menthyl acetate.

Mirza et al. (2011) reported the major constituents of essential oils in *M. piperita* at early, full and after flowering stages were menthol (27/7%, 26/9%, and 27/0%), menthon (37/0%, 21/9%, and 17/2%), and menthofuran (16/0%, 22/0%, and 25/3%), respectively.

Table 1. Chemical composition of the essential oil from *Mentha piperita* L.

Compounds [a]	RT [b]	%
α-Thujen	6.069	0.746
α-Pinene	6.182	4.743
β-Pinene	7.374	7.621
(+)-4-Carene	8.450	0.486
γ-Terpinene	9.876	4.081
α-Terpinolene	10.591	0.529
Menthone	12.932	13.893
α- Terpineol	14.835	1.491
Formaldehyde	15.048	0.902
n-Valeric acid cis-3-hexenyl ester	15.330	0.965
Pulegone	15.590	6.415
Piperiton	15.928	3.047
delat-Carane	16.270	3.816
Camphane	16.916	14.017
Menthyl acetate	17.138	1.640
Camphene	17.701	1.087
α-Cubebene	17.987	0.430
α-Copaene	18.655	1.293
β-Caryophyllene	18.919	3.422
Menthol	19.929	12.371
Germacrene-D	20.051	1.952
β- Cuvebene	20.337	1.050
α-Caryophyllene	20.575	2.351
β-Farnesene	20.645	1.560
(+)-*Epi*-bicyclosesquiphellandrene	20.788	1.011
β-Cubebene	21.291	4.950
α-Amorphene	21.629	2.457
delta-Cadinene	22.166	1.139
Viridiflorol	23.758	0.535

[a] Compounds listed in order of elution
[b] RT (retention time)

The Menthol content in peppermint of Chinese origin was lower whereas limonene was higher than USA origin (Aflatuni *et al.,* 2000). The major components of *M. piperita* essential oil analyzed in Serbia were menthol (37.4%), menthyl acetate (17.4%) and menthone (12.7%) (Iscan *et al.,* 2002). Menthol and menthone were the main components of *M. piperita* (Sokovic *et al.,* 2009). Menthol (64.0%), Menthyl acetate (9.2%) and Menthofuran were dominant in *M. piperita* collected from Italy (Ashok *et al.,* 1999). Menthanol (36.24%) and menthone (32.42%) also were the major compounds of the *M piperita* essential oil collected from Karaj (Iran) province (Behnam *et al.,* 2006). Similarly, menthon (44.1%), menthol (29.5%), menthylacetate (3.8%) and menthofuron (0.9%) were the major compounds of M. *piperita* from Turkey (Arldogan *et al.,* 2002). However, the leaves of *M. piperita* grown in Korea had linalyl acetate (28.2%), menthol (33.4%), 1,8-cineole (46.1%), limonene (64.5 to 94.2%), and *p*-menth-2-en-ol (34.5%) (Seun-Ah *et al.,* 2010). The main components of the oils of *M. piperita* from east- Azerbaijan (Iran) province were α-terpinene (20.11%), pipertitinone oxide (17.10%), and *trans*-carveol (19.48%) (Eteghad *et al.,* 2009). The chemical composition of *M. piperita* L essential oil from Tehran (Iran) province, contained α-terpinene (19.7%), isomenthone (10.3%), *trans*-carveol (14.5%), pipertitinone oxide (19.3%), and β-caryophyllene (7.6%) as the major compounds (Yadegarinia *et al.,* 2006). Intensive research on the chemical characteristics has been conducted on this species (Carla & Decorti, 2009). Different medicinal plant species show a marked variation in active ingredients during different seasons; these have been widely attributed to variations in environmental variables such as temperature and rainfall (Ahmad *et al.,* 2009).

4. Conclusion

A comparison of our results with different reports, differences in the volatile composition of the plants could be attributed to genetic (genus, species, and ecotype), chemotype, distinct environmental and climatic conditions, seasonal sampling periods, geographic origins, plant populations, vegetative plant phases, and extraction and quantification methods.

5. Acknowledgement

This research project has been supported by Islamic Azad University, Isfahan (Khorasgan) branch, Isfahan, Iran.

6. References

Aflatuni, A., Heikkinen, K., Tomperi, P., Jalonen, J. and Laine, K. 2000. Variation in the extract composition of mints of different origin cultivated in Finland. *Journal of essential oil Research.*, 12: 462–466.

Ahmad, I., Ahmad, M.S.A., Hussain, M., Hameed, M., Ashraf, M.Y. and Koukab, M.Y. 2009. Spatio-temporal effects on species classification of medicinal plants in Soone Valley of Pakistan. *International Journal of Agriculture & Biology.*, 11: 64-68.

Arldogan, B.C., Baydaf, H., Kaya, S., Demirci, M., Ozbaw, D. and Mumcu, E. 2002. Antimicrobial activity and chemical composition of some essential oils. *Archibes of Pharmacal Research.*, 25(6): 860-864.

Ashok, K., Chandra, S., Dutt, P., Lal Kaul, B., Tava, A. and Avato, P. 1999. Essential oil composition of *Mentha piperita* L. from different environments of north India. *Journal of Agriculture & Biology* 14(1): 5-8.

Behnam, S., Farzaneh, M., Ahmadzadeh, M. and Tehrani, A. S. 2006. Composition and antifungal activity of essential oils of *Mentha piperita* and *Lavendula angustifolia* on post-harvest phytopathogens. *Communications in Agricultural and Applied Biological Sciences.*, 71(3): 1321-6.

Carla, D. and Decorti, D. 2009. Ultrasound-assisted extraction coupled with under vacuum distillation of flavour compounds from spearmint (carvone-rich) plants: Comparison with conventional hydro-distillation. *Ultrasonics Sonochemistry.*, 16: 795–799.

Derwich, E., Benziane, Z., Taouil, R., Senhaji, O. and Touzani, M. 2010. Aromatic plants of morocco: GC/MS analysis of the essential oils of leaves of *Mentha piperita. Advances in Environmental Biology.*, 4(1): 80-85.

Eteghad, S., Mirzaei, H., Pour, S. F. and Kahnamui, S. 2009. Inhibitory Effects of Endemic *Thymus vulgaris* and *Mentha piperita* essential oils on *Escherichia coli* O157: H7. *Research Journal of Biology Science.*, 4(3): 340-344.

Iscan, G., Demirci, F., Kirimer, N., Kurkcuoglu, M. and Baser, K.H.C. 2002. Antimicrobial screening: *Mentha piperita* essential oil. *Journal of Agriculture and Food Chemistry.*, 50: 3943- 3946.

Jaimand, K., Rezaii, M.B. and Asgari, F. 2001. Comparative of two distillation methods and plant growth stages on the essential oil content and composition of *Mentha piperita L. Iranian Journal of Medicinal and Aromatic Plants.*, 18: 11-21.

Ka, M.H., Choi, E.H., Chun, H.S. and Lee, K.G. 2005. Antioxidative activity of volatile extracts isolated from Angelica tenuissimae roots, peppermint leaves, pine needles, and sweet flag leaves. *Journal of Agriculture and Food Chemistry.*, 53: 4124 - 9.

Mirza, M., Ghoraishi, F. and Bahadori, A. 2011. Effect of harvesting time on essential oils content and composition of *Salvia officinalis* L. and *Mentha piperita* L. in Khuzestan province. *Iranian Journal of Medicinal and Aromatic Plants.*, 26(4); 531-543.

Mozaffarian, V. 1996. *A Dictionary of Iranian Plant Names*. Farhang Moaser, Tehran, Iran. pp. 542.

Murrray, M.T. 1995. The healing power of herbs: the enlightened person 's guhde to the wonders of medicinal plants. Rocklin, CA: Prima Pub., xiv, 410.

Nostro, N., Germano, M., Angelo, V.D. and Cannatelli, M. 2000. Extraction methods and bioautography for evaluation of medicinal plant antimicrobial activity. *Letters in Applied Microbiology.*, 30: 379-384.

Ormancey, X., Sisalli, S. and Coutiere, P. 2001. Formulation of essential oils in functional perfumery. *Parfums Cosmetiques, Actualites.,* 157: 30–40.

Seun-Ah, Y., Sang-Kyung, J., Eun-Jung, L., Chang-Hyun, S. and In-Seon, L. 2010. Comparative study of the chemical composition and antioxidant activity of six essential oils and their components. *National Products Research.*, 24(2): 140 - 151.

Sokovic, M.D., Vukojevic, J. and Molecules, M. 2009. Chemical composition of essential oils of *Thymus* and *Mentha* species and their antifungal activities. *Journal Molecules.,* 14(1): 238-249.

Soltani, F., Sharifi, M., Khajeh, K. and Yousefzadi, M. 2009. Study of essential oil composition, menthone reductase activity and antimicrobial activity of *Mentha piperita* in two stages of growth. *Iranian Journal of Medicinal and Aromatic Plants.*, 21(5); 62-70.

Tucker, A.O. 1992. The truth about mints. *The Herb Companion.*, 4: 51–52.

Yadegarinia, D., Gachkar, L., Rezaei M. B., Taghizadeh, M., Alipoor, S. and Rasooli, I. 2006. Biochemical activities of Iranian *Mentha piperita* L.

and *Myrtus communis* L. essential oils. *Journal Phytochemistry*., 67: 1249–1255.

Yazdani, D., Jamshidi, A. H. and Mojab, F. 2003. Comparative essential oil and menthol of *Mentha piperita* L. different origin cultivated in Iran. *Iranian Journal of Medicinal and Aromatic Plants*., 3; 73-78.

PERMISSIONS

All chapters in this book were first published in JHD, by Islamic Azad University, Shahrekord Branch; hereby published with permission under the Creative Commons Attribution License or equivalent. Every chapter published in this book has been scrutinized by our experts. Their significance has been extensively debated. The topics covered herein carry significant findings which will fuel the growth of the discipline. They may even be implemented as practical applications or may be referred to as a beginning point for another development.

The contributors of this book come from diverse backgrounds, making this book a truly international effort. This book will bring forth new frontiers with its revolutionizing research information and detailed analysis of the nascent developments around the world.

We would like to thank all the contributing authors for lending their expertise to make the book truly unique. They have played a crucial role in the development of this book. Without their invaluable contributions this book wouldn't have been possible. They have made vital efforts to compile up to date information on the varied aspects of this subject to make this book a valuable addition to the collection of many professionals and students.

This book was conceptualized with the vision of imparting up-to-date information and advanced data in this field. To ensure the same, a matchless editorial board was set up. Every individual on the board went through rigorous rounds of assessment to prove their worth. After which they invested a large part of their time researching and compiling the most relevant data for our readers.

The editorial board has been involved in producing this book since its inception. They have spent rigorous hours researching and exploring the diverse topics which have resulted in the successful publishing of this book. They have passed on their knowledge of decades through this book. To expedite this challenging task, the publisher supported the team at every step. A small team of assistant editors was also appointed to further simplify the editing procedure and attain best results for the readers.

Apart from the editorial board, the designing team has also invested a significant amount of their time in understanding the subject and creating the most relevant covers. They scrutinized every image to scout for the most suitable representation of the subject and create an appropriate cover for the book.

The publishing team has been an ardent support to the editorial, designing and production team. Their endless efforts to recruit the best for this project, has resulted in the accomplishment of this book. They are a veteran in the field of academics and their pool of knowledge is as vast as their experience in printing. Their expertise and guidance has proved useful at every step. Their uncompromising quality standards have made this book an exceptional effort. Their encouragement from time to time has been an inspiration for everyone.

The publisher and the editorial board hope that this book will prove to be a valuable piece of knowledge for researchers, students, practitioners and scholars across the globe.

LIST OF CONTRIBUTORS

Gita Amini, Saeed Irian, Ahmad Majd and Sedigheh Mehrabian
Deparment of Plant Biology, Faculty of Biological Sciences, Kharazmi University, Tehran, Iran

Mehrdad Jafarpour, Ahmad Reza Golparvar and Amin Lotfi
Agriculture Faculty, Isfahan (Khorasgan) Branch, Islamic Azad University, Isfahan, Iran

Saman Mahdavi
Department of Microbiology, Maragheh Branch, Islamic Azad University, Maragheh, Iran

Yousef Mehmannavaz
Department of Animal Science, Maragheh Branch, Islamic Azad University, Maragheh, Iran

Masoud Taheri
Department of Botany, Marand Branch, Islamic Azad University, Marand, Iran

Jafar Nikan
Plant Protection Research Department, Agricultural and Natural Resources Research Centre of Hamadan, Hamadan, Iran

Hadi Khavari
University of Applied Science and Technology of Hamadan, Hamadan, Iran

Hassan Nourafcan and Ahmad Khalighi
Department of Horticulture, College of Agriculture, Tehran Science and Research branch, Islamic Azad University, Tehran, Iran

Fatemeh Sefidkon
Research Institute of Forests and Rangelands, Tehran, Iran

Amir Mousavi
National Institute of Genetic Engineering and Biotechnology, Tehran, Iran

Mozaffar Sharifi
Department of Plant Sciences, Faculty of Biological Sciences, Tarbiat Modares University, Tehran, Iran

Ali Khalilipour and Mahmood Dejam
Department of Agriculture, Fasa Branch, Islamic Azad University, Fasa, Iran

Ardavan Ghorbani, Farzad Mirzaei Aghjeh Qeshlagh and Roghayyeh Valizadeh Yonjalli
University of Mohaghegh Ardabili, Ardabil, Iran

Amir Ali Shahbazfar and Seyyed Jamal Emami
Department of Pathobiology, Faculty of Veterinary Medicine, University of Tabriz, Tabriz-Iran

Reza Asadpour
Department of Clinical Sciences, Faculty of Veterinary Medicine, University of Tabriz, Tabriz-Iran

Ahmad Reza Golparvar and Arezoo Armin
Department of Agronomy and Plant Breeding, College of Agriculture, Isfahan (Khorasgan) Branch, Islamic Azad University, Isfahan, Iran

Amin Hadipanah
Department of Horticultural, Science and Research Branch, Islamic Azad University, Tehran, Iran

Ali Mehras Mehrabi
Department of Plant Breeding, Kermanshah Branch, Islamic Azad University, Kermanshah, Iran

Fatemeh Malekpoor and Azam Salimi
Department of Plant Biology, Faculty of Biology Science, Kharazmi University, 15719-14911, Tehran, Iran

Abdollah Ghasemi Pirbalouti
Medicinal Plants Department, Shahrekord Branch, Islamic Azad University, Shahrekord, 88146, Iran
Medicinal Plants Program, College of Natural Sciences, Massachusetts University, Amherst, 01003, MA, USA

Fahimeh Fallahpour and Narges Javadzade
Department of Fisheries, Khuzestan Science and research Branch, Islamic Azad University, Ahvaz, Iran

Mahdi Banaee
Aquaculture Department, Natural Resources and Environmental Faculty, Behbahan Khatam Alanbia University of Technology, Iran

Malek Taher Maghsoodlou
Professor, Department of Chemistry, University of Sistan and Baluchestan, Zahedan, Iran

Nasrin Kazemipoor
Associate Professor, Department of Agriculture, Shiraz University, Shiraz, Iran

Rohallah Jafarazad
Master of Science, Department of Chemistry, University of Sistan and Baluchestan, Zahedan, Iran

Nahid Rahneshan
Master of Science, Department of Chemistry, University of Sistan and Baluchestan, Zahedan, Iran

Hejraneh Azizi
Faculty of Biological sciences, Shahid Beheshti University, Tehran, Iran

Maryam Keshavarzi
Faculty of Biological sciences, Alzahra University, Tehran, Iran

Nasibeh Sharifi, Mohammad Hojjatoleslamy and Maryam Jafari
Department of food Science and Technology, Islami Azad University, Shahrekord branch, Shahrekord, Iran

Atena Eslami Farouji and Hamed Khodayari
Department of Biology, Faculty of Science, Lorestan University, 5Km Khorramabad toward Tehran, Khorramabad, Iran

Adel Poshtdar, Alireza Abdali Mashhadi, Seyed Ata Siadat and Abdolmehdi Bakhshandeh
Department of Agronomy, Ramin Agriculture and Natural Resources University of Khouzestan, Khouzestan, Iran

Foad Moradi
Agricultural Biotechnology Research Institute of Iran, Karaj, Iran

Majid Mohammadhosseini
Department of Chemistry, Shahrood Branch, Islamic Azad University, Shahrood, Iran

Fakhteh Zandpour and Mohammad Reza Vahabi
Department of Natural Resources, Isfahan University of Technology, Isfahan 84156-83111, Iran

Ali Reza Allafchian
Research Institute for Nanotechnology and Advanced Materials, Isfahan University of Technology, Isfahan 84156-83111, Iran

Hamid Reza Farhang
MSc of Range Management, Isfahan University of Technology, Isfahan 84156-83111, Iran

Zohreh Emami Bistgani, Seyed Ata Siadat and Abdolmehdi Bakhshandeh
Department of Agronomy (Physiology of Crop Plants). Ramin Agriculture and Natural Resources University of Khozestan, Iran

Abdollah Ghasemi Pirbaluti
Department of Medicinal and Aromatic Plants, Research Center for Medicinal Plants and Ethnoveterinary, Shahrekord, Iran

Masoud Hashemi
Stockbridge School of Agriculture, University of Massachusetts, Amherst, MA 01003-9294. U.S.A.

Jude E Okokon and Emem E. Umoh
Department of pharmacology and toxicology, Faculty of pharmacy, University of Uyo, Uyo, Nigeria

Koofreh O. Davies
Department of Physiology, Faculty of Basic Medical Sciences, University of Uyo, Uyo, Nigeria

Louis U. Amazu
Department of Pharmacology and Therapeutics, College of Medicine, Evans Enwerem University, Orlu Campus, Imo State

Forugh Mahdiyan and Abdollah Ghasemi Pirbalouti
Medicinal Plants Department, Shahrekord Branch, Islamic Azad University, Shahrekord, 88146, Iran

Isa Jafari Footami
Ph.D student of Gorgan University of agriculture and natural resources, Gorgan, Iran

Moosa Akbarlou
Associate professor of Rangeland management, Gorgan University of agriculture and natural resources, Gorgan, Iran

Amin Hadipanah
Department of Horticultural Sciences, Science and Research Branch, Islamic Azad University, Tehran, Iran

Mohammad Mehdi Gheisari
Toxicology Research Center, Isfahan (Khorasgan) Branch, Islamic Azad University, Isfahan, Iran

Davood Naderi
Department of Horticulture, Isfahan (Khorasgan) Branch, Islamic Azad University, Isfahan, Iran

Shima Rahmaniyan
Department of Horticultural Sciences, Yasouj Branch, Islamic Azad University, Yasouj, Iran

Mojtaba Khorrami
Department of Horticultural Sciences, Hormozgan University, Bandar Abbas, Iran

Arash Saeedi and Hossein Ali Asadi-Gharneh
Department of Horticulture, Islamic Azad University, Isfahan (Khorasgan) Branch. Isfahan, Iran

Mehrab Yadegari
Department of Agronomy and Medicinal Plants, Faculty of Agriculture, Shahrekord Branch, Islamic Azad University, Po.Box:166. Shahrekord, Iran

Behnaz Hajiuon
Department of Physiology, Islamic Azad University, Kazeroon Branch, Kazeroon, Iran

Jila Asghari Mohammad Salehi and Mohsen Mazaheri Tehrani
Department of Chemistry, Faculty of Science, Golestan University, PO. Box: 49138-15739, Gorgan, Iran

Ahmad Reza Golparvar
Department of Agronomy and plant Breeding, Isfahan (Khorasgan) Branch, Islamic Azad University, Isfahan, Iran

Index